PRAISE FOR *REFLECTIVE PRACTICE,* THIRD EDITION

"This provocative third edition of Reflective Practice *offers several elements absent in nursing textbooks:*

- *Thoughtful integration of Watson's Caring Science theory, the QSEN competencies, AACN's new Essentials, and ANA's revised definition of nursing*

- *Inclusion of helpful models such as design thinking, liberating structures, and others from diverse thought leaders such as Benner, Tanner, and Freire*

- *Numerous innovative strategies to deepen one's reflective practice*

While educators are the key audience, rich learning opportunities exist for any health professions leader."

–Joanne Disch, PhD, RN, FAAN
Professor ad Honorem
University of Minnesota School of Nursing

"The third edition of Reflective Practice *depicts the concept of 'reimagining' in such a brilliant way and is a must-have resource for nurses. Sherwood and Horton-Deutsch provide excellent insights on Caritas literacy and consciousness, moral courage, and building academic-practice connections and transformative learning frameworks, which is essential for the nursing profession. The relevancy of developing awareness for achieving social justice, diversity, and inclusion is timely and much needed for our complex situations."*

–Portia Janine Jordan, PhD, MBA, MCUR, RN, FANSA
Professor, Department of Nursing and Midwifery
Faculty of Medicine and Health Sciences
Stellenbosch University

"The pandemic left us in need of inner healing from varying personal, professional, and spiritual human experiences. This third edition is a coherent response that re-ignites and re-kindles human passion to transcend the remnants of the contextual aftermath. The book accesses inner stoicism, which emerges with re-bonding to our primordial sense of compassion. The takeaway message is that we must heal ourselves as a forerunner to refresh values in connecting to humanity and our environment."

–Mustafa Bodrick, PhD, RN, RPsyN, RNEduc, RNAdm, MSc, MPH, FFNM (RCSI), FAAN
Consultant Advisor, Saudi Commission for Health Specialties, Kingdom of Saudi Arabia
Adjunct Professor Nursing & Health Sciences, MAHSA University, Malaysia
Adjunct Faculty, Johns Hopkins University

T0291091

"This compendium is a rich, timely resource that expands contemporary literacy on reflective practice. Authentic, rigorous, and practical, this book is designed to nurture the intrinsic needs of learners, educators, and practitioners to meet societal and professional self-care needs. The editors and authors navigate the topic skillfully, helping us to humanize, refocus, reimagine, refuel, and regenerate our resilient capacities. This nursing text is destined to be the most important definitive reflective resource available on the subject."

–Jacqueline Whelan, MSc, MA, BNS (Hons.), Academic Associate in Logotherapy, RN, RNT, RCNAssistant Professor of Nursing, Faculty of Health Sciences, School of Nursing & Midwifery Trinity College Dublin

"Looking inward at ourselves and our practice can be one of the most difficult things that we do as nurses. It is also one of the most necessary in order for us to improve as individuals and improve how we care for our patients. This third edition of Reflective Practice: Reimagining Ourselves, Reimagining Nursing, by Sara Horton-Deutsch and Gwen Sherwood, takes reflection, the need for it, its potential, and how to use it to new heights. They teach us the concepts of reflective practice, guide us in integrating reflection into our practice, and energize us to share reflective practice with others. Every nurse could benefit from reading this book, but it should be a mandatory read for nurses in academia and education and nurses in formal and informal leadership roles."

–Beth Ulrich, EdD, RN, FACHE, FAONL, FAAN
Professor, University of Texas Medical Branch School of Nursing, DNP Program
Editor-in-Chief, *Nephrology Nursing Journal*

"Reflective Practice *should have multiple audiences. For educators, the book provides a wide lens to frame what nursing is, how nurses think, and why nursing matters. For those in practice, the book provides a provocative view of what it means to be entrusted with the care of others. In the tradition of Jean Watson, these authors draw from many disciplines to shed light on nursing knowledge, practice, and pedagogy."

–Kristen M. Swanson, PhD, RN, FAAN
Dean Emeritus and Professor
College of Nursing, Seattle University

"In this outstanding book, Sara Horton-Deutsch and Gwen Sherwood provide an invaluable resource for nurse educators and their students.* Reflective Practice: Reimagining Ourselves, Reimagining Nursing *takes a complex topic and makes it accessible for learners across all levels. This should be required reading in all nursing programs!"

–Pamela R. Jeffries, PhD, RN, FAAN, ANEF, FSSH
Dean of Nursing, Valere Potter Professor of Nursing
Vanderbilt School of Nursing

THIRD EDITION

REFLECTIVE
PRACTICE
REIMAGINING OURSELVES, REIMAGINING NURSING

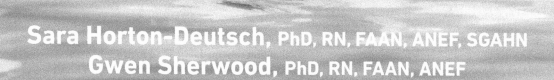

Sara Horton-Deutsch, PhD, RN, FAAN, ANEF, SGAHN
Gwen Sherwood, PhD, RN, FAAN, ANEF

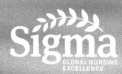

Sigma
GLOBAL NURSING
EXCELLENCE

Sigma Theta Tau International Honor Society of Nursing (Sigma) is a nonprofit organization whose mission is developing nurse leaders anywhere to improve healthcare everywhere. Founded in 1922, Sigma has more than 135,000 active members in over 100 countries and territories. Members include practicing nurses, instructors, researchers, policymakers, entrepreneurs, and others. Sigma's more than 540 chapters are located at more than 700 institutions of higher education throughout Armenia, Australia, Botswana, Brazil, Canada, Chile, Colombia, Croatia, England, Eswatini, Finland, Ghana, Hong Kong, Ireland, Israel, Italy, Jamaica, Japan, Jordan, Kenya, Lebanon, Malawi, Mexico, the Netherlands, Nigeria, Pakistan, Philippines, Portugal, Puerto Rico, Scotland, Singapore, South Africa, South Korea, Sweden, Taiwan, Tanzania, Thailand, the United States, and Wales. Learn more at www.sigmanursing.org.

Sigma Theta Tau International
550 West North Street
Indianapolis, IN, USA 46202

To request a review copy for course adoption, order additional books, buy in bulk, or purchase for corporate use, contact Sigma Marketplace at 888.654.4968 (US/Canada toll-free), +1.317.687.2256 (International), or solutions@sigmamarketplace.org.

To request author information, or for speaker or other media requests, contact Sigma Marketing at 888.634.7575 (US/Canada toll-free) or +1.317.634.8171 (International).

ISBN: 9781646481200
EPUB ISBN: 9781646481217
PDF ISBN: 9781646481224
MOBI ISBN: 9781646481231

Library of Congress Control Number: 2023038114

First Printing, 2023

Publisher: Dustin Sullivan
Acquisitions Editor: Emily Hatch
Development Editor: Rebecca Senninger
Copy Editor: Erin Geile
Cover Designer: Rebecca Batchelor
Indexer: Larry Sweazy

Managing Editor: Carla Hall
Publications Specialist: Todd Lothery
Project Editor: Rebecca Senninger
Proofreader: Todd Lothery
Text Designer & Compositor: Rebecca Batchelor
Illustrator: Malcolm Ribot

DEDICATION

We dedicate this book to our fellow educators and learners who courageously provided compassionate care and education through the COVID-19 pandemic and join in reimagining our profession with lessons learned as we continuously strive for wisdom and personal meaning through reflective and mindful practices that encourage openness, authenticity, compassion, and care for self and others.

We dedicate this book to those who have provided us with the encouragement, space, and confidence to grow through reflection—including our families, friends, colleagues, mentors, and coaches.

ACKNOWLEDGMENTS

The opportunity to reimagine this book has been sparked by the current forces impacting healthcare—rising costs, access, equity, professional workforce shortages, infectious disease, global warming, aging population, chronic-disease management, technological advances, and quality and safety to name a few. We attribute its co-creation to the dedication, insights, and contributions of reflective practitioners and educators, both present and past, who lead by example, as well as to the current generation of learners who inspire us to incorporate reflection, critical caring consciousness, and moral courage into our actions. Our experiences shape who we are, and we are all reimagining our ourselves and nursing as we have worked steadfastly through the COVID-19 pandemic—caring, learning, and growing towards a new future.

We add deep appreciation and gratitude to Sigma Theta Tau International for their innovative ideas and unwavering commitment to this project. We give special recognition to Carla Hall and Emily Hatch for their patient guidance throughout this process. We extend our thanks to Jill Leeper Sycamore for creating the supplemental materials and to the sales and marketing teams for their ongoing support in ensuring the success of this book.

ADDITIONAL BOOK RESOURCES

To download a sample chapter and other free book resources, visit the Sigma Repository at https://sigma.nursingrepository.org/handle/10755/23248 or scan the QR code below.

LEARNING GUIDE

A *Reflective Practice Learning Guide & Journal* is available for purchase from most online book retailers and for order from most brick-and-mortar book retailers.

SPECIAL NOTE TO READERS

Here at Sigma, we realize that language is constantly evolving. The meaning of a word often changes over time, some words become obsolete, and some terms that were once acceptable may become controversial or even offensive, depending on the context or circumstances. We have made every effort to make language choices that are inclusive and not offensive. Should you identify words in this book that you believe negatively impact a group or groups of people, please reach out to us at Publications@SigmaNursing.org.

ABOUT THE AUTHORS

SARA HORTON-DEUTSCH, PhD, RN, FAAN, ANEF, SGAHN, is a Caritas Coach & Leader, Professor, and Director of the University of San Francisco/Kaiser Permanente Partnership at the University of San Francisco School of Nursing and Health Professions. In this role she coordinates an RN-MSN specialty track for nurse leaders working at one of the 21 Kaiser Permanente hospitals in the Bay Area and collaborates with the Kaiser Permanente Scholars Academy to ensure relevant and quality continuing education programming grounded in Unitary Caring Science. She is also a Faculty Associate at the Watson Caring Science Institute, where she serves as the Co-Director of the Caritas Leadership Program, designed to engage participants in deep study and personal mastery of Caritas leadership, guided by Watson's Caring Science literacy and the 10 Caritas Processes.

Her work in reflective practice has been published in three co-edited books with Gwen Sherwood: *Reflective Practice: Transforming Education and Improving Outcomes* (2012 & 2017) and *Reflective Organizations: On the Front Lines of QSEN and Reflective Practice Implementation* (2015). The second was recognized as an AJN Book of the Year. Clinical nurses and academic programs around the world use the scholarly contributions found in these books to support deep learning—learning that leads to intentional, effective, and thoughtful action. It was through the iterative process of reflection that Horton-Deutsch deepened her own work in reflective practice, resulting in the integration of Caring Science. Like reflective practice, Caring Science calls healthcare professions to action—sacred actions that honor all living things—to health, healing, and wholeness.

In 2022 she co-edited *Visionary Leadership in Healthcare: Excellence in Practice, Policy, and Ethics* with Holly Wei, which received a first-place AJN Book of the Year Award. The textbook is directed towards those who believe centering care and compassion as the foundation for leadership is a worthy endeavor. It invites readers to explore leadership from a holistic perspective, including the knowledge and skills needed but also the social and emotional literacy required. It guides readers on how to be more self-aware, present, engaged, and connected with others to co-create new ways of being and doing our work together.

She continues to influence the scholarship and teaching-learning mindset of nurse educators around the world through her scholarly publications; international, national, and regional presentations; leadership in Caring Science; and service to the profession. She has served as a Research Fellow at the University of South Africa since 2016. In 2022, she was recognized as a Scholar in the Global Academy of Holistic Nursing. Horton-Deutsch currently serves on the board of directors of Sigma.

GWEN D. SHERWOOD, PhD, RN, FAAN, ANEF, has a distinguished record in advancing nursing education locally and globally. She is Professor Emeritus at the University of North Carolina (UNC) at Chapel Hill School of Nursing. She is an expert in patient safety, teamwork, and interprofessional education, and her work focuses on transforming healthcare environments by expanding the relational capacity of healthcare providers. Her work has examined patient satisfaction with pain management outcomes, the spiritual dimensions of care, and teamwork as a variable in patient safety spanning education and practice.

Sherwood was a pioneer in integrating quality and safety in health professions education. She was co-investigator for the award-winning Quality and Safety Education for Nurses (QSEN) project to transform education and practice to prepare nurses to work in and lead quality and safety in redesigned healthcare systems. Funded by the Robert Wood Johnson Foundation from 2005–2012, the QSEN Steering Team received the Sigma Theta Tau International Nursing Media Award, and its website (www.QSEN.org) received the Information Technology Award.

Sherwood has been engaged in multiple interprofessional projects including co-investigator for the UNC-Chapel Hill and Duke University Interprofessional Patient Safety Education Collaborative, patient safety leader at the University of Illinois at Chicago School of Medicine and the Academy for Emerging Leaders in Patient Safety (formerly the Telluride Project), and adjunct faculty in the Master of Science in Patient Safety Leadership program and now the MedStar Patient Safety Institute.

Her professional service includes the Research Committee of the National Patient Safety Foundation, the Technical Expert Panel of TeamSTEPPS, the QSEN Advisory Board, past President of the International Association for Human Caring, faculty and mentor in the Sigma Nurse Faculty Leadership Academy, and advisor for the Technical Expert Panel for the Patient Centered Care AHRQ Task Order at MedStar Health.

Sherwood's distinguished service to Sigma includes Distinguished Lecturer, Virginia Henderson Fellow, Chair of the global task force for the Scholarship of Reflective Practice position paper, and Vice President of the board of directors. She chaired the Research Scholarship Advisory Council and speaks frequently for chapters around the world. Her hospital research team received the 2001 Regional Research Utilization Award for implementing relationship-centered care.

Her work bridges US and global organizations to expand nursing undergraduate and graduate education capacity to serve developing regions. Formerly Executive Associate Dean at the University of Texas Health Science Center at Houston's School of Nursing, she bridged academia and practice through a joint appointment as Co-Director of the Center for Professional Excellence at The Methodist Hospital. She led numerous educational outreach programs in developing areas both on the Texas-Mexico border and around the world. A global ambassador for nursing, she has worked with nurse educators in Kazakhstan, Sakhalin, Macau, Thailand, Taiwan, and Kenya and helped lead the nursing education renaissance in China. Widely published, she is co-editor of three other books: *International Textbook of Reflective Practice in Nursing, Quality and Safety in Nursing: A Competency Approach to Improve Outcomes* (AJN Book of the Year), and *Reflective Organizations: On the Front Lines of QSEN and Reflective Practice Implementation* (second place AJN Book of the Year). Among many honors, she was awarded Outstanding Alumnus at Georgia Baptist College of Nursing and the University of Texas Austin in addition to the Special Award for International Interprofessional Education from the Prince Madhidol Conference, Sigma's Mary Tolle Wright Leadership Award, an Honorary Doctorate from Jonkoping University, and Fellowship Ad Eundem from the Royal College of Surgeons Ireland.

CONTRIBUTING AUTHORS

JENNIFER ALDERMAN, PhD, MSN, RN, CNL, CNE, CHSE, is an Associate Professor at the University of North Carolina-Chapel Hill School of Nursing. She holds administrative roles in the undergraduate program and as the School of Nursing's Director of Interprofessional Education and Practice. Alderman's areas of expertise include simulation, interprofessional education, leadership, quality and safety, and maternal/newborn nursing. Alderman has presented nationally and internationally on reflective practice and its role in leadership and transition to practice for new graduate nurses.

GAIL ARMSTRONG, PhD, DNP, RN, ACNS-BC, CNE, FAAN, has been in nursing higher education for more than 20 years. Armstrong has enjoyed a long-standing interest in reflective practice as her first two degrees are in literature. Early in her career, she was a med/surg bedside nurse where an interest in illness narratives united her work as a nurse and her foundation in Caring Science. Much of Armstrong's career focused on quality and safety and the integration of quality and safety content into early pre-licensure curricula. Armstrong found reflective practice to be fertile pedagogy for pre-licensure students to reflect on and respond to system gaps they were observing in their clinical rotations. In her current work as Faculty Development Coordinator, Armstrong supports the growth and development of CU Nursing faculty in all phases of their careers.

ANNA BILEY, Dip N, MSc, Doctorate of Caring Science, has worked across a range of specialties in clinical, leadership, and educational roles in the UK's National Health Service and in the voluntary sector. At the heart of her work has been understanding and developing Watson Caring Science and Human Caring Theory. Recent years brought personal change and challenge as Biley became a full-time mum and carer for close family members. During this time, she undertook the doctoral program at the Watson Caring Science Institute (WCSI) and as faculty now supports the Caritas Coach and Leadership programs. Grief, loss, and recovery are the focus of her most recent work and writing. A book based on her doctoral research, entitled *Birds Hold our Secrets: A Nurse's Story of Grief and Remembering*, was published in 2019 by Lotus Library (WCSI).

DAWN FRESHWATER, PhD, RN, FRCN, FRCSI, MAE, GAICD, is Vice-Chancellor of the University of Auckland. She was the first female Chair of the G08 Research Intensive Universities in Australia and the past Chair of the Partnership Board of the World University Network (WUN). Freshwater is currently Chair of UNZ Research Committee and Deputy Chair and Board Director of Research Australia. She was awarded her PhD at the University of Nottingham (1998). Her contribution to the fields of nursing, public health (specifically mental health and forensic mental health), and research on leadership practices won her the highest honor in her field—the Fellowship of the Royal College of Nursing (FRCN).

Freshwater is an elected Member of the Academia Europea and a Fellow of the Royal College of Surgeons Ireland. As an academic, she has contributed to more than 200 publications, including peer-reviewed papers, research reports, books, editorials, and media contributions, and she continues to supervise PhD students. Freshwater maintains strong professional ties with key figures in education and industry in Asia, Europe, and the United States. She is known for her advocacy and action for equity and inclusivity.

EILEEN FRY-BOWERS, PhD, JD, RN, CPNP-PC, FAAN, is Dean and Professor at the University of San Francisco School of Nursing and Health Professions. Her academic experience includes faculty and leadership appointments in Schools of Nursing, Medicine, and Public Health, and her extensive clinical experience spans multiple healthcare settings, including acute care facilities, specialty and community-based clinics, and military institutions. She is a certified pediatric nurse practitioner (CPNP), a licensed attorney, and a veteran of the US Navy Nurse Corps. Fry-Bowers is an elected Fellow of the American Academy of Nursing and former Chair of the Expert Panel on Child, Adolescent, and Family. She was named a Faculty Policy Fellow for the American Association of Colleges of Nursing and served two terms on AACN's Health Policy Advisory Council. Fry-Bowers is committed to transforming nursing education and practice to support the promotion, development, and maintenance of optimal mental, physical, and spiritual health for all, including the nursing workforce.

CHRISTINE GRIFFIN, PhD, RN, NPD-BC, CPN, is the Director of Caring Science and Nursing Practice at Queens Medical Center in Honolulu, Hawaii. In her PhD program, "Compassion Without Fatigue," Griffin studied how the theory-guided practices within Caring Science can inform effective compassion fatigue interventions to decrease burnout for healthcare providers. As faculty for the Watson Caring Science Institute and a Caritas Coach and leader, she hopes to bring Caring Science practices to nurses and nurse leaders so they have the capacity to flourish as they bring their authentic care and compassion to the bedside. Griffin has contributed to Caring Science and leadership chapters in *Caritas Coaching: A Journey Toward Transpersonal Caring for Informed Moral Action in Healthcare* (2018), *Nursing Theories and Nursing Practice,* 5th Edition (2020), and *Leadership Roles in Promoting a Resilient Workforce* (2022).

CAROLE HEMMELGARN, MS, is the Director of the Executive Master's program for Clinical Quality, Safety & Leadership at Georgetown University and the Senior Director of Education for the MedStar Health Institute for Quality & Safety. Hemmelgarn graduated from Colorado State University with a degree in Speech Communication. She received a master's degree in Patient Safety Leadership from the University of Illinois at Chicago and a second master's degree in Health Care Ethics from Creighton University. Hemmelgarn is involved in patient safety work across the country. She sits on the Leapfrog Patient & Family Caregiver

Expert Panel; the Board of Quality, Safety, and Experience at Children's Hospital Colorado; the Clinical Excellence Council for Colorado Hospital Association; ABIM Foundation; the Patient Advisory Committee and the board of directors for the Collaborative for Accountability and Improvement; and is a founding member of Patients For Patient Safety US.

ERICA HOOPER, DNP, RN, CNL,CNS, PHN, is a Regional Program Manager for Academic Relations and Community Health for the Kaiser Permanente Scholars Academy in Northern California and adjunct faculty at the University of San Francisco School of Nursing and Health Professions. She has nursing experience working in the areas of geriatrics, pediatrics, primary care, public health, leadership, program development, and education. She has a BSN and DNP in Health Care Systems Leadership from the University of San Francisco and an MSN in Advanced Community Health and International Nursing with a minor in Education from the University of California San Francisco. Hooper is a Caritas Coach, HeartMath certified trainer, healing circle facilitator, massage and reiki practitioner, yoga instructor, personal trainer, and life coach. She has a passion for alternative healing practices as well as promoting the health and wellness of vulnerable populations. Hooper has a personal mission in life to use her gifts to help others achieve their greatest potential and healthiest version of themselves.

ASHLEY A. KELLISH, DNP, RN, CCNS, NEA-BC, is an academic and clinical practitioner dedicated to the future of nurses in healthcare. Her experience has allowed her to provide mentorship to over 20 DNP and MSN candidates through the University of North Carolina (UNC) Medical School of Chapel Hill, North Carolina. She is a sought-after consultant with a propensity for implementing change and improving healthcare systems. She has formally presented and led workshops throughout the United States and globally on continuing education and shifting protocols. Kellish earned her DNP from Duke University, an MSN from Georgetown University, where she was awarded Performance Improvement Nurse of the Year, and a bachelor's degree in nursing from Boston College. She is a board-certified Critical Care Clinical Nurse Specialist. In 2022, she was honored by UNC as a member of the third cohort of Anne Belcher Interprofessional Faculty Scholars. She also holds many certifications and has authored publications on nursing, systems, and practices.

JENNIFER MANEY, PhD, is the Director of the Center for Teaching and Learning at Marquette University. Her role is to support all faculty/instructors in promoting a welcoming learning environment through their pedagogical practices, including the infusion of Ignatian principles into their teaching. She is responsible for helping to build inclusive, equitable, and justice-focused learning experiences across campus, and facilitating faculty exploration of the impact of implicit biases. Maney currently teaches in the first-year honors program at Marquette

University, is adjunct faculty for Mount Mary College, and is the board chair of St. Joan Antida Catholic High School. Prior, she was responsible for the coordination of the Greater Milwaukee Catholic Education Consortium in support of Milwaukee K-12 Catholic schools. She has experience directing a federal grant at the Milwaukee Area Technical College, helping to create the first bilingual early childhood credential program in the state of Wisconsin. She holds a doctorate in Educational Policy and Leadership with a minor in diversity education, a master's in counseling, and a bachelor's degree in journalism.

MEG MOORMAN, PhD, RN, CNE, ANEF, is the Coordinator of the MSN in Nursing Education Program and the Director of the Faculty Innovating for Nursing Education (FINE) Research Center at Indiana University School of Nursing. Prior to teaching, she worked as a labor and delivery nurse and nurse practitioner. Her research has focused on interactive teaching strategies, mostly focused on Visual Thinking Strategies (VTS) and the use of art to teach communication, observational skills, ethics, and diversity. Moorman has been the recipient of several teaching awards including the IU Trustees Teaching Award, Sigma Theta Tau Excellence in Nursing Education (Alpha Chapter) Award, and the Mosaic Teaching Fellowship. She has presented and consulted internationally with schools of nursing, medicine, education, and palliative care groups. Her research has been disseminated in Hong Kong, South Africa, Spain, Ireland, and Australia, and she has worked with several hospital systems to introduce VTS into nurse residency programs.

CRYSTAL MORALES, MS, BSN, RN, is the Director of Nurse Wellbeing at MedStar Health. Dedicated to nurses' well-being, she has the privilege of developing and implementing strategies aimed at improving professional, emotional, physical, and social well-being. Morales has a strong and extensive background in healthcare management, operations, and education. Most recently she served as the Senior Director of Education at the MedStar Institute for Quality and Safety. In that role, she was the acting Program Director for Georgetown's Executive Master's in Clinical Quality, Safety, and Leadership program. Prior to that, Morales held various roles at MedStar, where she skillfully led the development and implementation of system-wide strategies for high reliability and patient safety. Morales is exceptionally passionate about her work and enjoys making connections and working on diverse teams.

DANIEL J. PESUT, PhD, RN, FAAN, is a nurse educator, academic, researcher, consultant, and coach. He is an Emeritus Professor of Nursing at the University of Minnesota School of Nursing and Emeritus Katherine R. and C. Walton Lillehei Chair in Nursing Leadership at the University of Minnesota. He has held academic and administrative positions at the University of Michigan, the University of South Carolina, and Indiana University. He served as the Director of the Katharine J. Densford International Center for Nursing Leadership from 2012 until his retirement in 2021. He is a past President (2003–2005) of Sigma Theta Tau International. His Presidential Call to Action was "Create the Future Through Renewal." The Sigma Daniel J. Pesut Spirit of Renewal Award honors his leadership and legacy contributions to the nursing profession.

MELISSA SHEW, PhD, is a Senior Faculty Fellow in Marquette University's Center for Teaching and Learning, Faculty Director of the Executive MBA Program, and Co-Director of Marquette's Institute for Women and Leadership. She works in the history of philosophy, feminist philosophy, philosophy of education, and issues related to women at work. Her recent scholarship includes *Philosophy for Girls: An Invitation to the Life of Thought* (with Kim Garchar, Oxford University Press, 2020); *On the Vocation of the Educator in This Moment* (with Jennifer Maney, Marquette University Press, 2021); a TEDx Talk, "Women and Intellectual Empowerment" (2021); a white paper, "The Power of Intellectual Joy for the Future of Women at Work" (2023); and a creative public-facing research initiative, *The Persephone Project* (https://thepersephoneproject.org/).

GISELA H. VAN RENSBURG, DLitt et Phil, RN, RM, RPN, RCN, RNE, RNA, ROrthN, FANSA, obtained her DLitt et Phil at the University of South Africa, where she is a Professor in the Department of Health Studies. She serves as the Master's and Doctoral Program Coordinator and member of the Human Sciences Research Ethics Committee. She holds a grant for a Women in a Research project on psycho-educational support strategies for postgraduate supervisors and students to facilitate mental well-being. van Rensburg has engaged in a variety of research projects on research capacity development and teaching research methodology. She is an editor of two research books. Her current international research partnership involves reflective practices and Caring Science related to teaching and learning. As an educator, van Rensburg focuses on health sciences education, student support, and reflective practice. Her clinical interests are in orthopaedic nursing, in which she holds a specialist nursing qualification. She mentors members of the nursing community in research capacity development, with a special interest in supporting novices and emerging researchers.

ROBIN R. WALTER, PhD, RN, CNE, is contributing faculty in the DNP and PhD nursing programs at Walden University. She is a nurse educator with experience in health and public policy, committed to developing nurses as leaders in equity policy advocacy and as social justice allies. Her research on health disparities and inequities is anchored in understanding the political determinants of health that create inequities in the social determinants of health. Walter has developed curricula and courses conceptually grounded in social justice, diversity, equity, and inclusion at the baccalaureate, master's, and doctoral levels of nursing education. She co-led a grant-funded initiative in Florida to prepare nurse leaders across the state to engage in equity policy advocacy. Walter earned a BSN from Towson University, an MS in nursing/health policy from the University of Maryland at Baltimore, and a PhD in nursing from Barry University.

AMBER YOUNG-BRICE, PhD, RN, CNE, is an Assistant Professor in Nursing and Program Director of the Teaching Certificate for Nurse Educators program at Marquette University. She holds a master's degree in nursing education, PhD in nursing, and is a certified nurse educator. She has taught at the undergraduate, graduate, and post-graduate levels since 2008. Additionally, Young-Brice does educational development across the university and within her college of nursing as a new faculty mentor and conducts programming for onboarding all new faculty. Young-Brice's program of pedagogical research explores the relationship between the influence of non-cognitive factors and the successful trajectory of students. She studies ways to foster these factors through theoretically derived and evidence-informed pedagogical innovations. Her research is grounded in her expertise as an educator and underpinned by theories from nursing, education, and cognitive and social sciences. She is the 2018 NLN Ruth Donnelly Corcoran Research Award recipient and principal investigator on a 2023 NSF-funded study integrating human-centered teaching practices in engineering education.

TABLE OF CONTENTS

About the Authors xi

Contributing Authors xv

Foreword.. xxix

Introduction xxxi

PART I THE DEVELOPMENT AND EVOLUTION OF THE NURSE THROUGH REFLECTIVE PRACTICE 1

1 REIMAGINING OURSELVES: THE ROLE OF REFLECTION ON CRITICAL CARITAS CONSCIOUSNESS AND KNOWLEDGE DEVELOPMENT.................... 3

Overview 4

Supporting Theoretical Frameworks and Other Evidence 5

The Time Is Now: Reimagining Moral Courage 8

Reflection and Relationship: The Antidote for Learning Through Complexity and Uncertainty.. 10

Coming to an Understanding 12

Application for Personal and Professional Practice 12

Reflective Summary 13

Learning Narrative... 14

Reflective Questions.. 15

For Individual Reflection and/or Group Discussion.. 16

References 16

2 REIMAGINING REFLECTION TO DEVELOP AND SUSTAIN PERSONAL AND PROFESSIONAL PRACTICE 19

Overview 20

Theoretical Frameworks and Supporting Evidence 21

Developing Caring Reflective Practitioners 30

Engaging Learners in Practice Development 32

The Intersection of Reflective Practice, Transformative Learning, and Unitary Caring Science 33

Application for Personal and Professional Development 36

Reflective Summary 38

Learning Narrative 38

Reflective Questions...39
References 40

**3 REIMAGINING CREATIVE SPACE FOR REFLECTION
IN A CARING SCIENCE PARADIGM** 43

Overview..44
Supporting Theoretical Frameworks and Evidence...........................45
Ethics and Values of a Practice-Based Discipline.............................46
The Caritas Processes 47
Creating Space for Caring, Reflective Practice................................48
Application for Personal and Professional Practice 58
Reflective Summary 59
Learning Narrative...59
Reflective Questions..61
References 61

**PART II SELF-REFLECTION: BUILDING OUR CAPACITY
FOR INTROSPECTION AND INTENTIONAL
PRACTICE IN ACADEMIC AND CLINICAL
SETTINGS** 65

**4 SELF-REFLECTION THROUGH THE LENS OF UNITARY
CARING SCIENCE: LEARNING TO LISTEN AND LISTENING
TO LEARN** 67

Overview..68
Supporting Theoretical Frameworks and Evidence...........................68
Learning to Listen 71
Listening in the Clinical Environment 78
Listening in the Learning Environment 81
Reflective Summary 83
Learning Narrative...84
Reflective Questions..87
References 87

5   DEEPENING OUR FOUNDATIONS: REIMAGINING
     OURSELVES, REIMAGINING NURSING IDENTITY 89
         Overview 90
         Supporting Evidence and Theoretical Frameworks 91
         Knowing and Navigating the Context of Work Environments 93
         Attending to Self as Nurse 95
         Reflective Narratives: Reimagining Self and Nursing 99
         Rethinking Self-Care Towards Well-Being 103
         Application for Personal and Professional Development 109
         Reflective Summary 110
         Learning Narrative 110
         Reflective Questions 111
         References 111

6   THE ROLE OF REFLECTION IN GUIDING THE
     EVOLUTION OF CARE, COMPASSION, AND
     SOCIAL CHANGE 115
         Overview 116
         Reflection as a Central Component of Nursing Practice 116
         Supporting Theoretical Frameworks and Other Evidence 117
         Reflexive Pedagogies for Guiding the Development of Care and
             Compassion 121
         Reflective Questions 127
         Moving From Safe to Brave Learning Spaces to Guide Social Change 131
         Application for Personal and Professional Practice 132
         Reflective Summary 134
         Learning Narrative 134
         Reflective Questions 135
         References 135

PART III   REFLECTING WITH OTHERS 139

7   SHARING OUR STORIES: CO-CREATING LEARNING
     THROUGH NARRATIVE PEDAGOGY, SILENCE,
     AND LISTENING. 141
         Overview 142
         Supporting Theoretical Frameworks and Evidence 143

Narrative Pedagogy: Recreating Nursing Education..148

Narrative Medicine: Stories Improving Practice 150

Reflective Summary 156

Learning Narrative..157

Reflective Questions...158

References 159

8 REIMAGINING PRACTICING TOGETHER: REFLECTION IN SIMULATION-BASED LEARNING ...161

Overview..162

Supporting Theoretical Frameworks and Evidence.......................................163

Rethinking Nursing Education Across the Professional Continuum: Simulation-Based Learning..166

Application in Personal and Professional Practice 172

Reflective Summary 173

Learning Narrative..174

Reflective Questions 176

References 176

9 REFLECTIVE LEARNING: RECALIBRATING COLLABORATION AND EVALUATION FOR SAFETY AND QUALITY COMPETENCIES 179

Overview..180

Supporting Theoretical Frameworks and Evidence 181

Recalibrating Collaboration: Structuring Reflection in Clinical Learning 184

Micropractices: Connecting Quality and Safety and Reflective Practice 187

Critical Reflection: Reconsidering Practice Development Among Learners and Nurses 189

Reflective Practice: Developing Collaborative Relationships 191

Recreating Educator Evaluations or Annual Nurse Evaluations....................196

Application for Personal and Professional Practice: Reimagining Reflection and Self-Assessment 197

Reflective Summary 198

Learning Narrative..199

Reflective Questions...201

References 201

PART IV   REFLECTIVE PRACTICE IN ORGANIZATIONS AND COMMUNITIES 205

10 RETHINKING HOW WE WORK TOGETHER: REFLECTIVE PRACTICES USING EMERGENT STRATEGY, LIBERATING STRUCTURES, AND CLEARNESS COMMITTEES 207

Overview 208

Supporting Theoretical Frameworks and Other Evidence 208

Complexity Science: Rethinking Organizational Relationships 210

Emergent Strategy for Shaping the Futures We Want to Live 211

Liberating Structures: Recreating How We Interact and Reflect 214

Liberating Structures: Reflecting-in-Action and Reflecting-on-Action 216

Clearness Committees for Enabling Discernment and Courageous, Wise Actions 220

Application to Personal and Professional Practice 222

Reflective Summary 223

Learning Narrative 224

Reflective Questions 225

References 225

11 PLURALISTIC POSSIBILITY: REFLECTIVE PRACTICES TO REFRAME OUR WORLD 227

Overview 228

Supporting Theoretical Frameworks and Other Evidence 229

Complexities of "Diversity of Thought" 231

Redefining Language: Moving to a Caring Way of Being and Doing 237

Application in Personal and Professional Development 238

Learning Narrative: Creating Self-Awareness Through STEAM 244

Reflective Questions 245

Reflective Summary 245

References 246

12 REDESIGNING ACADEMIC AND PRACTICE PARTNERSHIPS: REFLECTIVE COMMUNITIES THAT LEARN AND PRACTICE TOGETHER 249
Overview 250
Hindsight, Insight, and Foresight Learning Perspectives on Academic-Practice Partnerships 250
Theoretical Frameworks and Supporting Evidence 255
Academic-Practice Partnerships as Reflective Relationships 259
Application for Personal and Professional Practice 260
Reflective Summary 262
Learning Narrative 262
Reflective Questions 263
References 263

PART V REGENERATION AND RENEWAL 267

13 THE VALUE OF EMANCIPATORY NURSING PRAXIS AND CARING SCIENCE IN AN ERA OF LEGISLATIVE CENSORSHIP 269
Overview 270
The Precarious State of Social Justice in Higher Education 270
Emancipatory Nursing Praxis: Overview of the Theory 272
Using Relational Emancipatory Pedagogy to Develop Emancipatory Nursing Praxis 275
Reflective Summary 282
Learning Narrative 283
Reflective Questions 284
References 284

14 REIMAGINING LEADERSHIP: A LEGACY PERSPECTIVE 287
Overview: A Personal Reflection 288
Theoretical Frameworks to Support Legacy Leadership Reflection 288
Principles and Practices of Legacy Leadership 291
The Be-Attitudes of Legacy Leadership 292
Creating Legacy Insights Through Strengths, Values, and Contributions Appraisals 295

Application for Personal and Professional Practice 297
Reflective Summary 297
Learning Narrative...298
Reflective Questions 299
References 300

15 REFLECTIVE PRACTICE, UNITARY CARING SCIENCE, AND WISDOM: THE HEART OF THE CAPACITY TO GROW 303

Overview...304
Supporting Theoretical Frameworks and Evidence 304
Reflective Practice and Unitary Caring Science...307
Relational Practices 311
Application for Personal and Professional Practice 317
Reflective Summary 318
Learning Narrative...318
Reflective Questions 319
References 320

INDEX 321

FOREWORD

This third edition of *Reflective Practice* not only expands the worldview of self and nursing but also summons and evokes an awakened consciousness and questioning of "Being Human/Being Nursing." What unfolds is a methodical, comprehensive tome of advanced reflective, Caring Science scholarship and praxis from authors around the world. The authors invite and engage readers in elational–contemplative disciplinary scholarship through reimaging self/nursing via a reflective, evolved unitary paradigm. These reflective thematic approaches, systematically organized throughout each chapter, serve as conceptual theoretical guides to recalibrate dominant thinking, informing and transforming mindsets. In entering this intensive and extensive book, you are invited into an inner world, opening space for self-creativity and new revelations for personal/professional development/expansion.

Each section of the book embraces a Caring Science lens toward core values, ethics, and context to support ontological reflective caring praxis. Content-specific, diverse, and inclusive grounding exercises are included for self, relationship, organization, and community. Learning narratives and reflective questions follow each chapter, serving as personal interactive guides toward theory-guided, Caring Science scholarship. Contemporary, pressing, moral social justice politics and social change are critiqued and reframed within a Caring Science praxis. Supporting evidence and theoretical context encompass visionary leadership possibilities, such as emancipatory praxis, reflective communities, and new forms of learning together to form academic and clinical partnerships. Ways to liberate and deepen the foundation for care and compassion are addressed as vibrant and vital dynamics requiring an emancipatory, literate lens for shared human–learning communities. Reflective approaches toward safety, quality, simulating learning, and common nursing–institutional, educational–practice phenomena are revisited within a larger vision of what might be, perhaps what ought to be, and ironically, what can be, with new imaginary consciousness.

Each standard, taken-for-granted nursing practice no longer works; the contemplative lens in this third edition requires revisioning. Static nursing approaches necessitate reimagining, moving from orthodox expectations of conformity with mainstream institutional compliance to compassionate critiquing, reflecting, reframing, and rethinking—opening to new possibilities for self/system/society. An evolved model of Caring Science is included throughout this edition, providing deep theoretical reflection for inner growth and foundational insights to underpin mature nursing praxis leadership and future vision. Whether educator, clinician, researcher, or executive administrator, *Reflective Practice*, Third Edition, transcends roles, positions, and settings; it encompasses, invites, informs, and instructs each reader into reimagining a new hopeful legacy for self and nursing.

–Jean Watson, PhD, RN, AHN-BC, FAAN, LL (AAN)
Founder, Watson Caring Science Institute

INTRODUCTION

Nurses' work is complex and often heavy. As a result, nurses and their work environments often suffer. At the same time, the future of nursing and its leadership depends on nurses' ability to recognize and address issues with bravery and determination. As agents of change, nurses must courageously confront and rectify inequities and promote healthier work environments. It is imperative we are part of the solution and create a better future for the nursing profession and those needing our care.

This third edition, *Reflective Practice: Reimagining Ourselves, Reimagining Nursing,* is particularly timely considering the current context of healthcare settings following the acute phase of a global pandemic. The public is aware that nursing is the heart, soul, and backbone of the healthcare profession. Nurse suffering is widespread, some nurses are stepping away, and both healthcare education and practice settings are called on to respond. This book provides a road map for how nurse educators and nurses can reimagine learning environments and guide learners in developing literacies and competencies for building effective relationships, psychologically safe inclusive environments, and meaning and purpose. Educators, learners, and nurses are invited to connect through meaning, purpose, ethics, and theory that ground them in caring consciousness. Nurse educators and nurses who engage students through reflective practice and create safe spaces to explore what it means to be a nurse lay a foundation for learners to find their voice and engage in courageous caring actions to secure the future of nursing and global health. A key feature is melding these concepts into a reimagined model of reflective practices as nurses reenvision the balance between their personal and professional lives.

Specifically, this book guides educators and nurses on how to facilitate learners at all levels for digging deeply into themselves to cultivate a critical awareness of who they are and their values, beliefs, and assumptions as the beginning point for engaging in caring relationships with others. Reflective practices facilitate each of us in understanding how personal knowing informs our moral, ontological, and intellectual practice as a nurse, developing awareness for achieving social justice, diversity, and inclusion. Teaching and practicing nursing are relational endeavors; thus, relationships play a crucial role in understanding the complexity of nursing practice and the way we work together inter- and intra-professionally.

Reflective Practice, Third Edition, pulls together multiple approaches for self-development individually and collectively through adaptable exercises and micropractices, bringing awareness of invisible biases contributing to microaggressions. This book also incorporates Unitary Caring Science, quality and safety, and the new American Association of Colleges of Nursing (AACN) Essentials with a reflective lens, emphasizing lifelong learning and the significance of being in a community with others.

Like the earlier editions of this textbook, which were published in 2012 and 2017, we continue to see multiple forces converging to influence nursing education and practice. The American Nurses Association's (2021) revised definition of nursing emphasizes the art and science of care, human functioning, compassionate presence, and recognition of all humanity. It emphasizes the need for nurses to be advocates for all individuals. This more expansive definition invites nurses to consider the who, what, where, when, and why questions related to nursing practice. Likewise, the AACN's new Essentials for nursing education (2021) redefines quality in nursing education and outlines the necessary curriculum content and expected outcomes of graduates from undergraduate and graduate nursing programs. The emphasis is to move toward a new model and framework for nursing education using a competency-based approach intended to prepare nurses for entry and advanced-level roles in a changing healthcare environment, foster lifelong learning, and promote innovation and excellence in nursing practice.

The ongoing convergence of these forces makes clear that to improve healthcare quality, we must be responsible for changing how we prepare and support those who deliver patient care. Together, the ANA revised definition of nursing and the Essentials are intended to help nurses provide safe, effective, patient-centered, and evidence-informed care; collaborate with other health professionals; and lead change and innovation in nursing practice. Reflective practices help nurses meet these demands by enabling nurses to develop a deeper understanding of their practice, identify areas of improvement, and make informed decisions based on their experience.

REFLECTIVE PRACTICE: REIMAGINING OURSELVES, REIMAGINING NURSING

The third edition of this book, *Reflective Practice: Reimagining Ourselves, Reimagining Nursing*, offers educators, nurses, and learners an expanded path to transform nursing education and practice. As a guide for academic institutions and healthcare organizations, the book provides models and strategies for addressing complex issues in healthcare.

The emotional labor of nursing takes a demanding toll on nurses as they cope with workforce issues, increasingly complex patients, and the impact of human factors. Still, for the vast majority of nursing programs, little is incorporated into nursing education to help nurses with compassion fatigue, the demands of working with multiple providers across multiple settings, and increasingly complex workplace issues that deplete energy and motivation. Nursing is a value-based profession; the motivation to make a difference in the lives of people is the chief reason nurses enter the profession. When work is counter to values, nurses are disenfranchised and become disengaged, and work becomes rote, cynical attitudes become pervasive, and quality of care suffers. And, following the COVID-19 pandemic, some nurses have chosen to leave the profession. To sustain nurses in the profession and improve patient care outcomes requires incorporating innovative pedagogies that engage and involve learners, reshape educational processes, and consider new ways to assess and evaluate outcomes. For these reasons, Watson's Unitary Caring Science model permeates this third edition to provide a lens for learners and practitioners to balance care for self with the care they provide others (Hills et al., 2021). The 10 Caritas Processes are listed in Chapter 1 and integrated throughout this text (Watson, 2008). They provide a path for learners to reimagine themselves—who they are and what they need to be the nurse they aspire to be.

CHANGING THE LEARNING PARADIGM

It is timely to transform nursing education. The ever-evolving healthcare landscape, driven by advancements in medical technology, changes in healthcare policies, and shifting healthcare needs of patients, requires all healthcare professionals to be adaptable and continuously learning. There is also a growing call for more person-centered and relational care, which requires nurses to develop a more holistic understanding of patients' needs and values, as well as authentic communication and collaboration skills (Hills et al., 2021). This translates into an imperative for change in these developing areas. Healthcare delivery is shifting towards team-based approaches, and this means nurses need skills for working effectively in interprofessional teams, which means education needs to focus more on interprofessional collaboration and communication (Sherman, 2023).

Significant healthcare disparities among different populations include those based on race, ethnicity, sexual orientation, and socioeconomic status (ANA, 2021). Nursing education needs to address these disparities and prepare nurses to be culturally aware and responsive. There are also significant burnout and mental health issues among college students, nurses, and educators. A transformative pedagogy that is responsive to those who experienced trauma requires we not only change our pedagogy but also the practice of our pedagogy (hooks, 1994; Thompson & Carello, 2022). All these factors overlay an industry that is being called to reduce costs and increase efficiency. Changing nursing education is crucial to ensure nurses are prepared to meet the evolving healthcare landscape and provide high-quality, person-centered care.

However, healthcare professionals are limited in their ability to provide person-centered care if they are not socialized and encouraged to attend to their own needs. Where do we incorporate the self-care practices and deep thinking time required for the integration of rational knowledge with person-centered aspects of care? How do nurse educators integrate other forms of knowledge that derive from aesthetics, ethics, personal reflection, and other ways of knowing? How do these converge for making sense of practice and understanding the broad dimensions of humanness relevant to health? This book describes how reflective practice can guide nurses to make sense of their practice and build resiliency to sustain them within their practice. Teaching boxes provide exemplars and instructions to help nurses with practical applications.

How we teach is as critical as what we teach. Lecture alone rarely achieves behavior change. Reflective practice is part of a new paradigm for nursing education that is learner-centered to help develop the person who comes to work as a nurse. Reflection provides a systematic way to integrate knowledge from experience with continued learning from multiple sciences—that is, developing the practical tacit knowledge important in developing clinical judgment.

REFLECTIVE PRACTICES: EMPHASIZING QSEN, CARING SCIENCE, THE NEW ESSENTIALS, AND DIVERSITY, EQUITY, AND INCLUSION

Each iteration of this textbook evolves to respond to societal needs. The first edition incorporated the work of the Robert Wood Johnson Foundation project Quality and Safety Education for Nurses (QSEN) as a vehicle for transforming nursing education to integrate a quality and safety framework (Cronenwett et al., 2007, 2009; Sherwood & Barnsteiner, 2021). To further engage learners in reflective practice and aid in tapping into the deeply human aspects of care, in the second edition we integrated Caring Science (Watson, 2018, 2021) as a foundation for how learners connect with self and others—to be more present, authentic, and intentional in their practice. This third edition continues to incorporate the QSEN competencies, expands Caring Science, addresses the new AACN Essentials (2021) and the revised ANA definition of nursing, and threads diversity, equity, and inclusion throughout.

By expanding on our earlier editions, this third edition further establishes the pedagogy of reflection by providing frameworks with specific applications and micropractices of reflective thinking and learning in learner-centered environments, implications for reflective educators, futuristic complexity science, and pluralistic possibility. This new edition extends and incorporates complementary paradigms that emphasize the desire to learn, to grow, and to be in community with others, including critical caring consciousness and social justice and issues related to diversity, equity, and inclusion. Diversity, equity, and inclusion are crucial to nursing and all health professions to create a more equitable, culturally responsive, and effective healthcare system. It also helps to improve the quality of care and health outcomes for all patients.

WAYS TO USE THIS BOOK

This book was designed keeping you in mind.

You may be a learner using this book for class. The first three chapters focus on the development, evolution, and need for reflective practice in nursing education and as a lifelong learning tool to help you intentionally respond to and balance the professional challenges we face in healthcare. Reflective practice learning activities incorporated throughout the book aim to establish a strong foundation and serve as a source of renewal. Each chapter features text boxes and ends with learning narratives and reflective practice questions to prompt you to scrutinize your thoughts, feelings, and behaviors and evaluate how they affect your personal and professional growth.

You may be an educator who has passion but limited time. You may be seeking tools for redesigning class or clinical learning to ensure learners engage in a systematic and structured approach to thinking about and analyzing experiences, actions, and knowledge gained in order to gain insights, develop new understanding and knowledge, and improve future performance. *Reflective Practice: Reimagining Ourselves, Reimagining Nursing* helps educators, nurses, and learners become more self-aware, develop a deeper understanding of their own values and beliefs, identify areas for improvement, and enhance their ability to learn from experiences.

You may be leading a book club. Reflective practice questions at the end of each chapter can guide rigorous dialogue, individual journaling, small group breakout sessions, or large group discussions.

The following descriptions provide a glimpse into the book's contents and structure to help visualize ways to utilize the book.

WHAT'S IN THIS BOOK

This third edition is a well-timed resource; despite the resurgent interest in reflective learning experiences, few resources focus on reflective learning strategies. The book is an inspiration and informative companion for nurse educators in both academic and clinical settings, learners eager to deeper their professional practice model, nurses and graduate students who are interested in developing leadership capacity, and nurses seeking to advance professional development from novice to expert. The five parts of this book assemble multiple approaches to reflective pedagogy for self-improvement through exercises adaptable to nurses' personal lives and professional work. It serves independent learners seeking meaning through their personal and professional growth and development. It is designed to use both individually and in group discussions, or with a coach, preceptor, or mentor. Each chapter begins with learning objectives and, for the first time, subjectives to emphasize the importance of fully integrating affective learning. To create optimal learning environments, we encourage educators to pay attention to emotions and the whole of the situation in acknowledging responses of the learner, as learning cannot take place in the absence of emotions (Immordino-Yang, 2016; Thompson & Carello, 2022).

PART I: THE DEVELOPMENT AND EVOLUTION OF THE NURSE THROUGH REFLECTIVE PRACTICE

Part I introduces reflective practice with three chapters. The opening chapter examines the converging societal and technological issues impacting knowledge development and the theoretical frameworks that guide reflection, critical caring consciousness, and caring literacy, thereby directly addressing the need to balance advancing technologies with a caring and relational imperative. Critical and reflective frameworks are introduced to encourage learners to examine various perspectives and create transformational learning opportunities where they integrate their experience into their knowledge and become active agents of change. Reflection is critical in expanding personal and professional leadership, developing self-awareness, promoting individual accountability, and changing behavior. Through the lens of Caring Science, nurses learn to deepen their reflective ability in and on practice and balance the "doing" task components of care with a way of "being" in right relation with self and other. Chapter 2 examines models of reflective practice to develop and sustain personal and professional practice. These models are an important part of redesigning nursing education to ensure students are prepared for practice and for rebuilding the academic-practice connection. Changing education is the first step to achieving new competencies in the nursing profession. The application of reflective methods is a model of change agency that can help to uncover gaps in the system for improvement. A chapter on the relationship between reflection and Caring Science, Chapter 3, completes this part by applying reflective practices to the care of self as the foundation of caring for others. Educators who see this aspect of disciplinary knowledge as an integral part of all levels of nursing education prepare nurses who seek meaning and relevance in their personal and professional lives.

PART II: SELF-REFLECTION: BUILDING OUR CAPACITY FOR INTROSPECTION AND INTENTIONAL PRACTICE IN ACADEMIC AND CLINICAL SETTINGS

The three chapters in Part II focus on building the learners' capacity for introspection and intentional practice in academic and practice settings. Self-awareness and mindfulness are considered from multiple perspectives as a cornerstone for reflection. Our presence, our being, is the most powerful teacher introduced in Chapter 3 and further explored in Chapter 4. This chapter explores how deep listening is nurtured through authentic presence. Together, authentic presence and deep listening can create a powerful communication dynamic that fosters trust, understanding, and meaningful connections. When we are authentically present and deeply listen to others, we create a safe space for open and honest communication, which can lead to better relationships and improved outcomes in education and healthcare settings. Chapter 5 deepens the foundations of what it is to be nurse, explores reflective pedagogies addressing nursing as a practice based discipline, and includes tools and strategies addressing self-care, wellness, and person-centered care. Chapter 6 explores the role of reflection in guiding care, compassion, and social change. It offers strategies and exercises to develop self-awareness and self-care and expand the capacity for compassion for self and others. From this foundation, the chapter explores how to create safe and brave spaces to address social change. Through this process, learners begin to see the necessity and value of self-care and compassion and are poised to carry these behaviors into their professional practice, becoming reflective practitioners committed to patient-centered care.

PART III: REFLECTING WITH OTHERS

The three chapters in Part III examine reflecting with others in both didactic and clinical practice. Sharing our stories is the focus of Chapter 7, and the chapter emphasizes learning through silence and listening. Narrative pedagogy as a research-based approach for educators and mentors to enhance reflective practice learning experiences is explained and exemplified throughout. In addition, the chapter explores developing and practicing listening and interpretative skills to envision new possibilities for understanding and working with one another and those receiving care. Of interest, this chapter is full of rich audio/video resources applied to learning. Chapter 8 illustrates the role of reflection within simulation-based learning practice, which uses the simulation experiences in an unfolding way to help learners with complex knowledge integration. It describes how reflection is applied to simulation learning using reflection-before-, -in-, -on-, and -beyond-action. Next, reflective learning, collaboration, and evaluation of safe, quality care are explored in Chapter 9. The importance of matching learning methods and objectives, reflection as learning, and reflection as assessment are explored. Engaging learners in co-creating reflective, learner-centered classroom and clinical environments and using reflective course evaluation and appreciative inquiry, educators help instill habits of the mind that reinforce lifelong learning.

PART IV: REFLECTIVE PRACTICE IN ORGANIZATIONS AND COMMUNITIES

Part IV explores the use of reflective practices in organizational and community settings as a way to deepen professional practice and expand the capacity to work effectively with others. Chapter 10 is about working together in groups, a key to transformation in healthcare. Through the use of emergent strategy, liberating structures, and clearness committees, reflective methodologies derived from complexity theory, we demonstrate how to create more effective and reflective ways of working together, whether in nursing or interprofessional teams. Building capacity for interprofessional practice through addressing diversity, equity, and inclusion is the focus of Chapter 11. This chapter explores the theoretical model of pluralistic possibility, a way of thinking about the world that emphasizes openness, inclusivity, and diversity of perspectives and experiences. The model focuses on consciousness-raising and how this can help to name, identify, and transform problems to meet future needs. As a reflective practice, it encourages learners to embrace complexity and diversity and seek out and engage with the richness of varying human experiences. The final chapter in this part, Chapter 12, focuses on designing academic-practice partnerships as reflective learning communities that can learn and grow together. When academia and practice settings co-design learning processes, they each inform the other through collaborative inquiry, reflective learning, and deliberative action.

PART V: REGENERATION AND RENEWAL

Part V poses future perspectives on reflective practice through the lens of regeneration and renewal. Reflective practice is a powerful strategy for regeneration and renewal because it allows individuals and organizations to learn from their experiences and make positive changes. The chapters in this part explore ways to reimagine goals, develop new strategies, enhance creativity, and build resilience. Through the lens of emancipatory nursing praxis and Caring Science, Chapter 13 explores thoughtful, evidence-informed approaches to address the seismic shift in college student demographics and the urgent need for inclusion and equity in higher education. Through inclusive and engaging teaching and learning practices, this chapter guides educators and learners in how to create communities of belonging and to become social justice allies to disrupt systems and spaces of oppression and exclusion. The next chapter, Chapter 14, explores how to reflect on your personal and professional legacy by identifying your unique strengths, values, and contributions. Chapter 14 emphasizes how to use this self-knowledge to guide decision-making and actions to inspire and mentor others to achieve their own legacies. Reflective practice and Caritas Processes help leaders to continually evaluate and refine their legacy leadership approach to ensure that they are making a positive and lasting impact on the nursing profession. Exercises, tools, and assessment activities are provided to support leaders in discerning their personal strengths, values, and contributions and in identifying areas for growth and development. The concluding chapter, Chapter 15, creates an emotional space within learners where they can further explore their individual gifts, talents, and wisdom. The chapter does not offer any definitive solutions but instead provides additional exercises, tools, processes, and insights on life to encourage a personal quest for wisdom that can positively impact your relationships and the organizations you belong to. Based on the principles of Unitary Caring Science, the chapter encourages learners to connect with their deepest and most insightful selves as a powerful tool for social change.

Wherever you are in your nursing journey, there is a message for you in this book. The power of reflective practice lies in the joy derived from meaningful work. The micropractices that drive reflective practice threaded throughout these chapters help you refocus, reimagine, and regenerate your human spirit so that you are sustained in this critical profession, making a difference to yourself and to others.

–Sara Horton-Deutsch, PhD, RN, FAAN, ANEF, SGAHN
–Gwen D. Sherwood, PhD, RN, FAAN, ANEF

REFERENCES

American Association of Colleges of Nursing. (2021). *The essentials: Core competencies for professional nursing education.* https://www.aacnnursing.org/Portals/42/AcademicNursing/pdf/Essentials-2021.pdf

American Nurses Association. (2021, June 11). *Journey of racial reconciliation: Racial reckoning statement.*

Cronenwett, L., Sherwood, G., Barnsteiner, J., Disch, J., Johnson, J., Mitchell, P., Sullivan, D. T., & Warren, J. (2007). Quality and safety education for nurses. *Nursing Outlook, 55*(3), 122–131. https://doi.org/10.1016/j.outlook.2007.02.006

Cronenwett, L., Sherwood, G., Pohl, J., Barnsteiner, J., Moore, S., Sullivan, D. T., Ward, D., & Warren, J. (2009). Quality and safety education for advanced nursing practice. *Nursing Outlook, 57*(6), 338–348. https://doi.org/10.1016/j.outlook.2009.07.009

Hills, M., Watson, J., & Cara, C. (2021). *Creating a caring science curriculum: A relational pedagogy for nursing* (2nd ed.). Springer.

hooks, b. (1994). *Teaching to transgress: Education as the practice of freedom.* Routledge.

Immordino-Yang, M.H. (2016). *American Educational Research Association Ed-Talk: Learning with an emotional brain* [Video]. YouTube. https://www.youtube.com/watch?v=DEeo350WQrs

Sherman, R. (2023). *A team approach to nursing care delivery: Tactics for working better together.* Rose Sherman. www.emergingleader.com

Sherwood, G., & Barnsteiner, J. (2021). *Quality and safety in nursing: A competency approach to improving outcomes* (3rd ed.). Wiley Blackwell.

Sherwood, G., & Horton-Deutsch, S. (2015). *Reflective organizations: On the front lines of QSEN and reflective practice implementation.* Sigma Theta Tau International.

Thompson, P., & Carello, J. (2022). *Trauma-informed pedagogies: A guide for responding to crisis and inequality in healthcare.* Palgrave Macmillan.

Watson, J. (2008). *Nursing: The philosophy and science of caring.* University Press of Colorado.

Watson, J. (2018). *Unitary caring science: The philosophy and praxis of nursing.* University of Colorado Press.

Watson, J. (2021). *Caring science as sacred science* (Rev. ed). Lotus Library.

PART I
THE DEVELOPMENT AND EVOLUTION OF THE NURSE THROUGH REFLECTIVE PRACTICE

1   Reimagining Ourselves: The Role of Reflection on Critical Caritas Consciousness and Knowledge Development 3

2   Reimagining Reflection to Develop and Sustain Personal and Professional Practice 19

3   Reimagining Creative Space for Reflection in a Caring Science Paradigm 43

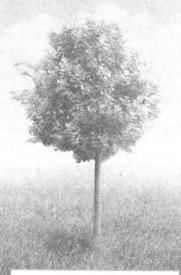

REIMAGINING OURSELVES: THE ROLE OF REFLECTION ON CRITICAL CARITAS CONSCIOUSNESS AND KNOWLEDGE DEVELOPMENT

–Dawn Freshwater, PhD, RN, FRCN, FRCSI, MAE, GAICD
Sara Horton-Deutsch, PhD, RN, FAAN, ANEF, SGAHN
Gwen Sherwood, PhD, RN, FAAN, ANEF

LEARNING OBJECTIVES/SUBJECTIVES

- Identify converging societal and technological issues impacting knowledge development.

- Explore theoretical frameworks that guide reflection, critical Caritas consciousness, and Caritas literacy.

- Explain the role of reflection, critical Caritas consciousness, and Caritas literacy in addressing complex issues in nursing.

- Appraise the value of relational learning for the development of more socially and culturally conscious and morally courageous nurses.

OVERVIEW

Humanity is at a critical juncture. We are facing multiple and extraordinarily complex issues of vital importance, most recently revealed in the COVID-19 pandemic, that—combined with an accelerated pace and scale of change—are bringing our commitment to the development, dissemination, and impact of knowledge to the fore. Digitization of information has fundamentally altered its distribution and the depth of how it is analyzed, understood, responded to, and acted upon. Moreover, Wallace et al. (2022) in their text, *Checkmate Humanity: The How and Why of Responsible AI,* challenge us to consider what it means to be human amid the acceleration of artificial intelligence (AI) and the potential benefits of AI in healthcare and education. The explosion of AI fuels the caring and relational imperative that is the foundation of nursing practice as we navigate AI and the challenges to empathy and reflection (Watson, 2018).

The infodemic (misinformation and disinformation spread rapidly through digital and physical means) we're currently experiencing means that individuals (patients, learners, health professionals, or communities) have access to an enormous amount of information to sift. At the same time, we have more choices and autonomy over our lives. Knowing the right course of action is ever more fraught, no matter your frame of reference. Ethical and moral dilemmas abound.

Nurses have always faced moral and ethical questions; matters related to the right course of action surface daily, including such questions as "How might I think about this?" "How can I assist in ensuring decisions are made in the best interest of the patient?" "How do I balance patient safety and quality with the limitations of my own humanity and self-care?" and so on.

Identification of ethical problems necessitates a degree of critical consciousness, underpinned by a discipline of reflection and a commitment to *moral courage* (the ability to act ethically and authentically in the face of challenges, risks, or opposition), along with sensitivity and an awareness of ethical principles. Khoshmehr et al. (2020) argue that possessing moral sensitivity and knowledge is key for nurses to be able to deal with moral and ethical dilemmas. Moreover, they state that nurses also have to develop moral courage in order to "perform based on what is considered ethically right, provided personal values and criteria correspond to the accepted healthcare values" (Khoshmehr et al., 2020, p. 1).

Right action is not always comfortable; sometimes it requires courage in the face of potential alienation from peers and colleagues. Negative consequences that can be created through moral courage include stress, anxiety, fear of being scolded, rejection by colleagues, and seclusion. Nevertheless, moral courage is also a motivating force that helps nurses to overcome many fearful barriers, enabling them to care for and protect the patient effectively.

We have seen this writ large in recent years as nurses and health professionals not only faced directly into the COVID-19 pandemic but actively walked straight towards the challenging, dynamic, and emergent nature of the experience of self and others at one of the most unprecedented times of fear and uncertainty in many of our lives.

COVID-19 not only overwhelmed nursing practices but also disrupted academic institutions and other settings within which nursing education and nursing research are undertaken. Within the health field, schools of nursing have faced and are preparing for novel and unique challenges related to their role in helping to develop the next generation of care providers. Societal interest in patient safety is growing, with consumers of healthcare services more likely to obtain healthcare information from multiple unchecked sources, increasing the demand for high-quality, well-informed healthcare.

Academic nurse educators were quick to adapt in light of the COVID-19 pandemic; many very quickly moved to emergency remote/online course delivery. Junior nursing students had their clinical placements postponed due to shortages of supervisory staff and rapid changes within the clinical environment, while more senior nursing students were being called upon to integrate into the healthcare workforce. During this period, nursing education continued the process of cultivating nursing students to become nursing professionals, with the capacity for self-reflection and critical thinking.

There has, however, been little time or energy for reimagining ourselves during this recent time of "immediacy"; it is critical for the future of our profession that we now make the time, and take the time, to reflect, learn, and identify ways to rejuvenate, refresh, revitalize, and reframe nursing, nursing education, and nursing practice. In this first chapter, we focus on reimagining ourselves through the prism of reflection, critical Caritas consciousness, and Caritas literacy. We agree with Brindley (2020) that in these unprecedented times, new opportunities to reflect on practice have emerged. We argue that critical caring consciousness, Caritas literacy, and moral courage are fundamental to this reimagination and are at the heart of high-quality, evidence-informed nursing care that uses the development of knowledge situated in a relational ethic.

SUPPORTING THEORETICAL FRAMEWORKS AND OTHER EVIDENCE

Theoretical frameworks serve as the foundation for reimagining ourselves through the lens of reflection, critical caring consciousness, and Caritas literacy. Theories guide our understanding and advance knowledge for both scholarship and practice by providing a set of concepts and principles to help us understand, explain, and make sense of the complex issues before us. These frameworks serve as lenses through which we view and interpret the world around us and guide our thinking, feeling, and actions. In this chapter, the broad theoretical frameworks that support reflection and critical consciousness include critical theory, transformative learning theory, and Caritas literacy.

Critical theory is a philosophical approach that emphasizes the need for individuals to question the social, political, and economic systems that create and perpetuate oppression. At the heart of critical theory is the belief that power relations are embedded in social structures and that these power relations are often hidden from view (Horkheimer, 2007). This is where *Pedagogy of the Oppressed,* a book written by Brazilian educator Paulo Freire (2000), comes into play. Freire argues that traditional education perpetuates existing power structures by presenting knowledge as something that is given by those in authority. Instead, he proposes a model of education that promotes critical consciousness, in which through the development of critical literacy, individuals become aware of how they are oppressed and develop a critical awareness of the world around them (Freire, 2000). Critical literacy integrates active learning within socio-cultural settings where reading extends to interpreting, reflecting on, theorizing, investigating, and questioning (Watson, 2017). This approach empowers individuals to take action to change oppressive systems and work toward social justice through emancipatory learning. Through critical theory and the goals of emancipatory learning developed from *Pedagogy of the Oppressed,* individuals challenge the status quo and gain a deeper understanding of the social structures that shape their lives to work towards a more equitable and just society.

Building on the work of theorists like Paulo Freire, Jack Mezirow developed the theory of *transformative learning,* emphasizing the role of critical reflection that questions deeply held beliefs and assumptions to experience transformation into new ways of thinking (Mezirow & Taylor, 2009). According to transformative learning theory, learning involves more than simply acquiring new knowledge or skills; it also involves a process of critically reflecting on one's experiences, beliefs, and assumptions resulting in personal transformation into new perspectives and ways of thinking. This process is often uncomfortable because it requires individuals to confront and question deeply held beliefs that they may have previously taken for granted. However, the result of transformative learning leads to personal growth and development, as individuals gain new insights and understandings that can help them navigate the complexities of the world around them. By emphasizing critical reflection and personal transformation, transformative learning theory provides a powerful framework for individuals to develop new skills, gain new insights, and become more effective and engaged in the world (Van Schalkwyk et al., 2019).

Watson (2017) translates critical theory and literacy into the lifeworld of the nurse by critiquing inconsistencies between institutional settings dominated by a medical-scientific-clinical view composed of concrete tasks and cognitive skills alone with a more holistic, humane, caring, and relational worldview as a way of being/becoming. Within her theory of Unitary Caring Science, Watson (2017) translates critical literacy to Caritas literacy, calling for the development of ontological competencies. *Ontological competencies* or *Caritas literacies* focus on developing people skills including consciousness, intentionality, centering, authentic presence, deep listening, reflection, and so forth. Described as an antidote to nursing burnout (Lee, 2017), Caritas literacy guides nurses toward a deeper practice that is more life-giving, life-sustaining, and joy-filled, and that comes from deep human connection. Caritas literacy elevates nurses' work to the highest level of consciousness—Caritas consciousness—through a moral-ethical-philosophical connection with humanity. As an inner practice of expanding awareness through reflection, Caritas consciousness involves being more aware of the energy and vibration that come from caring and love (Horton-Deutsch, 2018).

CARITAS CONSCIOUSNESS

"Caritas Consciousness and relationship call for authenticity of Being and Becoming—more fully human and humane, more open-hearted, compassionate, sensitive, present, capable, more competent as a human; more able to dwell in silence, to engage in informed moral actions, with pain, discomfort, emotional struggle and suffering without turning away" (Watson, 2008, p. 80).

CARITAS LITERACY

"Caritas, from Latin, refers to that which is precious and cannot be taken for granted; conveys charity in the sense of the use of self in compassionate service to humankind. Caritas literacy requires an understanding of being and becoming as an ontological form of literacy—that is, being literate in ways that relate to critical reflection; the capacity to deepen and critique culture, ethical, and humane social views and policies; and affecting what it means to be fully human" (Watson, 2017, pp. 4–6).

THE TIME IS NOW: REIMAGINING MORAL COURAGE

It is well documented that nurses, the largest of any occupational cohort in the healthcare and medical field, experience stress and emotional exhaustion related to their work. This can lead to detrimental mental and physical health outcomes for some in these professions (Kim & Chang, 2022; World Health Organization, 2020). Healthcare workers have higher incidence of both physical and psychological illnesses; given the size of the healthcare workforce globally, this is a significant drain on healthcare systems with an associated economic burden (Freshwater, 2023).

Nurses' increasing vulnerability to stress and anxiety is attributed to many factors (Freshwater & Cahill, 2020), including external environmental factors creating instability, organizational contexts, workload, constant change and high levels of uncertainty, inadequate resourcing and skill levels, and long-term emotional consequences of exposure to acute and chronic suffering and dying. This latter point is more poignant in the context of the recent pandemic, with recent studies pointing both to the impact on nursing staff (Khodaveisi et al., 2021; Kim & Chang, 2022) and to the need to rethink nursing education and the underpinning pedagogies (Neuwirth et al., 2020).

The short- and long-term impacts of exposure to suffering and dying are referred to as the burden of *emotional labor*; it is the effort required for the "emotional management" of the self to be achieved (Zaghini et al., 2020). Framed as a way of meeting the expectations and the demands experienced within the work environment, it is perhaps a way of presenting a convincing professional facade. Emotion suppression or emotion management results in emotional discomfort and stress (Kim & Chang, 2022). Emotional labor is further linked with the concepts of death anxiety, moral courage, and empowerment (Freshwater, 2023; Khoshmehr et al., 2020). Contemporary nursing literature shifts our thinking in foregrounding death anxiety through the incidence of COVID-19, with its high morbidity and mortality. The pandemic caused nurses and other caregivers to experience unprecedented levels of fear and death anxiety. Norouzi et al. (2022) reported results of a systematic review of factors associated with death anxiety among nurses including job stress, exhaustion, and psychological hardiness, concluding that healthcare systems should address ways to support nurses in developing resilience and moral courage to mitigate this important job risk. Anxiety and particularly death anxiety can have a deleterious impact on the moral courage of nurses. Moral courage and moral decision-making are closely aligned with the discipline and capacity to reflect critically on practice and in practice (Freshwater, 2023). Reflection enables nurses to overcome fear and anxiety and provide safe and principled care for their patients, thereby leading to a more purposeful and meaningful professional life.

Resilience is a positive adaptation to adverse situations combined with the ability to manage life-threatening situations successfully and courageously and correlates with moral courage; Khodaveisi et al. (2021) linked resilience and moral courage to providing patient care during COVID-19. Developing resilience helps nurses deal with adversity and attenuate the effects of job demands, thereby reducing emotional exhaustion and fostering work engagement, ultimately achieving personal and professional growth (Moloney et al., 2020; Yu et al., 2019). Developing resilience carries corresponding accountability for employers to improve the work environment (Moloney et al., 2020).

Studies demonstrate that moral courage requires acting ethically even when experiencing sensitivity to justice or control over one's emotions and performance such as emotional self-regulation and self-efficacy (Abdollah et al., 2021; Khoshmehr et al., 2020; Kleemola et al., 2020). Moral courage is doing the right thing even when you are not being watched. Observing and feeling the anxiety and fear that comes with doing the right thing and taking the leap to act demonstrates moral courage. When nurses struggle to act according to the nurses' code of ethics (International Council of Nurses [ICN], 2021), moral courage helps them to apply their best effort to achieve their ultimate goal, regardless of the consequences. In doing so, they consider moral principles and perform a correct act that is not easy to do. We refer to this as the *right action*.

This leads us to consider how nurses develop moral courage in the face of workplace pressures. Unitary Caring Science provides a framework for nurses to explore the concepts of moral courage through Watson's philosophy of human caring (Watson, 2018). It emphasizes the wholeness, uniqueness, and interconnectedness of human beings and their environment within a unitary field of energy and consciousness. Unitary Caring Science also recognizes the sacredness, dignity, and value of every person and their potential for healing and growth. To practice nursing from this perspective, nurses need to cultivate moral courage, which is fostered by applying the 10 Caritas Processes—values and actions that express caring, compassion, respect, and reverence for self and others (Watson, 2008):

1. Sustaining humanistic-altruistic values by practice of loving kindness, compassion, and equanimity with self and others.

2. Being authentically present, enabling faith/hope/belief system; honoring subjective inner, life-world of self/other.

3. Being sensitive to self and others by cultivating own spiritual practices; beyond ego-self to transpersonal presence.

4. Developing and sustaining loving, trusting-caring relationships.

5. Allowing for expression of positive and negative feelings—authentically listening to another person's story.

6. Creatively problem-solving "solution-seeking" through caring processes; full use of self and artistry of caring-healing practices via use of all ways of knowing/being/doing/becoming.

7. Engaging in transpersonal teaching and learning within context of caring relationship; staying within other's frame of reference-shift toward coaching model for expanded health/wellness.

8. Creating a healing environment at all levels; subtle environment for energetic authentic caring presence.

9. Reverently assisting with basic needs as sacred acts, touching mind-body-spirit of spirit of other; sustaining human dignity.

10. Opening to spiritual, mystery, unknowns—allowing for miracles.

Reflective practices applying the 10 Caritas Processes are threaded throughout this book. By reimagining nursing through the lens of Unitary Caring Science, nurses can transform their practice into a sacred moral praxis that honors the human spirit and contributes to the well-being of humanity.

REFLECTION AND RELATIONSHIP: THE ANTIDOTE FOR LEARNING THROUGH COMPLEXITY AND UNCERTAINTY

While it is true that nursing education has been disrupted because of the COVID-19 pandemic, we need to remind ourselves that education and learning practices were changing rapidly before the advent of COVID-19, with learner environs and learner expectations responding to the commensurate shifts in healthcare provision, advances in technology and AI, models of care, and the future of work. Nevertheless, there remains an enormous challenge for educators in integrating pre- and post-pandemic practices into a form of hybrid and blended learning that facilitates excellence in competencies and Caritas literacies (ontological competencies) for learning. These ontological competencies provide an essential path to renewal for professional nurses with highly attuned reflective and relational skills.

As Wittenberg et al. (2021) commented on the sudden pivot to online education during the COVID-19 pandemic, students no longer had access to traditional activities for learning communication skills. The gap created a critical demand for open educational resources available to both faculty and students, yet few existed, with even less pedagogical content. Even so, evidence demonstrates that transpersonal caring relationships can be modeled, practiced, and affirmed in online learning environments (Gdanetz, 2019).

Learner experiences and ways of learning have been impacted in remarkable ways, creating further complexities and compounding educator workload. These changes add to the feelings of exhaustion overwhelming both educators and learners with negative impacts on quality, safe care. Naturally, there are consequential sequelae on recruitment and retention in nursing, noted as a global crisis (ICN, 2022). The education and learning environment has shifted markedly, as expectations of what education should be and should do are changing, and students, employers, professionals, communities, and academics insist those expectations be met. These expectations also arise from how we live our professional and institutional values, who we are as a professional community, how and to whom we connect, and how we go about our work. This translates to how we as nurses and people show up in all our personhood. Acting with or without our values, open to learning or closed off, we strive to survive the system and our own difficult and often contradictory feelings about our daily nursing practice. In this, then, we are all called to act with moral courage.

Controversial at the time, Menzies' research exposed some of the social systems and active negatives that nurses constructed to avoid thinking about the psychological difficulties associated with their work; a way of avoiding anxiety created through being a part of the system per se, the social system being a part of the solution (Menzies, 1960). Deconstructing the authentic self, emotionally and physically, to construct the professional nurse self was experienced as not only personally beneficial but institutionally and educationally encouraged. Her work showed how the stresses of nursing and the intimate relationship it demanded with patients left those closest to patients exposed to emotional pressures that administrators at the upper levels may not see.

Menzies' essays reported the dysfunctional outcomes for staff and patients when employing institutional defenses that served to routinize and depersonalize human contact. In this sense it was a decisive work, first postulating that nurses coped with the frequent exposure to suffering and dying within a social system through supported objectification of both their patients and themselves. Later works further comprehended that experiencing both caring ("good") and hating ("bad") feelings for the same patient, an ambiguity that is difficult for most nurses to tolerate, required constant recalibration for even the most conscious and emotionally mature nurse (Briant & Freshwater, 1998).

Through a Unitary Caring Science framework, nurses develop a Caritas consciousness by embracing universal values of humanistic altruism. It offers a personal-professional path of authenticity, bringing universals of love, energy, spirit, the infinity of purpose, and meaning back into the lives of nurses and their work. Unitary Caring Science guides nurses to deconstruct the authentic self by introducing the concept of praxis as an informed moral practice. *Praxis* involves a critical reflection on one's actions and values, as well as creative use of self and a sense of belonging. Praxis also requires a deepening of self-awareness and self-consciousness, as well as nurturing interpersonal and intersubjective connections and relations. Nurses enhance their resilience and compassion as caring-healing practitioners and strengthen their relations with others by practicing praxis, which involves aligning their actions with their purpose and fulfillment (Watson, 2018; Wei et al., 2021).

COMING TO AN UNDERSTANDING

German philosopher Hans-Georg Gadamer (1960) argues that understanding is something that comes to us or happens to us when we are *prepared* for it. In this sense, understanding is always also *an act of understanding ourselves*—an act of reflection, related and relational to our positioning. As Damsgaard and Phoenix (2022, p. 178) comment, "Understanding depends on ourselves and consequently also what we as human beings have brought with us, formed through upbringing, formative education and culture and the prejudices and expectations that we have adopted—for example from schools and practice." An important part of understanding is produced from being open and receptive to all that we have brought with us and all that we will become.

APPLICATION FOR PERSONAL AND PROFESSIONAL PRACTICE

As exemplified in the previous section, *relational learning* emphasizes the importance of relationships and social interactions in shaping individuals' understanding of themselves and the world around them. While relational learning is distinct from critical theory, transformative learning theory, and Unitary Caring Science, there are complementary connections and overlap among these approaches. First, relational learning emphasizes the importance of understanding the social and cultural contexts in which learning occurs. This is similar to the focus of critical theory and Unitary Caring Science on recognizing and examining power relations and social structures that may impact individuals' ability to learn, heal, and grow. These approaches recognize the importance of considering the broader social and cultural contexts that shape individuals' experiences and extend to a global worldview.

Next, transformative learning theory and Unitary Caring Science emphasize the importance of agency and personal transformation in the learning process. Similarly, they all recognize the importance of individuals taking an active role in their own learning and personal growth and emphasize the potential for relationships and social interactions to support this process. These approaches recognize the need for individuals to have a sense of self-awareness and agency, while also emphasizing the importance of social connections and supportive relationships in promoting positive outcomes.

Nurses who learn to apply relational learning, critical theory, transformative learning, and Unitary Caring Science to their personal and professional lives cultivate a greater sense of self-awareness, relational competence, and agency and are prepared to navigate complex social and cultural contexts with greater confidence, courage, and resilience. Begin by:

- **Reflecting on social and cultural contexts:** Using critical theory and relational learning, reflect on your own social and cultural contexts and how they may impact your learning and growth. What power structures and dominant cultural narratives influence your perspectives, values, and beliefs? How may these factors shape your relationships and interactions with others?

- **Engaging in dialogue and authentic communication:** Apply relational learning, transformative learning, and Unitary Caring Science to engage in meaningful dialogue and authentic communication with others. By actively listening and responding to others' perspectives and experiences, you can deepen your understanding of self and the world around you and develop greater compassion and relational literacy.

- **Embracing growth and transformation:** Transformative learning theory and Unitary Caring Science emphasize the potential for individuals to undergo significant personal/professional growth and transformation through their learning experiences. Use these theories to embrace new challenges and experiences and view setbacks and failures as opportunities for learning and development.

REFLECTIVE SUMMARY

The process of reflective learning and learning through relationships is characterized by the notion of growth, even through trauma. This is a crucial capacity for health professionals and learners and their communities alike. The chapters that follow will guide you in reflective practices to expand your critical Caritas consciousness, exploring values, intentions, listening, self-care, caring for others, transpersonal relationships, and ultimately compassionate actions in the world that come from moral courage. It may seem paradoxical, but as many are now saying, if as a profession we can understand this traumatic period and seize the moment, the crisis inflicted by the pandemic may function globally as a vision for a more humanized world—a world marked by social justice and an awareness of the importance of the other.

It may rehabilitate the urge to learn and understand other practices and to truly understand through reflection—to create what Nussbaum (1998) referred to as competent and wise health professionals.

LEARNING NARRATIVE

Putting it into practice: Knowledge development through a reflective curriculum model of relational learning.

The University of Auckland's novel curriculum framework recognizes that excellence in teaching and research is necessary for, and provides a means of, engendering transformation in the lives of many people. Putting the learner at the center of learning and teaching, it recognizes and values their social and emotional selves alongside their academic contributions and through the intersectionality of their often complex lives.

It seeks to create an individual, personalized experience for students in a collective environment, while also supporting staff to innovate purposefully to meet the changing demands of tertiary education and of healthcare settings. The curriculum framework reflects the underpinning principles and approaches highlighted in the university strategy, *Taumata Teitei,* including the role of indigenous knowledge; Te Tiriti o Waitangi principles and accountabilities; Māori pedagogies; research-led and research-informed teaching; sustainability; transdisciplinarity, innovation, and entrepreneurship; and work- and community-integrated learning and practices. It also reflects academic, cultural, social, and emotional strengths and needs within the curriculum; fundamentally, it is built on the foundation of relational learning.

Relational learning (and teaching) refers to practices that invite both learners and educators to enter a dialogue about learning. Key aspects include relationships, interactivity, interactions, connections, communication, and learners' interests. Relational learning recognizes the differences—across culture, gender, physicality, and neurodiversity—as strengths in understanding knowledge from diverse, situated perspectives.

Importantly, relational learning demands an education model that goes beyond the transmission of information, requiring learners to take an active role in the learning process, and encompasses a range of different practices. There is no necessary binary between online and in-person learning in terms of delivering relational learning.

Relational learning is also aligned with *technology-enhanced learning* (TEL), used to describe the application of technology to teaching and learning activities, signaling the value that technology adds to learning in both practice settings and the formal learning environment. TEL is an umbrella term covering all types of teaching and learning delivery, including blended, flexible, multimodal, online, and face-to-face learning. It can foster rich online and in-person experiences, opening new avenues for learning, and helps educate nurses and professionals for the present while empowering them for lifelong learning.

Like many institutions of higher education, the University of Auckland has an aspiration for learners to make the world better tomorrow than it is today. To this end, the university's graduate profile articulates students' educational journey toward this goal through several themes. One theme, *Waipapa ki Uta: The Landing Place,* is highly relevant to sustainability ambitions, speaking as it does to connecting to place for sustainable and enduring partnerships and fostering a range of related capabilities.

With a curriculum that is underpinned by principles of cultural identity, social justice, ecological awareness, and civic duty and which demonstrates sustainable practices and positive outcomes for our communities, we foster graduates who are interculturally aware and connected to their local and global communities. This has essential benefits for our health professionals and for nurses, who practice culturally competent care in one of the most diverse cities in the world.

Many hospital settings and public health environs now have carbon zero and sustainability strategies, some focused on energy and many focused on food waste, reducing admissions, pushing back to community care, and telehealth, with TEL being critical to nursing education and also to preparing nurses for new ways of working as they will develop the skills of helping patients to access increasingly digital healthcare services.

REFLECTIVE QUESTIONS

1. In what ways has the pandemic highlighted the necessity for transformative and relational learning in academic and practice settings?

2. Why are ontological competencies (Caritas literacies) vital to the future of nursing and other healthcare professions?

3. What new insights have emerged through nurses' relationships with patients and colleagues during the pandemic, and how can these insights inform future approaches to nursing practice and education?

4. How can nurses use the principles of Caring Science to shape their personal/ professional development and growth in response to the pandemic, and in doing so, enhance their sense of self-awareness and strengthen relationships with others?

5. What are examples of moral courage you have demonstrated or have observed in advocating for patients and their families during the pandemic, particularly in situations where patients' rights and dignity were at risk?

6. How can nurses foster a culture of moral courage and ethical decision-making within their healthcare teams, and what strategies can they use to encourage others to speak up and take action in the face of ethical challenges?

FOR INDIVIDUAL REFLECTION AND/OR GROUP DISCUSSION

1. In what ways can the principles of Unitary Caring Science, such as presence, intentionality, and mutual respect, be applied to relational learning in education to foster more holistic and authentic learning experiences for students?

2. How does relational learning inform and guide individual and organizational responses to urgent and complex issues such as food waste, reducing admissions, expanding community care, telehealth, and technology-enhanced learning?

3. How can relational learning be used in academic and practice settings to reach and reconcile with marginalized and vulnerable groups and improve access to digital healthcare and improve culturally appropriate care?

4. How can culturally diverse and indigenous knowledge systems inform and help to solve the world's greatest sustainability challenges?

5. How does relational learning in education share similarities with the principles of Unitary Caring Science in healthcare, such as the importance of connection, relationship-building, and compassion in promoting learning and healing?

REFERENCES

Abdollah, R., Iranpour, S., & Ajri-Khameslou, M. (2021). Relationship between resilience and professional moral courage among nurses. *Journal of Medical Ethics and History of Medicine, 14,* 3. https://doi.org/10.18502/jmehm.v14i3.5436

Briant, S., & Freshwater, D. (1998). Exploring mutuality within the nurse–patient relationship. *British Journal of Nursing, 7*(4), 204–211. https://doi.org/10.12968/bjon.1998.7.4.204

Brindley, J. (2020). Reflecting on nursing practice during the COVID-19 pandemic. *Nursing Standard.* https://doi.org/10.7748/ns.2020.e11569

Damsgaard, J. B., & Phoenix, A. (2022). World of change: Reflections within an educational and health care perspective in a time with COVID-19. *The International Journal of Social Psychiatry, 68*(1), 177–182. https://doi.org/10.1177/0020764020979025

Freire, P. (2000). *Pedagogy of the oppressed.* The Continuum Publishing Company.

Freshwater, D. (2023). Anxiety and moral courage: The path to authentic nursing? *Handbook of Philosophy in Nursing.* Routledge.

Freshwater, D., & Cahill, J. L. (2020). Care and compromise: Developing a conceptual framework for work-related stress. *Journal of Research in Nursing, 15*(2), 173–183. https://doi.org/10.1177/1744987109357820

Gadamer, H. G. (1960). *Truth and method.* Continuum.

Gdanetz, L. (2019). *Transpersonal caring relationships as a part of an online nursing education environment.* [Doctoral Dissertation, University of Colorado].

Horkheimer, M. (2007). *Dialectic of enlightenment.* Stanford University Press.

Horton-Deutsch, S. (2018). The ever-evolving, introspective, and morally active life of the Caritas coach. In S. Horton-Deutsch & J. Anderson (Eds.), *Caritas coaching: A journal toward transpersonal caring and informed moral action in healthcare.* Sigma Theta Tau International.

International Council of Nurses. (2021). *The ICN code of ethics for nurses.* https://www.icn.ch/system/files/2021-10/ICN_Code-of-Ethics_EN_Web_0.pdf

International Council of Nurses. (2022). *Sustain and retain in 2022 and beyond.* https://www.icn.ch/system/files/2022-01/Sustain%20and%20Retain%20in%202022%20and%20Beyond-%20The%20global%20nursing%20workforce%20and%20the%20COVID-19%20pandemic.pdf

Khodaveisi, M., Oshvandi, K., Bashirian, S., Khazaei, S., Gillespie, M., Masoumi, S. Z., & Mohammadi, F. (2021). Moral courage, moral sensitivity and safe nursing care in nurses caring of patients with COVID-19. *Nursing Open, 8*(6), 3538–3546. https://doi.org/10.1002/nop2.903

Khoshmehr, Z., Barkhordari-Sharifabad, M., Nasiriani, K., & Fallahzadeh, H. (2020). Moral courage and psychological empowerment among nurses. *BMC Nursing, 19,* 43. https://doi.org/10.1186/s12912-020-00435-9

Kim, E. Y., & Chang, S. O. (2022). Exploring nurse perceptions and experiences of resilience: A meta-synthesis study. *BMC Nursing, 21,* 26. https://doi.org/10.1186/s12912-021-00803-z

Kleemola, E., Leino-Kilpi, H., & Numminen, O. (2020). Care situations demanding moral courage: Content analysis of nurses' experiences. *Nursing Ethics, 27*(3), 714–725. https://doi.org/10.1177/0969733019897780

Lee, S. (2017). Advancing caring literacy in practice, education, and health systems. In S. Lee, P. Palmeire, & J. Watson (Eds.), *Global advances in human caring literacy.* Springer.

Menzies, I. E. P. (1960). A case-study in the functioning of social systems as a defense against anxiety: A report on a study of the nursing service of a general hospital. *Human Relations, 13*(2), 95–121. https://doi.org/10.1177/001872676001300201

Mezirow, J., & Taylor, E. (2009). *Transformative learning in practice: Insights from community, workplace, and higher education.* Jossey-Bass.

Moloney, W., Fieldes, J., & Jacobs, S. (2020). An integrative review of how healthcare organizations can support hospital nurses to thrive at work. *International Journal of Environmental Research and Public Health, 17*(23), 8757. https://doi.org/10.3390/ijerph17238757

Neuwirth, L. S., Jović, S., & Mukerji, B. R. (2021) Reimagining higher education during and post COVID-19: Challenges and opportunities. *Journal of Adult and Continuing Education, 27*(2), 141–156. https://doi.org/10.1177/1477971420947738

Norouzi, M., Vajargah, P. G., Falakdami, A., Mollaei, A., Takasi, P., Ghazanfari, M. J., Miri, S., Javadi-Pashaki, N., Osuji, J., Soltani, Y., Aghaei, I., Moosazadeh, M., Zeydi, A. E., & Karkhah, S. (2022). A systematic review of death anxiety and related factors among nurses. *Omega.* Advance online publication. https://doi.org/10.1177/00302228221095710

Nussbaum, M. (1998). *Cultivating humanity. A classical defense of reform in liberal education.* Harvard University Press.

Van Schalkwyk, S. C., Hafler, J., Brewer, T. F., Maley, M. A., Margolis, C., McNamee, L., Meyer, I., Peluso, M. J., Schmutz, A. M. S., Spak, J. M., Davies, D., & Bellagio Global Health Education Initiative (2019). Transformative learning as pedagogy for the health professions: A scoping review. *Medical Education, 53*(6), 547–558. https://doi.org/10.1111/medu.13804

Wallace, C., Vidgen, R., Kirshner, S., Caetano, T., Sepasspour, R., & Weatherall, K. (2022). *Checkmate humanity: The how and why of responsible AI.* Global Stories.

Watson, J. (2008). *Nursing: The philosophy and science of caring.* University Press of Colorado.

Watson, J. (2017). Global advances in human caring literacy. In S. Lee, P. Palmieri, & J. Watson (Eds.), *Global advances in human caring literacy.* Springer.

Watson, J. (2018). *Unitary Caring Science: The philosophy and praxis of nursing.* University Press of Colorado.

Wei, H., Hardin, S. & Watson, (2021). A Unitary Caring Science resilience-building model: Unifying the human caring theory and research–informed psychology and neuroscience evidence. *International Journal of Nursing Science, 8*(1), 130–135. https://doi.org/10.1016/j.ijnss.2020.11.003

Wittenberg, E., Goldsmith, J. V., Chen, C., Prince-Paul, M., & Capper, B. (2021). COVID-19-transformed nursing education and communication competency: Testing COMFORT educational resources. *Nurse Education Today, 107.* https://doi.org/10.1016/j.nedt.2021.105105

World Health Organization. (2020, April 6). *State of the world's nursing 2020: Investing in education, jobs and leadership.* https://who.int/publications/i/item/9789240003279

Yu F., Raphael D, Mackay L, Smith M, King A. (2019). Personal and work-related factors associated with nurse resilience: A systematic review. *International Journal of Nursing Studies, 93,* 129–140. https://doi.org/10.1016/j.ijnurstu.2019.02.014

Zaghini, F., Biagioli, V., Proietti, M., Badolamenti, S., Fiorini, J., & Sili, A. (2020). The role of occupational stress in the association between emotional labor and burnout in nurses: A cross-sectional study. *Applied Nursing Research, 54.* https://doi.org/10.1016/j.apnr.2020.151277

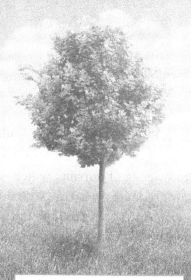

CHAPTER 2

REIMAGINING REFLECTION TO DEVELOP AND SUSTAIN PERSONAL AND PROFESSIONAL PRACTICE

–*Gwen Sherwood, PhD, RN, FAAN, ANEF*
Sara Horton-Deutsch, PhD, RN, FAAN, ANEF, SGAHN

LEARNING OBJECTIVES/SUBJECTIVES

- Examine models of reflective practice to develop and sustain personal and professional practice.

- Reimagine reflective practices for bridging real-world experiences with theory-guided learning to engage learners in practice development.

- Explore emancipatory learning by guiding nurses in connecting personal experiences with authentic being as a nurse.

- Develop tools and strategies to instill habits of reflective practice.

OVERVIEW

New graduate nurses often struggle as they transition from academic learning to new roles in clinical settings. A 2020 survey revealed that only 20% of new nurses reported they felt very strongly about their general knowledge of nursing, which is the same level of confidence for starting practice reported by new graduates in 2012 (Wolters-Kluwer, 2020). Nurses in practice echo this finding, with 66% stating that today's nurse graduates lack the same preparedness as those graduating five to 10 years ago. The recent COVID-19 pandemic exacerbated the problem, as new graduates report the lack of onsite clinical learning stymied their practice readiness (McMillan et al., 2023). Practice mirrors education: What happens in one impacts the other. *Educating Nurses: A Call for Radical Transformation* (Benner et al., 2010) revealed the urgency for transforming nursing education if we are to better prepare nurses to be fit for 21st-century healthcare. Yet, more than a decade later, education outcomes for practice-ready graduates are not dramatically changed.

There is urgency in redesigning nursing education with new paradigms for reframing the academic-practice connection. Nurse educators have reconceptualized academic curricula centered on competency-based education across all levels of education becoming more commensurate with competency assessments in practice settings (American Association of Colleges of Nursing [AACN], 2021; National League for Nursing, 2019). Redesigning pedagogical approaches and rethinking clinical learning experiences can guide nurses in their development to consider what they know, make interpretations, and determine thoughtful action; engagement and reflexivity bring the presence of mind to recognize potential gaps in care and thereby improve outcomes.

How do nurse educators and mentors help learners and new graduates transition and adapt so they are more equipped to apply what they learned in their formal academic work in the real world of nursing practice? Reflective practice can be an effective learning strategy to help bridge the chasm that sits between theory and nursing as a practice-based discipline through emancipatory learning focusing on inquiry. Tanner (2006) developed a multistep model of clinical judgment—including reflection-on-action and reflection-in-action—which helps learners process information to make decisions about their work and develop clinical reasoning to "think like a nurse." It is nurses' critical thinking and analyses that provide the foundation for a practice-based discipline ready to address 21st-century health problems (Benner et al., 2010) and is reinforced as a competency statement in the Knowledge domain in the 2021 AACN Essentials (AACN, 2021).

This chapter explores a new vision for nursing education to develop transformative learners who cultivate self-awareness and apply a critical reasoning process that both questions actions and reassesses what is known. In this exploration, we aim to examine how reflective practices can encourage learners to engage in both formal and self-directed learning activities. This chapter illustrates how reflection can facilitate transformative learning and provide guidance to foster a supportive and nurturing environment for reflective practice. In this environment, critical thinking and authentic dialogue are promoted to encourage the exchange of ideas. Tools and micropractices for instilling habits of reflective practice are examined in the context of emancipatory learning to guide nurses in connecting personal experiences with authentic being as a nurse.

THEORETICAL FRAMEWORKS AND SUPPORTING EVIDENCE

Theory informs education and practice. We present theoretical perspectives that inspire experiential interactive pedagogies so that clinical application becomes the focus of nursing education. We examine transformative and emancipatory learning theories, changing paradigms in nursing education, models of reflective practice, and how each intersects with Unitary Caring Science.

TRANSFORMATIVE LEARNING THEORY

Transformative learning is a learner-centered process that involves critical reflection and discourse to question assumptions and expectations. It stimulates nurses to think independently and creatively. Transformative learning can lead to deep structural changes in the basic aspects of thinking, feeling, and behavior of nurses and enhance their professional competence and ethical sensitivity (Tsimane & Downing, 2020). Transformational learning often results in a more holistic and integrative view of the world, where individuals can see the interconnectedness of various social, economic, and political issues. It can also lead to greater agency and empowerment, as individuals become more aware of their own values, assumptions, and biases and are better able to advocate for themselves and others (Van Schalkwyk et al., 2019).

Transformational education engages learners in the deeper meaning and application of what they are learning to meld theory and content with real-world clinical application to challenge learners to think like a nurse. Interactive learning can help learners develop critical reasoning and judgment skills that allow them to understand the underlying causes of different diseases and to make informed decisions about how to treat the signs and symptoms associated with those diseases based on available evidence. Questions framed to integrate the classroom with a clinical application for co-creating learning reinforce that taxonomies require more than memorization; they are real with someone's life depending on the ability to sift through this array of knowledge to inform patient intervention (Day & Sherwood, 2022).

Transformational learning is a necessary aspect of practice development. Developing practice derives from critical reflection on the assumptions that often lie under the surface yet guide decisions and actions (Sherwood & Horton-Deutsch, 2015). Transformation is a process of both personal and professional growth; it is said that who we are is who we bring to practice. Development inherently moves beyond the acquisition of new knowledge and skills to our capacity to question the assumptions, values, and perspectives influencing the decisions we make in practice and our choices in how we treat others.

Transformative education undergirds emancipatory learning. *Emancipatory education* integrates interactive pedagogies encouraging learners to increase their self-awareness. Emancipatory learners question what they do, the ways they act, and the assumptions guiding their thinking to stimulate what they accept as the reality for proposing changes to the status quo.

Freire (2000) first described emancipatory education as more than simply transferring knowledge but bringing a questioning attitude toward the dominant ways of doing something while exploring whether better alternatives may improve outcomes. To raise consciousness of the real world, emancipatory education guides learners in co-producing knowledge together with educators, co-workers, and patients while also developing respect of those who have values differing from theirs (Winarti, 2018). Emancipatory learning is generated from lived experiences, much as Dewey has said learning comes from reflecting on the experience, not the experience itself. In emancipatory education, the educator does not hold dominant power but co-creates learning together with engaged learners in the critical examination of values and relationships of influence, freeing the learners' restrictive mindsets.

TRANSFORMATIVE LEARNING

Transformative learners apply critical reasoning by constantly asking questions to reassess what is known—in concert with a well-developed emotional intelligence—to improve their work.

Transformation is the conversion that comes from a change in behavior, attitudes, and skills for improved performance.

Similarly, but more specifically, emancipatory learning aims to empower learners to become advocates for social justice and human rights on behalf of their patients, especially the vulnerable and marginalized (Synder, 2014). It involves students examining and questioning the systems and structures of oppression that affect their own and their patients' lives and collaborating with them to bring about change. Emancipatory learning also encourages learners to engage in critical reflection and action informed by caring and ethical practice.

EMANCIPATORY LEARNING

Emancipatory education designs learning experiences for developing learners to identify and seek to change restrictive systems around them.

Emancipatory and transformational learning can help learners develop a sense of agency, autonomy, and responsibility while building a commitment to lifelong learning and social transformation. Emancipatory learning is like transformative learning in that both aim to foster deep structural changes in the basic aspects of thinking, feeling, and behavior of learners through critical reflection and discourse. However, emancipatory learning is more explicitly oriented toward social action and change, while transformative learning may focus more on personal development and understanding (Synder, 2014).

At a point in human history when we are facing multiple crises such as the climate crisis, structural racism, and the COVID-19 pandemic, there is a need to transform taken-for-granted ways of knowing and being in the world and create a more equitable and sustainable future for all. Transformative and emancipatory learning can help to achieve this goal by fostering a sense of agency, responsibility, and civic engagement among learners, as well as by honoring their diverse cultures and experiences. Transformative and emancipatory approaches to education offer a way of teaching and learning as well as a way of living and leading future approaches to the crises we currently experience (European Society for Research on Adult Education, 2017).

MODELS OF REFLECTIVE PRACTICE

Multiple models of reflective practice apply in nursing education and are effective across a nurse's professional career regardless of setting, rank, or position. Reflective practice helps us access and build on experiential or tacit knowledge as well as other forms of knowledge development (Johns, 2022; Tanner, 2006). Historical debates about whether nursing is an art or a science are outdated in reality (Freshwater, 2008; Hills et al., 2021). The processes of reflection help practitioners move between the seeming opposites, helping articulate and make evident all ways of knowing. This in turn contributes to the full understanding of nursing.

The views of reflection and its use in personal and professional contexts have been evolving since Dewey (1933) defined it as the active, persistent, and careful consideration to determine beliefs supported by knowledge and resulting conclusions. The goal was to learn how to recognize which beliefs are based on tested evidence. Schön (1987) described a different perspective; instead of a rational view of reflection, Schön included the intuitive and open. Professional growth is initiated with a critical reflection that asks questions about how one goes about their work or

TACIT KNOWLEDGE

Knowledge that is subconsciously understood or implied and difficult to articulate objectively but may be shared through interactive conversation or narrative. It is the integration of knowledge with experience for new understanding and operation related to specific situations in practice.

relationships. Questioning opens a way of thinking that reframes situations to think about alternatives. Learners consider the tacit norms that underlie decisions, the theories that guide practice, and their feelings that lead to reframing the problem. Through reflection, they explore a detailed view of a situation, opening multiple dimensions. The process of rational thinking delays action until the situation is understood, a goal for action is determined, alternatives are considered, and a plan is developed (Cranton, 2006). However, this view of thinking did not account for the affective domain; thus, Cranton expanded the definition to include feelings and beliefs through the reflective process, transformative learning, in which the learner changes behavior, attitudes, and skills for a new way of thinking and acting.

Johns (1995, 2016, 2022) as well as Freshwater (2008) and Taylor (2000) are early pioneers in applying reflective practice within nursing. They describe reflection as a focused way of thinking about practice, whatever that practice or work is. Taylor includes any type of attentive consideration such as thinking, contemplation, or meditation that helps make sense of cognitive acts and leads to contextually appropriate changes. In this way, reflection potentiates change. Freshwater further distinguished critical reflection as thinking not just about current practice but also questioning the underlying political, ethical, historical, and cultural traditions.

Many have developed reflective practice frameworks and models to guide learners and nurses in the process of reflection to be able to consciously think deeply about their choices (Patel & Metersky, 2021). Three phases are part of most frameworks:

- **Noticing:** Aware of inner discomfort about feelings or thoughts about something of importance

- **Reflecting:** Critical analysis of the particulars of a situation, past experience, or understanding; remaining open to new information and perspectives; deep immersion in the situation

- **Action/intervening:** Developing a new perspective from a range of options, deciding whether and how to take action; perspective transformation; cognitive, affective, and behavioral changes that result in action

In working with nurses in practice, Johns (1995, 2016, 2022) applied a classic definition of reflective practice as one's ability to access, make sense of, and learn by analyzing one's work experiences to access more desirable, effective, and satisfying work experiences. Conflict or cognitive dissonance arises in practice between the ideal and the actual when people act differently from their stated beliefs, thus creating a contradiction between attitudes and actions. These contradictions create dissonance between theories of practice and actual practice such as foregoing evidence-based practice by taking shortcuts that introduce risk. Exposing contradictions in practice demands nurses confront themselves and the practice conditions that limit achieving "good" work in which one "does the right thing." The potential for "creative tension" evolving from the uncomfortable experience of contradiction can propel practice improvement as the resolution is realized (Johns, 2016).

Johns described a reflection exercise for examining contradictions (Johns, 2016):

- Identify and understand the goal of ideal practice.

- Examine the many and varied factors that are either hindering or enhancing the ability to achieve ideal practice.

- Consider alternative actions for the future.

Freshwater (2008) describes three models of reflective practice as *descriptive, dialogic,* and *critical,* which build on each other:

- **Descriptive reflection:** Practice becomes conscious. Clinicians engage in reflection-on-action. Mentors encourage nurses to develop descriptive reflection-on-action through reflective journals and to share critical incidents through narratives.

- **Dialogic reflection:** Practice becomes deliberative. Clinicians develop dialogic reflection through formal clinical supervision or through discourse with peers, coaches, supervisors, or other experts to gain feedback on how they are thinking.

- **Critical reflection:** Engage in self-questioning by applying critical reasoning to reframe how one acts, thinks, or knows and connect it to adult learning characteristics (emotional maturity, awareness, empathy, and control). Engaging in continuous improvement of practice leads to caring for the full dimension of humanness and innovations that transform practice.

The Clinical Judgment Model developed by Tanner (2006) is referred to as a reflective approach. The four stages shown in Figure 2.1 explain how learners develop the skills to construct or deconstruct an experience, by moving back and forth in a fluid and circular pattern and gaining insights through the reflective process.

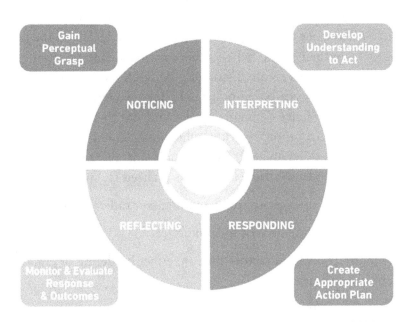

FIGURE 2.1. Clinical Judgment Model based on Tanner, 2006.

REDESIGNING NURSING EDUCATION PARADIGM FOR CONTEMPORARY HEALTHCARE

Educators are agents of change. Promoting learning and thinking to achieve both personal and professional development has long been a hallmark of nursing; these habits are developed during formative academic programs. The challenges and opportunities of preparing nurses for practice have never been greater. Advances in science and technology, patient-shared decision-making, market-driven healthcare, and the changing nature and setting of nursing practice have changed practice environments. Education and practice are like mirrors; practice changes affect nursing education and vice versa. Education paradigms to prepare nurses for 21st-century healthcare require more than simply applying learned knowledge content in practice. Nursing is a high-stakes profession that requires developing multiple types of knowledge, with the capacity to sift through the evidence and make critical decisions in complex situations. Benner et al. (2010) describe how the teacher can lead an ongoing dialogue between information and practice needs, between the particular and the general, that helps build a multiplicity of knowledge applied within one's experiences to develop a sense of *salience* (i.e., the ability to recognize what is urgent and important in particular clinical situations). We circle back to the importance of nurses knowing how to make critical judgments in the middle of practice dynamics (Tanner, 2006).

CRITICAL REASONING

Critical reasoning is a form of learning that raises consciousness and supports all healthcare professionals to more carefully examine and purposefully enact the care they provide.

CLINICAL JUDGMENT

Clinical judgment is the reasoning process under uncertainty when caring for patients combining empirical evidence, personal experience, patient perspectives, and other insights.

REFLECTIVE INQUIRY

Reflective inquiry is using the process of reflection to ask questions, challenge assumptions, and investigate one's practice.

Structured, objective-based nursing education delivered via PowerPoint slides does not assure understanding the dynamics of practice that lead to personal transformation. Changes in knowledge, skills, and attitudes—competencies—develop when learners are engaged in both informational and transformational learning experiences through which they experientially apply what they know, what they know how to do, and how they align attitudinal adjustments in making critical decisions. The level of inquiry, of engaging in the moment, of asking critical questions, creates a synergy through which nurses actively think and reason in changing situations and act to work for the good of the patient.

Practice—however it is defined—is by its very nature not linear but unfolds with multiple dimensions. Learners need guidance in knowing how to apply the knowledge, skills, and attitudes from formal, didactic learning; application provides informal learning that helps them go deeper into understanding what they know to apply in the real world. All professional situations have learning potential. "Reflection enables a continuum of learning and development in which the practitioner grows in and through their practice" (Freshwater, 2008, p. 9). Reflection is a means of formalizing informal learning and development through practice and can be a component of professional development or a learning portfolio (referred to in Chapter 9).

ENGAGING LEARNERS: CONNECTING TO AUTHENTIC SELF

Unprecedented changes in healthcare delivery have contributed to evolutionary professional practice models, and by corollary, expectations for new graduates are changing. Traditional nursing education program outcomes are often incongruent with market needs. The historical education focus on technical, instrumental knowledge is insufficient to provide safe, quality care in the dynamics of post-pandemic healthcare (Day & Sherwood, 2022). Instrumental or empirical knowledge is certainly vital to learn to predict and control the environment—to assess cause-and-effect relationships. Instrumental knowledge by itself, however, does not account for the full range of competencies and human caring literacies needed to manage the complexities of 21st-century practice and intersubjective human interactions and connections. Current practice incorporates other ways of knowing that help practitioners consider the social norms, traditions, and values underlying their work culture and influence decisions in practice (Johns, 2016).

Benner et al. (2010) reviewed the historical roots of nursing education, noting the major nursing education paradigm has changed little in the past four decades—students have didactic classes, go to clinical learning experiences in small groups with an instructor, care for one or two patients, and participate in post-clinical conferences. Content-based curricula expect recitation of disease taxonomies without deep integration into the context of real-world clinical investment in the patient's perspective. Further, nursing education that illuminates the human condition as part of the care process prepares learners for merging theory with patients' lived experience of illness, enriching both nurse and caregiver.

Educators have the dilemma of finding ways to teach an ever-increasing knowledge base balanced with helping learners know how to implement it in practice. Benner et al. (2010) describe three apprenticeships for transforming how we educate nurses:

- **Knowledge base:** What we need to know and why

- **Skilled know-how and clinical reasoning:** What we need to be able to do

- **Ethical comportment:** Values and beliefs guiding choices and actions

Integrating these three apprenticeships guides learners in developing a moral sense of what it is good to be and good to do in a situation based on evidence-based knowledge; they develop skilled know-how (*competence)* and learn how to act within an ethical framework based on values and beliefs (human caring literacy; Watson, 2017).

Experiential Learning Theory (Kolb, 1984) guides how learners develop situated cognition (knowing), skills (what to do), and ethical comportment (attitudes and values). Developing a sense of salience and clinical reasoning prepares nurses for using evidence-based knowledge while cultivating habits of thinking, deepening their clinical judgment and increasing skilled know-how. Situated learning processes engage the learner in understanding the social learning processes in a specific context while also positioning within the community of practice, as befitting workplace learning in nursing (O'Brien & Battista, 2020). Teaching is integrative, learner-centered, and focused on the patient as the main idea, the subject; experience is melded with various knowledge forms to develop an approach to practice. Educators act as coaches, leading learners in professional identity formation, igniting their imaginations, and engaging them in learning from experiences, establishing a learning continuum across their career from novice to expert.

Acquiring skills for effective practice is a foundation of professional development. Yet it is the combination with professional artistry that distinguishes professions from skills-based, technical work (Schön, 1987). The uniqueness of a practice-based discipline is the capacity to respond in-action—that is, reflecting-in-action—to deal with complex and sometimes contradictory circumstances, moving toward professional maturity and proficiency. Mezirow (1991) asserted adults learn by developing skills and acquiring new knowledge informed by critical reflection and transformative learning; adults transform perspective as they reflectively reconstruct experiences that can lead to becoming expert clinicians (Sherwood & Day, 2022).

Creating a radical new vision to transform nursing education that prepares nurses fit for practice requires developing multiple advanced competencies, clinical judgment skills, caring literacies, and ethical standards with a patient-centered focus. Transformation happens as educators instill innovative pedagogical approaches strong in situated coaching and experiential learning to develop nurses who have a deep sense of professional identity and commitment to professional values.

Over the past 40 years, educators have become increasingly committed to redesigning content-heavy curricula to address rapid and continuous change arising in society, knowledge development, technology, and healthcare delivery. Benner et al. (2010) cited paradigm shifts catalyzing radical transformation to integrate learning across settings from classroom, clinical, and simulated lab experiences. It is imperative to:

- Replace the focus on decontextualized knowledge with a focus on teaching for a sense of salience, situated cognition, and action in particular clinical situations.

- Shift from the sharp separation of didactic and clinical teaching to integrative teaching in all settings.

- Reframe the emphasis on critical thinking to emphasize clinical reasoning and multiple ways of thinking, including critical thinking.

- Move away from an emphasis on socialization and role-taking to emphasizing professional identity formation.

UNITARY CARING SCIENCE

A Unitary Caring Science perspective emphasizes human caring literacies (Hooper & Horton-Deutsch, 2023; Watson, 2018) and proposes a more recent list demanding paradigm shifts:

- Emphasize health promotion and prevention and caring for the whole person in relation to their environment.

- Shift from the separation of nursing and other disciplines to integrative collaboration and interprofessional education that values the contributions of each profession to Caring Science.

- Reframe the emphasis on evidence-based practice to emphasizing caring-based practice that incorporates multiple ways of knowing, including empirical, aesthetic, ethical, personal, and spiritual sources of knowledge.

- Facilitate the development of caring consciousness and intentionality over role-taking that transcends the ego and connects with the universal field of love and care.

DEVELOPING CARING REFLECTIVE PRACTITIONERS

Reflective practice is inquiry-based, asking questions that examine theory-practice gaps; it fosters professional development and undergirds human caring (Goulet et al., 2016). Reflective practice is used to guide knowledge development, explore social change, and make sense of emotions and contradictions in practice. Reflection represents both the constructed experience and how we deconstruct it to reconstruct it. Practitioners apply the reflective process by asking questions about what they are doing, why, and how it can be improved; therefore, they can reconsider experiences or situations from multiple points of view to realign new perspectives into future responses. Reflective practice is an important process for novice nurses as they transition from carefully constructed academic learning to the clinical dynamics that welcome them as new graduates in practice (Spector et al., 2017).

When we reflect, we can question the assumptions on which we typically base our work or interactions so that we think more deeply beyond what the eye or mind sees on the surface. Reflection is an individual process of learning that reflects individual experience and meaning, but Cranton (2006) proposes that engaging in critical reflection with others helps the learner raise questions that surface assumptions as a first step in changing perspective. Critical reflection is at the core of co-creating learning in which educators learn with their students, exhibited in ways educators design and use unfolding case studies (Day & Sherwood, 2022).

Reflection is a process of asking relevant questions that instill habits of the mind essential for learning across the professional continuum. Building an environment that nurtures ideas and encourages constant questioning to improve and grow lessens overreliance on technical rationality and forms the foundation for developing professional maturity. Freshwater (2008) described critical reflection as examining the assumptions underlying content, processes, or premises to explore the situated context for a personal response grounded in theory and experience to guide actions and decisions in practice.

Reflection helps in developing self-awareness as part of emotional intelligence (Freshwater, 2008; Horton-Deutsch & Sherwood, 2008; Sherwood & Horton-Deutsch, 2008). Reflective practice is a necessary component of how learners understand nursing and caring (Horton-Deutsch, 2016).

Table 2.1 describes reflection-before, -in, and -on action. *Reflection-before-action* is the planning process or other preparation that aligns action with goals and purpose. *Reflection-in-action* requires presence and engagement to recognize the need for a huddle or to problem-solve when things are not going according to expectations. *Reflection-on-action* takes place after an event either individually or as a group to make sense of what happened, what went well, and what can be improved (Freshwater, 2008). The process of planning, acting, and debriefing—that is, reflecting before, in, or on action—does not mean reflective practice is a linear process, nor does it mean it occurs on a continuum, but it may occur in cycles of interpretation as one analyzes what happened.

TABLE 2.1 REFLECTIVE MODEL	
TYPE OF REFLECTION	DESCRIPTION
Reflection-before-action	Thinking through a particular situation before making decisions or taking actions
Reflection-in-action	Art of thinking in the moment; thinking on one's feet
Reflection-on-action	Retrospective thinking that occurs after an event

Dewey (1933) asserts that reflection is developed through the capacity for open-mindedness, wholeheartedness, and responsibility. Jacobs (2016) describes the importance of providing structure to student reflections to be able to process practice improvements.

As such, employing a variety of reflective approaches to facilitate learning supports adult development, transformational learning, and personal and professional growth (Bulman & Schutz, 2013; Burns & Bulman, 2000).

Reflection and reflective practice are vital to keeping the values and principles of Unitary Caring Science alive. Reflective practitioners are caring-conscious, ethical, aware, authentic, vulnerable, and compassionate. Reflection is a way of caring, a way of connecting with purpose. Reflective practice allows nurses to access the full spectrum of contemplative thoughts and feelings in their daily lives and caring actions. Unitary Caring Science comes out of a paradigm that opens the possibility to reflect on the past-present and present-future with hope, to identify the healing needs of humanity, and to reaffirm the commitment to protect its dignity (Horton-Deutsch & Rosa, 2019; Watson, 2018).

ENGAGING LEARNERS IN PRACTICE DEVELOPMENT

In teaching a reflective approach to practice, nurses recognize that contradictions exist because, for whatever reason, practitioners are unable to always act congruently with their beliefs (Johns, 2022). Reflective practice enables nurses to develop an awareness of contradictions in practice and thereby acknowledge the incongruities and develop skills to realign practice with their values. Nurses often become aware of contradictions between what they are taught and the realities of practice; thus, a creative tension builds between academic and workplace learning. Educators can use this tension for reflections on why nurses act the way they do and how they choose evidence-based practices versus shortcuts that compromise patient care. Being able to articulate these tensions in critical discourse with others can help novice nurses learn how to speak up to follow best practices, share new knowledge, and act in congruence with their values—lessons that can guide their professional continuum.

CREATIVE TENSION

Creative tension is experiencing uncertainty or conflict that leads to improved outcomes or ideas.

Expert nurses are able to act in a situated context; that is, they can understand the multiplicity of factors defining a situation, recall previous experiences, apply their background of knowledge, and choose a plan of action. *Tacit knowledge* is embedded knowledge developed in practice experiences that is highly pragmatic and situation-specific. Tacit knowledge is difficult to articulate as it lies in the subconscious. Benner (1984) identified access to tacit knowledge as a hallmark of expert clinicians; it develops over time through reflective learning on experience. As novices, early learners are less confident of their embedded knowledge and need guidance in recognizing the different ways of knowing to demonstrate that expertise is more than extensive content knowledge (Johns, 2016).

Clarifying the purpose of reflection creates a more deliberative learning experience. Reflective models foster dialogue between knowing and doing. Reflecting on beliefs, values, and norms leads to more conscious, deliberative, and intentional interventions (Scheel et al., 2021). Reflective questioning of the validity of previous learning can lead to regeneration of knowledge and melding experience with knowledge and can help avoid complacency and reliance on routine in everyday practice.

Guiding learners in deliberate reflective processes rather than random reflection processes provide more purposeful learning. Guided reflection is a distinct process for reliving experiences. Using a specific model to describe, deconstruct, and employ reflective practice in nursing education may lessen mindless circling on the learner's part; learners can get to the point more clearly to make an application (Armstrong et al., 2022). If a learner is spinning in the process—they circle around the subject without making any conclusions—educators can pose a potent question to move the learner along (Sherwood & Day, 2022). Constructive feedback combined with encouragement helps learners explore their own reflections in more depth (Yeh et al., 2019), staying with a question to its resolution.

Guided by beliefs, values, and norms to more conscious, deliberate, and intentional practice, educators and learners are ethically challenged to address new questions:

- How do we integrate facts with meanings?

- How do we demonstrate that the personal and professional are integral to one another?

- How do we create, develop, and engage in reflective, caring practice?

THE INTERSECTION OF REFLECTIVE PRACTICE, TRANSFORMATIVE LEARNING, AND UNITARY CARING SCIENCE

To illustrate the paradigm shifts, Day and Sherwood (2022) describe interactive classrooms as patient-centered, in which learning is situated in clinical contexts. Learners engage and interact, going beyond content acquisition, applying unfolding case studies to experience a real-world scenario. In dialogue with educator coaches, learners reveal how they are thinking and how they are processing knowledge to apply it to practice. Educator coaches provide feedback to guide their questioning and thinking through the case study, facilitating practice development whether in a clinical setting, high-fidelity simulated learning, or a didactic environment. Case studies provide an opportunity for contextualized learning that can spark clinical imagination to continually seek new approaches and integrate new evidence. This deliberate, ongoing interaction with the educator coach helps learners translate knowledge to clinical care and more adequately prepares learners fit for practice (Yeh et al., 2019).

Critical reflection is key to transformative learning that can lead to changes in practice. Not all reflection leads to transformation; we can question things without changing anything. Transformative reflection is a change process; transformation involves or leads to a change in perspective or way of doing or acting. It is a way of solving problems that arise in practice. Mezirow (1991) distinguished content, process, and premise reflection as three ways reflection leads to transformative learning:

- **Content reflection:** Focuses on the description of the problem or situation of interest

- **Process reflection:** Focuses on thinking about the strategies used to solve the problem rather than the content of the problem only

- **Premise reflection:** Leads to questioning assumptions, values, and beliefs underlying the situation

EDUCATORS AS CHANGE AGENTS

Educators are change agents propelling learners forward and not keepers of the status quo. Educators foster the growth and development of learners by serving as role models and mentors for practice through their own spirit of inquiry (Graham & Johns, 2019). Educators with a vision for continuous learning share a mutual commitment with the learner to constantly ask reflective questions that help integrate knowledge and experience, which develops a sense of salience as learners learn to make choices (Benner et al., 2010). Reflective practice helps create a world that more faithfully reflects our personal and professional values and beliefs, so the ideal and real-world practice are congruent (Taylor et al., 2008).

In this discussion, we are moving back and forth between the role of the educator and the learner; both are significant in reflection for transformative learning. Day and Sherwood (2022) explore the vital role of the nurse educator in situated coaching. Reflection is an individual activity—and we need to respect the privacy of learners' thoughts—but it is through dialogue, written or verbal, that learners develop the skill to critically appraise their own work and receive feedback from another in a way that is informative for professional development. The dialogue with the educator or coach can illuminate facets of the situation and bring them to the surface to build onto the evidence base guiding practice.

Then, reflective practice becomes a companion as well as a precursor to improving practice by helping to assess whether practice behavior is congruent with best practices or espoused values and beliefs. Benner (1984) and Benner and Wrubel (1989) demonstrate that reflection is a vital process in building competence along the novice-to-expert trajectory. Through reflection, nurses develop autonomy through self-monitoring and accountability toward professional maturity. Reflective learning as part of a professional development portfolio or course assignment can be part of assessment and evaluation by using rubrics or other dialogue in giving feedback, as discussed further in Chapter 9.

When educators consciously create the context, organization, and culture of a transformative, emancipatory learning environment, they position themselves for dialogue with learners to better understand the context, organization, and culture of the practice setting, thus erasing the silos separating academic and workplace learning. By including reflective processes in nurses' foundational education programs, educators facilitate the growth of reflective learners at all levels, reinforcing this habit of the mind across the professional continuum.

Educator development for their own self-awareness and the skills to shift to a mode of facilitator and coach is a current challenge that calls for the transformation of nurse educator preparation. Shifting to a facilitator model means redesigning the classroom from standard desks and fixed auditoriums to flexible seating to encourage teamwork and small group discussion and intellectual debate. Careful classroom design to replace the teacher as "sage on the stage" fosters a spirit of inquiry, shaping a lifelong, co-created learning philosophy that comes from habits of critical reflection. Educators become true change agents as learners transform their thinking as they grow toward professional maturity. Learners grow into influencers for change beyond their individual growth to improve the organization and community culture in which they live and work (Cranton, 2006).

Reflective practice is about tapping into things deeply human: our own as well as others' experience, knowledge, understanding, and wisdom. Transformative learning emphasizes the process of change in understanding ourselves as well as the revision of beliefs and behaviors. It also emphasizes that the words we use and how we use them carry much power to influence others. Similarly, Watson's *Nursing: Philosophy and Science of Caring* (2008) emphasizes self-knowledge, self-discovery, and shared human experiences. Combined with the study of human emotions and relations that reflect our shared humanity, these concepts provide a foundation for and guidance on how nurses and other healthcare professionals can more deeply reflect on their own practice, including their language (Watson, 2017), and how they use it to connect with self and others. Ultimately, reflective practice and Caring Science serve as a guide for transforming one's way of thinking, acting, and leading in a way that nurtures and sustains professional practice.

Reflective practice integrates art and science, revealing what is beyond the visible world, to "see" that which connects to the human spirit and bears witness to the joy, pain, suffering, love, and struggle defining the human experience. Caring Science focuses on educating learners for a values-based practice that is morally guided to create reflective practitioners. Transformative teaching and learning integrate a moral and scientific model for considering caring as an ethic, ontological, epistemic, and praxis endeavor (Watson, 2008). Transpersonal caring relationships are the foundation of Unitary Caring Science. Cultivating conscious caring intentions about others recognizes and focuses on the uniqueness of the self and other. This form of coming together supports the emergence of new possibilities for healing, wholeness, and health.

THE CARITAS PROCESSES

Transpersonal caring is cultivated through Caring Science or Caritas literacy and results in authentic caring moments with another. *Caritas* means to cherish, appreciate, and give special loving attention through compassion and generosity of spirit. Caritas is related to critical reflection on what it means to be human, deepening our understanding of culture, ethics, and human social views (Horton-Deutsch, 2016; Watson, 2016). Caritas literacy emphasizes an understanding of being and becoming. It involves being morally informed with the capacity— beyond task-conscious learning—toward an evolved, heart-centered consciousness of learning that recognizes the connection of all human beings to affirm and sustain humanity.

Watson (2008) has developed and refined 10 Caritas Processes to guide nurses and other healthcare professionals to cultivate transpersonal caring and reflection that support an in-depth exploration of humanity and what it means to be human. Applying the 10 Caritas Processes nurtures self-knowledge, self-discovery, and shared human experiences that are life-giving and receiving. These processes serve to model the way for others, support authentic dialogue, and affirm and confirm others by holding them in high ethical regard.

The 10 Caritas Processes form deep transpersonal caring, focusing on how to "Be" while "Doing" the work of nursing. Chapter 1 outlines all 10 processes. Micropractices detailing reflective practices based on the Caritas Processes are interspersed throughout the book.

APPLICATION FOR PERSONAL AND PROFESSIONAL DEVELOPMENT

We interpret the world around us based on deeply embedded assumptions. Assumptions are largely what we take for granted and (without critical reflection) likely would not be challenged. By drawing attention to how we base decisions and actions on assumptions, educators can coach learners to first pause to see more deeply to articulate the assumptions guiding their developing practice and explore their validity in written or oral dialogues with the educator, a preceptor, a coach, or a professional peer and to explore the utility of alternatives. A variety of learning strategies employed in classroom, clinical, or simulation provide opportunities for learners to engage in presentations, discussions, readings, brainstorming, debates, role-play, simulations, scenarios, unfolding case studies, narratives, storytelling, or aesthetic imaginations. A white paper, *The Scholarship of Reflective Practice,* developed by the Sigma Theta Tau International Task Force on Reflective Practice, explores these strategies in more depth and is posted at http://www.nursingsociety.org/docs/default-source/position-papers/resource_reflective.pdf?sfvrsn=4 (Freshwater et al., 2005).

Recognizing alternative perspectives through reflective analysis, learners can visualize and reconstruct their responses to how to act in a situation. Educators act as facilitators in both helping learners question assumptions and in coaching them toward alternative approaches. This duality of learning in the reflective dialogue between learners and educators requires educators to themselves adopt a reflective, mindful stance that lets go of the power dynamic common in higher education between learner and teacher.

Self-directed learning is the foundation for transformative learning. Mezirow (1991) developed the theory of transformative learning that permeates adult education—a reflective process in which the nurse or learner recognizes a disorienting dilemma and applies critical reflection to reach a changed meaning perspective. This form of learning builds the foundation for adult development to advance growth and development, moving from one stage to the other. Real change and growth in our practice results from ongoing processes of examining and questioning our assumptions, values, and perspectives. Critical reflection, whether written or verbal, is the central process toward transformative learning.

For reflective practice to become a deliberate conscious process, educators need to provide content and background about reflective practice, so learners develop schemata and language for deliberate reflective learning (Yeh et al., 2019). Reflective practice used systematically to "make sense of experience" can be the avenue to promote human connections, practice improvements, and work satisfaction. Educators can guide reflective learning by providing reflective prompts to learners to stimulate provocative exploration to heighten awareness and insights that can, in turn, lead to behavioral changes. Reflective practice becomes a transformative change process for improving practice, refocusing work, and fostering meaning and satisfaction from work well done—essential for nurse well-being and retention.

REFLECTIVE SUMMARY

Reflective practice pedagogy, whether in academic or clinical settings, provides important opportunities for nurses to explore their professional and individual commitment to quality and safety in their emerging practice. Written reflective dialogue with teachers, mentors, or other nurses provides systematic learning; this reflection-on-action is a process of sense-making of experience, thus building tacit knowledge to move toward professional maturity. Insights into improved systems begin in a nurse's own practice; improved systems are often the result of collaboration among professionals who are first committed to improving their own practice.

Learners need flexible and dynamic frameworks to guide their development as they move from content to application (practice). Therefore, applying what one knows in making clinical decisions does not necessarily unfold in a linear pattern: most likely, it occurs in back-and-forth deepening reflection as learners continually develop knowledge in situations. Deep learning can only be made known as it comes to the surface. Deep learning is more than content acquisition; classroom and clinical learning based on Kolb's (1984) Experiential Learning Theory positions learners to be able to apply content in an inquisitive way to learn how to make clinical choices and thus gain a sense of salience. Reflection enables that process through the ability to construct, deconstruct, and reconstruct an experience.

Reflection is sometimes referred to as critical thinking with the addition of the multiple ways of knowing that account for the affective domain. Reflection is a systematic way of thinking about our actions and responses that contributes to a transformed perspective, or the reframing of a given situation or problem, and it determines future actions and responses. It is learning from experience by considering what we know, believe, and value within the context of a particular situation in our work. Reflection contributes to working according to our sense of mission and purpose and as such helps develop spiritual resources for managing life. Reflection helps us make sense of events, develop leadership capacity, improve responses through emotional intelligence, develop mindfulness to engage in work activities, and thus improve quality and safety for patients. Caring Science deepens reflective practice by connecting reflection with caring and love as the basis for practice in a way that supports healing, health, and wholeness of self and other.

LEARNING NARRATIVE

Mrs. Garcia is a 45-year-old undocumented immigrant from Nicaragua who has been diagnosed with type 2 diabetes. She has been admitted to the hospital for complications related to her diabetes, including hyperglycemia and dehydration. Her nurse, Adrianne, is responsible for Mrs. Garcia's care. Adrianne recognizes that caring for Mrs. Garcia requires a culturally sensitive approach, appreciating she may have unique cultural beliefs and practices related to health and illness. In addition, as an immigrant herself, Adrianne is aware that her pain and guilt surface when Mrs. Garcia talks about missing her family whom she cannot visit due to being undocumented. She reaches out to you, the nurse educator, to guide her in processing her emotions and in how to use the Caritas Processes to guide her in caring for Mrs. Garcia.

1. What are you most concerned about in caring for Mrs. Garcia?

2. What emotional support would be most helpful to Mrs. Garcia?

3. Choose two Caritas Processes to apply to Adrianne's care of Mrs. Garcia. Explain their value to Adrianne in providing care based on cultural sensitivity, competence, and caring literacy.

4. Considering the overall learning experience, how would the Caritas Processes be part of Adrianne's reflection on the learning experience?

REFLECTIVE QUESTIONS

1. Evidence indicates many of us teach the way we were taught, which may mean we are preparing graduates for a healthcare system that no longer exists. How do the supporting theories in this chapter inform the discussion?

2. What are pedagogical strategies that engage learners and spark their imaginations in preparing for working in ever-changing clinical situations?

3. What are effective strategies as new graduates transition to the workplace?

4. What are ways to provide a welcoming, inclusive environment?

5. Describe how reflective practice enables one to examine an experience by first constructing, deconstructing, and reconstructing.

6. What is unique about the duality of academic and workplace learning that forms the core of nursing education within a practice-based discipline?

7. What is meant by saying education and practice are mirrors of each other?

REFERENCES

American Association of Colleges of Nursing. (2021). *The essentials: Core competencies for professional nursing education.* https://www.aacnnursing.org/Portals/42/AcademicNursing/pdf/Essentials-2021.pdf

Armstrong, G., Sherwood, G., Ironside, P., Cerbie Brown, E., & Wonder (2022). Reflective practice: Using narrative pedagogy to foster quality and safety. In G. Sherwood & J. Barnsteiner (Eds.), *Quality and safety in nursing: A competency approach to improving outcomes* (3rd ed., pp. 301–320). Wiley-Blackwell

Benner, P. (1984). *From novice to expert: Power and excellence in nursing practice.* Addison-Wesley Publishing Company.

Benner, P., Sutphen, M., Leonard, V., & Day, L. (2010). *Educating nurses: A call for radical transformation.* Jossey-Bass.

Benner, P., & Wrubel, J. (1989). *The primacy of caring: Stress and coping in health and illness.* Prentice-Hall.

Bulman, C., & Schutz, S. (2013). *Reflective practice in nursing* (3rd ed.). Blackwell Publishing.

Burns, S., & Bulman, C. (2000). *Reflective practice in nursing: The growth of the professional practitioner* (2nd ed.). Blackwell Science.

Cranton, P. (2006). *Understanding and promoting transformative learning: A guide for educators of adults.* Jossey-Bass.

Day, L., & Sherwood, G. (2022). Transforming education to transform practice: Integrating quality and safety using unfolding case studies. In G. Sherwood & J. Barnsteiner (Eds.), *Quality and safety in nursing: A competency approach to improving outcomes* (3rd ed., pp. 269–300). Wiley-Blackwell.

Dewey, J. (1933). *How we think: A restatement of the relation of reflective thinking to the educative process.* D.C. Heath.

European Society for Research on Adult Education. (2017). *Interrogating transformative processes in learning and education.* http://esrea.org/networks/transformative-and-emancipatory-adult-education/

Freire, P. (2000). *Pedagogy of the oppressed.* The Continuum Publishing Company.

Freshwater, D. (2008). Reflective practice: The state of the art. In D. Freshwater, B. Taylor, & G. Sherwood (Eds.), *International textbook of reflective practice in nursing* (pp. 1–18). Blackwell Publishing.

Freshwater, D., Horton-Deutsch, S., Sherwood, G., & Taylor, B. (2005). *The scholarship of reflective practice.* (position paper). Sigma Theta Tau International. http://www.nursingsociety.org/docs/default-source/position-papers/resource_reflective.pdf?sfvrsn=4.

Goulet, M.-H., Larue, C., & Alderson, M. (2016). Reflective practice: A comparative dimensional analysis in nursing and education studies. *Nursing Forum, 51*(2), 139–150. https://doi.org/10.1111/nuf.12129

Graham, M. M., & Johns, C. (2019). Becoming student kind: A nurse educator's reflexive narrative inquiry. *Nurse Education in Practice, 39*, 111–116. https://doi.org/10.1016/j.nepr.2019.07.007

Hills, M., Watson, J., & Cara, C. (2021). *Creating a caring science curriculum: A relational emancipatory pedagogy of nursing.* Springer Publishing.

Hooper, E., & Horton-Deutsch, S. (2023). Integrating compassion and the theoretical premises of caring science into health professions education. *Creative Nursing, 29*(1), 1–12.

Horton-Deutsch, S. (2016). Thinking, acting, and leading through caring science literacy. In S. Lee, P. Palmieri, & J. Watson (Eds.), *Global advances in human caring literacy* (pp. 59–70). Springer.

Horton-Deutsch, S., & Rosa, W. (2019). Reflective practice and caring science. In W. Rosa, S. Horton-Deutsch, & J. Watson (Eds.), *A handbook for caring science.* Springer.

Horton-Deutsch, S., & Sherwood, G. (2008). Reflection: An educational strategy to develop emotionally-competent nurse leaders. *Journal of Nursing Management, 16*(8), 946–954. https://doi.org/10.1111/j.1365-2834.2008.00957.x

Jacobs, S. (2016). Reflective learning, reflective practice. *Nursing, 46*(5), 62–64. https://doi.org/10.1097/01. NURSE.0000482278.79660.f2

Johns, C. (1995). Framing learning through reflection within Carper's fundamental ways of knowing in nursing. *Journal of Advanced Nursing, 22*(2), 226–234. https://doi.org/10.1046/j.1365-2648.1995.22020226.x

Johns, C. (2016). *Mindful leadership. A guide for the health care professions.* Palgrave Macmillan.

Johns, C. (2022). *Becoming a reflective practitioner* (3rd ed.). Wiley-Blackwell

Kolb, D. A. (1984). *Experiential learning: Experience as the source of learning and development.* Prentice-Hall.

McMillan, K., Akoo, C., & Catigbe-Cates, A. (2023). New graduate nurses navigating entry to practice in the Covid-19 pandemic. *The Canadian Journal of Nursing Research = Revue Canadienne de Recherche en Sciences Infirmieres, 55*(1), 78–90. https://doi.org/10.1177/08445621221150946

Mezirow, J. (1991). *Transformative dimensions of adult learning.* Jossey-Bass.

National League for Nursing. (2019). *Integrating competency-based education in the nursing curriculum.* National League for Nursing.

O'Brien, B. C., & Battista, A. (2020). Situated learning theory in health professions education research: A scoping review. *Advances in Health Sciences Education: Theory and Practice, 25*(2), 483–509. https://doi.org/10.1007/s10459-019-09900-w

Patel, K. M., & Metersky, K. (2021). Reflective practice in nursing: A concept analysis. *International Journal of Nursing Knowledge, 33*(3), 180–187. https://doi.org/10.1111/2047-3095.12350

Scheel, L. S., Bydam, J., & Peters, M. D. J. (2021). Reflection as a learning strategy for the training of nurses in clinical practice setting: a scoping review. *JBI Evidence Synthesis, 19*(12), 3268–3300. https://doi.org/10.11124/JBIES-21-00005

Schön, D. A. (1987). *Educating the reflective practitioner.* Jossey-Bass.

Sherwood, G., & Day, L. (2022). Quality and safety in clinical learning environments. In G. Sherwood & J. Barnsteiner (Eds.), *Quality and safety in nursing: A competency approach to improving outcomes* (3rd ed., pp. 321–348). Wiley-Blackwell.

Sherwood, G., & Horton-Deutsch, S. (2008). Reflective practice: The route to nursing leadership? In D. Freshwater, B. Taylor, & G. Sherwood (Eds.), *International textbook of reflective practice in nursing* (pp. 157–176). Blackwell Publishing.

Sherwood, G., & Horton-Deutsch, S. (Eds.). (2015). *Reflective organizations: On the frontlines of QSEN and reflective practice implementation.* Sigma Theta Tau International.

Snyder, M. (2014). Emancipatory knowing: Empowering nursing students toward reflection and action. *Journal of Nursing Education, 53*(2), 65–69. https://doi.org/10.3928/01484834-20140107-01

Spector, N., Ulrich, B., & Barnsteiner, J. (2017). Improving quality and safety with transition to practice. In G. Sherwood & J. Barnsteiner (Eds.), *Quality and safety in nursing: A competency approach to improving outcomes* (2nd ed., pp. 281–300). Wiley-Blackwell.

Tanner, C. A. (2006). Thinking like a nurse: A research-based model of clinical judgment in nursing. *Journal of Nursing Education, 45*(6), 204–211. https://doi.org/10.3928/01484834-20060601-04

Taylor, B. J. (2000). *Reflective practice: A guide for nurses and midwives.* Open University Press.

Taylor, B., Freshwater, D., Sherwood, G., & Esterhuizen, P. (2008). International perspectives in reflective practice: Global knowledge reservoirs. In D. Freshwater, B. Taylor, & G. Sherwood (Eds.), *International textbook of reflective practice in nursing* (pp. 71–96). Blackwell Publishing.

Tsimane, T., & Downing, C. (2020). A model to facilitate transformative learning in nursing education. *International Journal of Nursing Science, 7*(3), 269–276. https://doi.org/10.1016/j.ijnss.2020.04.006

Van Schalkwyk, S. C., Hafler, J., Brewer, T. F., Maley, M. A., Margolis, C., McNamee, L., Meyer, I., Peluso, M. J., Schmutz, A. M., Spak, J. M., Davies, D., & Bellagio Global Health Education Initiative. (2019). Transformative learning as pedagogy for the health professions: A scoping review. *Medical Education, 53*(6), 547–558. https://doi.org/10.1111/medu.13804

Watson, J. (2008). *Nursing: The philosophy and science of caring* (Rev. ed.). University of Colorado Press.

Watson, J. (2016). Global advances in human caring literacy. In S. Lee, P. Palmieri & J. Watson (Eds.). *Global advances in human caring literacy* (pp. 3–20). Springer Publishing Company.

Watson, J. (2018). *Unitary caring science: The philosophy and praxis of nursing.* The University of Colorado Press.

Winarti, E. (2018). Emancipatory education and the preparation of future teachers. *On the Horizon, 26*(2), pp. 113–121. https://doi.org/10.1108/OTH-08-2017-0068

Wolters-Kluwer. (2020, September 23). *How prepared are new nurse graduates for practice today? Clinical judgment skills identified as a primary gap in practice readiness according to Wolters Kluwer report.* https://www.wolterskluwer.com/en/news/how-prepared-are-new-nurse-graduates-for-practice-today

Yeh, V. J.-H., Sherwood, G., Durham, C. F., Kardong-Edgren, S., Schwartz, T. A., & Beeber, L. S. (2019). Designing and implementing asynchronous online deliberate practice to develop interprofessional communication competency. *Nursing Education in Practice, 35*, 21–26. https://doi.org/10.1016/j.nepr.2018.12.011

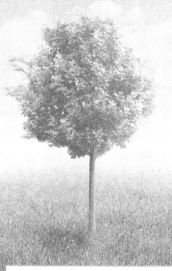

CHAPTER 3

REIMAGINING CREATIVE SPACE FOR REFLECTION IN A CARING SCIENCE PARADIGM

–Anna Biley, Dip. N, MSc, Doctorate of Caring Science, Caritas Coach

LEARNING OBJECTIVES/SUBJECTIVES

- Describe the ethics and values of Watson Caring Science.

- Examine the relationship between reflective practice and Watson Caring Science.

- Analyze what it means to hold space and be in authentic presence.

- Apply the Caritas Processes to support deep listening and nurture learning communities as a safe space for reflective practice.

"So, I continue to teach, to write about, to try to live that which I now see and yet still need to learn the most about."

–Watson, 2005, p. 73

OVERVIEW

The background and evolution of structured reflection are well documented, and its role and purpose are inextricably linked to nursing practice, education, and research (Horton-Deutsch & Rosa, 2019; Lombard & Horton-Deutsch, 2017; Schön, 1987). Johns (2022) described the theory of structured reflection as a means of "realizing one's vision of practice as a lived reality" and "a process of self-realization" (p. vii). The theory of structured reflection is by its nature complex and difficult to articulate. More than a task to be done or a skill set to be learned, reflective practice is an invitation to "bring the mind home" (Johns, 2022, p. 6) and deepen personal understanding of self.

The notion of reflective practice is not new. Humanity's existential quest to find meaning and purpose echoes ancient times (Giovannoni, 2019; Perkins, 2019). Rumbling through the texts of history, philosophy, science, art, and literature, the human instinct to reflect on what is, what was, and what is to come offers the discipline of nursing an invitation to ponder where and how the reflective practitioner may support modern healthcare practice. As a value-driven discipline with care and wholeness at its heart, nursing is concerned with the human experience (Watson, 2018). In a 21st-century world reeling from a global pandemic, climate emergency, and the chaos of war and injustice, humanity holds in its hand and heart unprecedented grief, pain, and anxiety. In a place of "dissolving certainties" (Wright, 2017, p. 18), the universal human experiences that emerge at such points, such as suffering, joy, hope, and bereavement, are the business of nursing and as such are best understood from a deeply reflective, disciplinary perspective (Biley, 2019b). In the milieu of an angst-ridden cauldron of fear and moral distress, the perpetual search for meaning, purpose, and understanding is the human story. Listening to that story, journeying alongside, and remembering who we are as a discipline is what humanity requires of the profession and, as such, is a moral imperative for nursing (Watson, 2021).

The instinct to fix, ease, bring comfort, and heal is traditionally what nurses endeavor to do. In a complex, post-pandemic, divided world, "doing to people is no longer appropriate, but participating knowingly with people in their well-becoming is" (Phillips, 2017, p. 226). However, holding space for the human values of care, healing, and compassion is becoming increasingly challenging. Stepping into the arena, Watson's Unitary Caring Science and the Theory of Human Caring invite a new paradigm for nursing (Watson, 2008, 2018).

Welcoming loving-kindness and compassion to self, Caring Science offers a heart-centered, heart-led approach to reflection. In essence, nursing practice is "a reflective journey of personal and professional growth, where learning is continual and always evolving" (Lombard & Horton-Deutsch, 2017, p. 73).

The purpose of this chapter is to utilize reflective practices in describing and applying the framework underlying Watson's Caring Science and delve into what it means to hold space and be within an authentic presence. The ethics and values of Watson Caring Science defined in the 10 Caritas Processes support deep listening and nurture learning communities as safe reflective practice spaces.

SUPPORTING THEORETICAL FRAMEWORKS AND EVIDENCE

Becoming a reflective practitioner from Watson's Unitary Caring Science point of view means deeply appreciating the uniqueness and oneness of the lived human experience in the unfolding moment. Offering an "ethical, philosophical and moral disciplinary foundation ... for value-centered 21st century nursing" (Watson, 2012, p. 18), deep reflection from a Caring Science perspective gently shifts the individual from a mode of "doing" and "fixing" to "being," "becoming," and "walking alongside." Inviting the individual to turn their attention inwards, embodying reflection through care, compassion, and loving-kindness to self transforms and transitions "process" and "practice" to a way of being. In a Caring Science paradigm, reflection is a way of being that includes presence, holding space, gentle listening, and nurturing learning communities. It is not role specific but an invitation to all— educators, students, researchers, practitioners, or leaders. In other words, it is about who you are and how you show up (Halifax, 2008). It is about being human.

Watson's Caring Science is rooted in philosophies that invite love, caring, and connection. "Becoming love is our true state of Belonging-Being-Becoming that we are all seeking to remember in our own way" (Watson, 2021, p. 123). Consistent with expanding scientific knowledge that exists beyond the limits of a linear, cause-and-effect view of the world (Phillips, 2017), Caring Science resides in a unitary paradigm whereby "human connection transcends time, space and physical presence" (Watson, 2018, p. 44). Awakening to the reality known by our ancestors (Perkins, 2019), Caring Science reminds us that we belong in a flowing, connected universe where all is living, vibrating energy, and the smallest of actions impact the whole. In the intrinsically dynamic web of life, wholeness is "not an ideal, but a given" and the experience of being human is "as an unbroken whole" (Cowling, 2012, p. 121). "In oneness of love with all," 650 years ago, the English medieval mystic anchorite

Julian of Norwich thought as she held in her hand a small hazelnut. "I looked at it with my mind's eye and thought, 'what can this be?' And the answer came to me, 'it is all that is made'" (Julian of Norwich, 1998, p. 47).

In the poem "Auguries of Innocence," William Blake saw "a world in a grain of sand and a heaven in a wildflower. Hold infinity in the palm of your hand and eternity in an hour" (Blake, 1863). Offering an invitation to reflect, reawaken, and remember the sacredness of living in the moment, where past experiences and future hopes and dreams meet, Watson Caring Science reminds us that nursing holds a gift of seeing the universality of each unique encounter, honoring and valuing the uniqueness and oneness of the unitary human being (Newman, 2008). Nurses are co-participants in an unfolding journey, being with each other with caring intentions and trust. Central to this perspective is the transpersonal human relationship, where the nurture and care of self are in a mutual, evolving pattern of connection.

ETHICS AND VALUES OF A PRACTICE-BASED DISCIPLINE

Based on a Levinasian worldview, "ethics is first philosophy" (Critchley & Bernasconi, 2002, p. 34) and "philosophy is the work of reflection that is brought to bear on unreflective, everyday life"—it is a reminder of what is already known (p. 7). From Levinas's philosophical position, in a connected universe, humanity has an innate and infinite moral responsibility and commitment to others (Critchley & Bernasconi, 2002). In the context of Caring Science, this is reflected in what Watson describes as the *Ethic of Face* and the *Ethic of Hand* (Watson, 2021). We belong in a connected universe and "literally and metaphorically, hold another person's life in our hands" (Watson, 2021, p. 89), and as we face the humanity of others, we cannot help but face our brokenness. But how, in a complex and cruel world, can nurses uphold these ethics and values and continue to show up every day with an open heart? Care, compassion, and healing; the human instinct to reach out and uphold dignity are the gifts that nursing has brought to the world. In the confusion, exhaustion, and sadness of a post-pandemic reality, that is a big ask, and it is not unreasonable to ponder how it is remotely possible to uphold this ancient covenant.

Through the leadership of Jean Watson, the Watson Caring Science Institute (WCSI), and Caring Science scholars, practitioners, educators, and researchers worldwide, an evolving circle of knowledge grounded in the values of caring and healing continues to unfold. Advancing the art and science of nursing, the notion of separation and disconnection is transcended, and wholeness and "energy spirit" (Phillips, 2017, p. 223) are coming to the fore. With a language of caring and self-care micropractices, Watson Caring Science offers a safe space for all to nurture the human instinct to reflect, find meaning, and deepen understanding of self and other.

THE CARITAS PROCESSES

For nursing to survive as a discipline, it must be grounded in philosophy and ethics with a moral base (Watson, 2018). Furthermore, it must own a language of caring proudly, thus making it visible and taking away the awkwardness and shame of admitting love. To pin down the essence of human caring and the universal values upheld by Caring Science, Watson defined the Caritas Processes as introduced in Chapter 1. Latin in origin, *caritas* means love of or charity for humankind, and processes denote that this is ongoing and unfolding. Thus, the Caritas Processes represent a flow of caring energy and are an invitation and challenge to be mindful of this love, not only in relationships with others but towards our planet and ourselves.

Expressed as self/other, like a pebble in a pond, in a unitary caring paradigm, all is a connected, rippling flow of energy. As Caritas Process 8 highlights, we are our own and each other's environment. With mindful intention and ministering actions of loving-kindness, compassion, and dignity, the invitation is to be and become an environment of caring in every unfolding moment. With a Caritas consciousness, the transpersonal caring moment may go beyond human-to-human connection to become the essence of who we are and want to be. Acting with compassion, kindness, and a mindful, intentional, caring presence, the authentic caring moment is a connection of souls, a manifestation of oneness and an appreciation of what it means to be human (Watson, 2021).

Being in caring consciousness is also a journey of becoming, and some transpersonal relationships and caring moments break through to a deeper level of consciousness and oneness with the universe. In the book *Grace and Grit*, Wilber (1993) shared the tale of Treya, his wife, and their journey with her terminal cancer. He witnessed a rebirthing of purpose and meaning through pain, frustration, and fear; deep personal transformation; and profound love, connection, and surrender. In a Unitary Caring Science paradigm, everyone is in the sacred circle of life and death (Watson, 2021). In a "unified reality" (Phillips, 2017, p. 223), there is no distinction between body and soul, living and dying, as "in reality, there is no separation, only interpretation, and unity" (Halifax, 2008, p. xviii). In an autoethnographic study of the experience of remembering purpose, the author described being alongside her husband as he lived his dying. Embodying the Caritas Processes as a framework for deep reflection, the story was analyzed and crafted to become autoethnographic data. The author wrote:

> Being genuinely present and holding caring intention in practice often meant absorbing hurt, frustration, and sadness. Frequently the self, as described in the Caritas Processes was invisible, as the world seemed to be asking more of me than I could ever give. However, amid all this, I had the profound sense of remembering my purpose and that everything I had ever done, felt, and experienced was to live those days. (Biley, 2019b, p. 633)

Caring Science does not limit knowledge development to the physical, as we know it, but creates space to embrace the unknown, to reflect and contemplate (Watson, 2021). Delving into the most intimate human experiences, the Caritas Processes offer a mode of reflective inquiry that invites curiosity, creativity, and healing. Deepening understanding of what we think we know, being in reflection, the Caritas Processes welcome the unfolding of fresh insights into "what brings us here," what it means to be human, and how we may serve (Wright, 2017). The Caritas Processes invite key questions for deep, transformative reflection. In an invitation to pause and to take a caring moment for ourselves, we may ponder, "When seeing, how do we see? When touching, how do we touch and when thinking, how do we think?" (Biley, 2010, p. 2; Biley, 2019a, p. 45). In doing so, we are reminded that "what we carry in our heart matters" (Watson, 2021, p. 135). Pausing to take a reflective moment of care for self creates an energy that ripples out to others, to all. It matters. *You matter.*

CREATING SPACE FOR CARING, REFLECTIVE PRACTICE

The values and ethics of Watson's Caring Science invite us to consider what it means to be our authentic selves and be in the right relationship, seeking "not to find definitive answers but to understand our own humanity" (Watson, 2005, p. xxxiii). As touchstones for ways of being and becoming, the Caritas Processes illuminate the true essence of nursing (Horton-Deutsch & Anderson, 2018) and offer a gentle guide to consider how we may embrace loving-kindness, inspire trust, and nurture loving, trusting, caring relationships. In a safe reflective space, we are invited to consider what it means to be authentically present and to listen deeply to our own story and that of others. How may we forgive and seek solutions when in pain and moral distress? How may we give voice to what we know and be open to the mystery of the unknown? Being in an authentic caring presence, how do we uphold human dignity in ministering the sacred act of caring? For some, these questions may stir a feeling of coming home and remembering the existential turning points that remind us who we are in our hearts and souls. They may be joyful, exciting, or challenging—yet, at the same time, all at once, push boundaries and raise uncomfortable, frustrating questions. Quoting Lourie (2020), Jean Watson reassures us to "give yourself permission to touch and honor those spaces and places we want to hide from:

- Be confused; it is where you begin to learn new things.

- Be broken; it's where you begin to heal.

- Be frustrated; it is where you start to make more authentic decisions.

- Be sad, because if we are brave enough we can hear our heart's wisdom through it.

- Be whatever you are right now." (Watson, 2021, p. 114)

With time and with the support of a nurturing, caring community of learners, creating space for reflection realigns "doing," "fixing," "task," and retrospection to "being" (Johns, 2022). Holding intentional space for reflective practice, taking small steps, and treading gently, the nurturing values of the Caritas Processes invite the shy, authentic self to come to the fore. In creating a mindful space for Caritas and reflective practice to flourish, moments of caring, vulnerability, and shared humanity may be illuminated. With loving, caring, and intentional repatterning of the energy field, balance and equanimity awaken deep listening, gentle understanding, and remembering (Watson, 2018).

BEING IN AUTHENTIC PRESENCE

Being in an authentic presence is the second of the Caritas Processes. But what does it mean to be in authentic presence? How do we show up, and how do we know? As a concept, presence is complicated and perhaps difficult to define. And yet it is foundational to personal and organizational human relationships (Phillips, 2020). Towards explaining the elusive nature of presence, Watson (2018) argues that it moves beyond the physical and psychological definitions of "being there" and "being with" (p. 91) toward caring, authentic presence:

> It is through being present and allowing constructive expression of all feelings that we create a foundation for trust and caring. When one is able to hold the tears or fears of another without being threatened or turning away, that is an act of healing and caring. (Watson, 2008, p. 102)

The invitation to create space to hold tears and fears is the sacred work of developing loving, trusting, caring relationships (Caritas Process 4). As we step into the Caritas Processes, the heart-centered universals of human caring find language and voice and carry intention and energy.

Being in an authentic presence is an act of compassion. Levine (1986, as cited by Rinpoche, 1992) explained that "when your fear touches someone's pain it becomes pity, when your love touches someone's pain it becomes compassion" (p. 200). Facing suffering and holding frail, raw humanity in our hands is a vulnerable place to be. Welcoming mindful, reflective presence is essential if the wisdom and strength to embody compassion are to manifest and the authentic self is to feel safe. Rooted in mindful intention, living Caritas honors and holds kindness and compassion for another's journey as well as our own. Remembering that "this one moment with this one person may be the reason you are here on earth at this time" (Watson, 2021, p. 69), being alongside moves us beyond empathy to equanimity and compassion, reconnecting and remembering spirit and heart.

Traditionally, nursing has been immersed in a medical model and a language of separation, duality, distance, and object (Giovannoni, 2019). Intimately linked to a language (of medicine) that is not even its own, this presents an awkward paradox. Turkel et al. (2012) point out that "language is more than the sum of its parts. Language is a way of looking at the world, an entire storehouse of knowledge, wisdom, stories and meaning" (p. 197). Watson's Caring Science offers the potential for the discipline of nursing to own its language, to give voice to caring and compassion, and in doing so, shine a light on the essence of nursing. As Frank (2013) stated, "from the popular culture that surrounds them, storytellers have learned formal structures of narrative, conventional metaphors and imagery and standards of what is and is not appropriate to tell" (p. 3). Reclaiming the nursing story, giving voice to the story of self through caring reflection, reaches out to listen, hear, and understand. Deepening the story of our shared humanity, authentic caring presence is an invitation to honor that we are part of each other's journey and in moments of caring intentionally connect to "the life history of each person" (Watson, 2008, p. 51).

Caring language or *caritas literacy* (Anderson, 2018, p. 12) is a gentle language of presence. Showing up with intention; bearing witness to another's story; belonging and connecting in a loving, trusting, caring relationship; creating and holding safe space; being alongside; and becoming the healing environment as it unfolds in the moment are all ways of being in authentic presence. As a conduit for energy, language and literacy realign us to Caritas presence. Furthermore, as a structure for reflection, the language and values of the Caritas Processes can repattern energy and offer fresh insight, understanding, and ways of being in authentic presence.

Alongside another in loving-kindness and compassion, authentic presence lets go of control and ego and invites acceptance. Open to mystery (Caritas Process 10), we no longer have to "fix" or offer rational explanations for everything. Inviting intuition and inner wisdom to come to the fore, the values of Caring Science welcome all ways of knowing (Caritas Process 6). Being in an authentic presence, you are open to and acknowledging the inner voice that says, "Something special is going on here," "There is a connection here," or maybe, "There is a block here." When we are in a safe place, ways of knowing manifest in feelings and the body:

> There's a part of me that I didn't even know I had until recently—instinct, intuition, whatever. It helps me and protects me. It's perceptive and astute. I just listen to the inside of me and I know what to do. (Belenky et al., 1997, p. 52)

In an early feminist study of women's ways of knowing, Maher and Tetreault (1996) argued that patterns of knowing coexist all at once:

> When I know something, it is just this inward sense of listening with all of me and when it comes out it does not come out in parts, it is like a big picture. This is what I think intuition is—the brain's more efficient way of being able to process all this amazing information from everywhere, from the whole universe, and bring it into this kind of full-blown moment, of like ah-ha. (p. 355)

Embracing all ways of knowing, Caring Science reminds us that we are the environment and the energy (Caritas Process 8), and we have huge potential to choose to show up with sensitivity (Caritas Process 3), loving-kindness, and compassion (Caritas Process 1).

Caring Science dwells in the human-to-human, transpersonal caring moment and uses the Caritas Processes to guide both values and actions. As touchstones for caring reflection, it is logical that the reflective practitioner may also be guided in this way. The ethic of face and hand, the moral responsibility, and "stewardship of self" (Francis, 2018, p. 97) to and for shared humanity are fundamental principles when engaging in Caritas reflection. Gently pondering the difficulties and challenges of being human in a pressurized world and work environment, deep Caritas reflection discerns what it means to be in an authentic caring presence. Teasing out ego agendas, personal drama, and unconscious bias, and alert to organizational buzzwords or box-ticking tasks as evidence for care and compassion, the Caritas Processes invite curiosity and seek solutions (Caritas Process 6). Giving voice to the inner teacher, Caritas inquiry asks, what ways of knowing come to the fore (Caritas Process 6)? It is a means of reawakening, returning to the center, and remembering. To be in an authentic presence is an invitation to trust in the transformative process and risk being changed.

G.R.A.C.E. MICROPRACTICE

The WCSI Caritas Coach Education Program (CCEP) is a six-month immersion into Watson Caring Science (www.watsoncaringscience.org). In the context of loving, trusting, caring relationships, it is a process of deep sharing and personal reflection. Students (or coaches) post reflections on an internet learning platform discussion board. A dynamic connection and flow of energy emerge as all listen to and share their stories. In response to a post in which the author shared some personal, negative self-talk, a fellow coach responded, "Anna, allow yourself some grace." Those words touched my heart and were transformative in my CCEP journey and personal grief.

Here is a short meditation/micropractice. Based on the acronym G.R.A.C.E., it is a tool to cultivate compassion (www.upaya.org). Use it to find center, find stillness, and remember your authentic self:

- **G—Gather attention. Focus on breathing and being physically present. Still the mind.** *How is my body?*
- **R—Recall intention and commitment to act with integrity.** *Why am I here?*
- **A—Attune to the flow of self/other energy. Create gentle space, inviting a remembering.** *Who am I?*
- **C—Consider the wise and compassionate path.** *What do I see, sense, and learn? How may I serve?*
- **E—Engage in compassionate action. Acknowledge what has taken place. End the interaction by breathing, releasing, and letting go.**

Source: Halifax, 2015, p.241; www.upaya.org

HOLDING INTENTIONAL SPACE FOR CARING REFLECTION

Being alongside in authentic presence, we are "reminded and remember our most authentic human self and service" (Watson, 2005, p. 96) and uncover and recognize patterns that no longer serve us. Nurses spend their days holding the "tears and fears" of others (Watson,

2008, p. 102) and in doing so, create space for healing. And yet, "space is an interesting concept to ponder" (Lombard & Horton-Deutsch, 2017, p. 74). The yearning for "space" when stressed, tired, or in need of reflection and restoration is something we are all familiar with. It may manifest physically, for example in gazing at the stars or returning to a special place in nature. Space may be an emotional or spiritual endeavor of journeying inwards to find stillness and peace, perhaps through self-development micropractices such as art, poetry, music, journaling, or meditation (one micropractice you might find helpful is in the sidebar above, "G.R.A.C.E. Micropractice"). It may be some or all these or something unique, just for you. Whatever it is, the notion of "space" echoes a shared human experience. Explaining what it means to hold space for another, Einion (2022) states:

> To hold space means to be physically, mentally, and emotionally present for another person, creating the conditions for them to feel safe, explore their feelings, experience whatever is happening at that moment, and suspend judgment for that period of time. Regardless of what we might perceive, think, or believe about a particular situation, action, decision, or opinion, to hold space means to be lovingly present without preconditions, presuppositions, and without preconceptions. (p. 7)

The notion of "holding space" is not new. From Heidegger's philosophical perspective, "space is the medium through which relationships flow" (Lombard & Horton-Deutsch, 2017, p. 74). Offering kindness, empathic listening, sharing stories, or holding deep space for others when they can't do it for themselves are all manifestations of holding space (Plett, 2020). For millennia, humanity has held space in the life and death transition (Andrews, 2017). Midwives at the beginning and end of life, nurses, and nurturers have created deep spaces to hold each other in the rawness of our humanity, bearing witness to fear, joy, hope, loss, and broken hearts. As natural as a smile and as instinctive as a hug, holding deep space in anticipation of the first and last breath is "in our bones" (Warner, 2013, p. 32). Holding space then is intuitive (Plett, 2020). At all levels, it is what we do because we are human, because we are connected, and because "walking alongside is what you are here to do" (Biley, 2019a, p. 4).

Holding space begins with loving-kindness and compassion for self (Halifax, 2015). The Caritas Processes hold this space by inviting gentle self-care and "compassion for ourselves, for others and humanity" (Horton-Deutsch & Rosa, 2019, p. 167). As unitary, interconnected beings, holding space for self is a mindful act that creates a healing environment for all (Caritas Process 8). Still, silent, and connected with our deepest sense of knowing (Caritas Process 6), holding space is an invitation to pause, breathe, listen, and "bring the mind home" (Johns, 2022, p. 23). Holding space for caring and healing in authentic caring presence, Watson (2008) detailed Caring Science touchstones as daily microbpractices for reflection and presence in the beginning, middle, end, and continuing (see Table 3.1).

TABLE 3.1 TOUCHSTONES: SETTING INTENTIONALITY AND CONSCIOUSNESS FOR CARING AND HEALING
CARING IN THE BEGINNING
• Begin the day with silent gratitude; set your intentions to be open to give and receive all that you are here to give and receive this day; intend to bring your full self, in the day-to-day moments of this day, cultivating a loving, caring consciousness toward yourself and all others who enter your path.
CARING IN THE MIDDLE
• Take quiet moments to "center," to empty out, to be still with yourself before entering a patient's room or when entering a meeting; cultivate a loving-caring consciousness toward each person and each situation you encounter throughout the day; make an effort "to see" who the spirit-filled person is behind the patient/colleague.
• Return to these loving-centered intentions again and again, throughout the day, helping yourself to remember why you are here.
• In the middle of stressful moments, remember to breathe; ask for guidance when unsure, confused, and frightened; forgive and bless each situation.
• Let go of that which you cannot control.
CARING IN THE END
• At the end of the day, fold these intentions into your heart; commit yourself to cultivating a loving-caring practice for yourself.
• Use whatever has presented itself to you this day as lessons to teach you to grow more deeply into your own humanity and inner wisdom.
• At the end of the day, offer gratitude for all that has entered the sacred circle of your life and work this day.
• Bless, release, and dedicate the day to a higher, deeper order of the great sacred circle of life.
CARING CONTINUING
• Create your own intentions and your own authentic presence to prepare your *Caritas Consciousness*; find your individual spiritual path toward cultivating caring consciousness and meaningful experiences in your life and work and the world.

Source: Watson, 2008, p. 51

We are often our own worst self-critic; it is helpful to be starkly reminded that cruel words do violence to self and others. Speaking with gentleness and truth is a deliberate act of non-violence—an intention to be in the right relationship and to do no harm (Kumar, 2013). Likewise, being in conscious Caritas reflection invites mindful presence, compassion, equanimity, and a nonjudgmental stance. Holding space for self takes courage in facing our own, complex humanity. Embraced by the Caritas Processes, Watson (2018) reminds us that if we are to sustain human dignity (Caritas Process 9), we cannot at the same time hold ourselves or others in judgment and shame. Holding brave, intentional space for Caritas reflection gently touches our innate sense of unworthiness and honors vulnerability. Being in an authentic presence opens space to hold, touch, and honor dignity. Repatterning mindsets of "fixing" to modes of being, we may listen wholly and without judgment. Knowing we are in a safe place, held by caring and wholehearted intention for self/other, fear and vulnerability may show themselves (Horton-Deutsch & Rosa, 2019), and in loving, trusting, caring relationships (Caritas Process 4), dignity may flourish.

CO-CREATING INTENTIONAL LISTENING

The ethics and values of Watson Caring Science and the Caritas Processes are an invitation to embody ways of being that support growth, transformation, repatterning, and healing. As we turn toward/face the humanity of ourselves and others with loving acceptance, honor, calmness, and equanimity, we can connect and communicate in ways that are caring, healing, and authentic. Holding space, one may appreciate presence as deep listening (Watson, 2018). Allowing for the expression of positive and negative feelings—authentically listening to another person's story—is the essence of Caritas Process 5 and is at the heart of Caring Science practice. Gentle questions of self and others hold space to reflect and explore feelings, decisions, actions, and life patterns. Using open-ended questions that are gentle, thoughtful, and deep encourages authentic expression and curiosity.

Being in mindful reflection, the Caritas Processes mold tender questions for co-creating intentional listening that comes from a consciousness of care and compassion. For example: What do I need in this moment? How can I give myself some loving-kindness today? What would love have me do? What moments of caring (however small) did I witness today? What moments of compassion did I witness today? What words of gratitude did I hear? Seeing all interactions with others as an honor and privilege, how did I uphold human dignity for myself and others? How did I show up today? What did I know? How did I know? What did I learn? What is my story?

To illustrate how a consciousness of care and compassion may create space for intentional listening, the following short narrative offers a reflection of how the author came to be in caring presence with a friend.

> Recently, a close friend was going through a traumatic time in her life. She went to the ground, ignoring my texts and emails. I was worried and wondered if I had done something wrong. After three months she eventually reached out. She had indeed been avoiding having a conversation with me. Acknowledging that "I had been through so much" because my mother had died, she said, "I want to be positive when I see you and not offload negativity as that doesn't feel right." When the time was right for her, we met for a dog walk, and she shared her story. We talked about how there was no positive or negative for either of us. There was only our shared life experience, listening, and friendship. What she was going through was as real and painful as my loss. By sharing, she was not offloading negativity but releasing something that could repattern her distress and create a healing space for us both. Where loving-kindness and compassion are shared in a transpersonal caring moment, sacred space is invited in.

Listening to our story, or holding space for another's, may give rise to pause and silence. As "doers" and "fixers," silence can be awkward and stressful, creating pressure to fill the void with words. In contrast, Watson (2021) teaches the importance of nurturing silence when creating space for mindful Caritas reflection. In authentically listening to the positive and negative, we can pause and be still and silent. We don't have to speak, "fix," or find answers. We can hold silence and, in doing so, honor the inner teacher as a source of insight and wisdom. Quoting the poet Rainer Maria Rilke, Francis (2018) reminds us that "some questions cannot be answered on the spot but must be lived into over time" (p. 128). As Watson's touchstones (refer to Table 3.1) reveal, stillness is the essence of reflection, and it is from that place that all ways of knowing/being/doing/becoming flow (Caritas Process 6). We are our own teachers if only we had the time to be still, listen to our heart, and hear our inner voice. Speaking of teaching in *The Prophet*, the poet Kahlil Gibran (1926/1991) contemplates: "No man can reveal to you aught but that which already lies half asleep in the dawning of your knowledge."

The inner teacher that lies at the heart of all ways of knowing described in Caritas Process 6 may be likened to the concept of the clearness committee (Francis, 2018). It is based on the principle that individual wisdom lies within each of us. Co-creating space for intentional, deep listening, the role of the clearness committee is to ask open, honest questions with the sole intent of supporting an individual to unravel complexities, discover their wisdom, and let the right actions emerge. Chapter 10 further explores the clearness committee.

In search of mindfulness, Biley (2010, p. 2) reflected on the words of the ancient philosopher Lao Tzu: "Do you have the patience to wait till your mud settles and the water is clear? Can you remain unmoving until the right action emerges by itself?" And so once again we see how the Caritas circle of reflection comes to the fore. As a way of being in an authentic presence, asking open, honest questions is a way of holding a safe, sensitive space for self/other to grow in loving-kindness and compassion. Watson Caring Science reminds us that what we do for others we do for self, and what we do for self is part of the whole (Christopher et al., 2020), and in "helping to move toward a more humane and caring moral community and civilization, we move from caritas to communitas" (Watson, 2018, p. 46).

NURTURING COMMUNITIES OF REFLECTIVE LEARNING

In traditional educational structures, reflective practice frameworks are a means of system organization, supervision, and safeguarding. Reflection is an individual, inner experience, but in it isolation may be difficult to sustain (Johns, 2022). Nurturing, curious learning groups offer the equanimity of "individual introspection and supportive community" (Francis, 2018, p. 23). In a Watson Caring Science learning community/communitas, there is no expert, hierarchy, or power structure. In our shared humanity, the Caritas Processes hold nonjudgmental, safe, reflective spaces in which new insights are co-created, creative solution-seeking is nurtured (Caritas Process 6), and new beginnings emerge. Remembering that Watson's Unitary Caring Science resides in a unitary transformative paradigm where all is connected and care begins with self, it radiates from self to other, "widening the field" (Watson, 2021, p. 128) to the entire infinite field of humanity and planet earth. Once a strange and abstract concept in relationship to nursing, the concept of the quantum universe, spoken of by nursing theorist Martha Rogers in the 1970s, is now mainstream science (Phillips, 2017). And so we are reminded that nurturing and growing reflective communities is transformational, compassionate human service, and "what we carry in our heart matters" (Watson, 2021, p. 135).

The CCEP is one such learning space that has grown as a reflective community (Horton-Deutsch & Rosa, 2019). Making conscious choices to work together to develop loving, trusting, caring relationships, faculty educators teach what they need to learn (Watson, 2005), and all are supported to "hold another in your heart space with unconditional compassion, kindness, dignity and regard" (Watson, 2018, p. 84). As individuals giving voice to our raw humanity, we are all at times vulnerable, yet "when we hold space for someone, we need to be prepared to hold the whole of them, not just the parts that are easy and straightforward" (Plett, 2020, p. 50). Nurturing reflective Caritas communities permits us to show up in the whole of our complexity and to trust that to be honored without shame. In a dynamic process of "energyspirit" filled relationships (Phillips, 2022b), power is relinquished, voices are heard, and energy is repatterned to bring equanimity and healing.

The art of building reflective, caring communities will be explored in further chapters. Watson's Unitary Caring Science perspective defines being and belonging in communitas as an all-at-once journey of deep, inner personal work and shared humanity. Held by the Caritas Processes, communitas in action is about showing up in an authentic presence with caring and compassionate intentions. It is about the courage to hold space for listening deeply and for nurturing curiosity, creativity, understanding, and knowing (Watson, 2018). Phillips argues that "everything in the universe is imbued with beauty" (2022a, p. 49), and its place in the "well-becoming" (p. 50) of all should never be underestimated. Consistent with this approach, Caring Science honors the daily practice of nurturing self/other as "an act of power and an act of beauty" (Watson, 2021, p. xxix). In personal, reflective space, or in community, to seek creative solutions through the art and beauty of caring micro-practices is an act of remembering and honoring who we are and why we are here.

MICROPRACTICE

"At the deepest level, ours is not to make ourselves heard but to be still enough to hear. During your day, take five minutes and stop making, stop doing, stop thinking ... and just listen" (Nepo, 2020, p. 353).

APPLICATION FOR PERSONAL AND PROFESSIONAL PRACTICE

"All we have in life are moments" (Watson, 2018, p. 52). Cultivating "loving-kindness, compassion, joy, and equanimity ... can strengthen their presence within us. As that presence grows stronger, so does their boundless quality" (Halifax, 2008, p. 38). Being in an authentic presence, holding space for co-creating intentional listening, and nurturing reflective communities is the Caritas circle of reflection. Becoming mindful of being in the moment, in the energy of transpersonal, connected relationships, gently reminds us that we are "part of the life history of each person and the larger complex pattern of life and the universe" (Watson, 2018, p. 54). May we pause, be still, and ask (Biley, 2010, p. 2):

- When seeing, how do we see?

- When touching, how do we touch?

- When thinking, how do we think?

REFLECTIVE SUMMARY

COVID-19, climate change, social and cultural injustices, health and mental health crises—how do we navigate our way in the world? At the front line, accepting the unacceptable requires courage, authenticity, and vulnerability. As the value of "being-with-another-in-the world" has been acutely brought into focus by the pandemic (Silva et al., 2021), care and learning environments have transitioned to virtual spaces, and physical touch has repatterned into a hug of energy and intention (Phillips, 2022b). In facing our shared humanity in new ways, the Caritas Processes and the values of care, compassion, and dignity are the constants that connect us and make us who we are. The language and values of Watson Caring Science and the scope for nurses to own their vulnerability continue to resonate with the reality of practice. In uncertain times, the Caritas circle of reflection may keep the ship steady for self/ others in the now and in the future. In wisdom and stillness "holding sacred space for loving kindness, peace, and understanding, creates an energetic field for creative solutions that benefit all of humanity" (Giovannoni, 2019, p. 363).

LEARNING NARRATIVE

The following learning narrative is the author's personal experience of being alongside her husband as he lived his dying.

When my husband was first diagnosed with terminal cancer, I was offered what was to become the most helpful advice I had ever received. My brother, an intensive care nurse for many years, said to me, "Be the listener." He told me that my husband would not have the capacity to take in all the complex information thrown at us at the time. Some things were just too hard to hear. Of course, as a nurse myself I knew that, but living it when it was my life partner's death sentence was another matter. And so I learned to listen deeply. To become still. To read silence, hands, faces, and to hear the buried muffles of unspoken truths.

In the following weeks he lived his dying, and death came to us as destiny took its inevitable and heartbreaking course. Through long days and even longer nights, I held space and silence and I listened. And something began to happen. So often in the past I had doubted the authority of my own experience and yet, at the still point, at the center of the chaos that was our cancer-dominated reality, I began to hear my inner voice telling me again and again, "You know what to do. Trust what you know." Being with dying brought to the fore the deepest human instinct to bring compassion, care, and dignity to the moment.

It is said that Caring Science starts with self. But in truth, at that time, there was no sense of self—only instinct, intuition, and a visceral calling to nurture and protect my loved ones. Over time, the inner voice became stronger and would not be silenced. Scrambling back from the abyss of bereavement in the months beyond my husband's death, safe ground slowly revealed itself, and it was there in snatched spaces of reflection that Caring Science offered a guiding hand to steady the fledgling feet of a newly anointed widow and single mum. Somehow, I had to survive because my kids needed me, and the only way I could do that was to begin caring for and listening to self.

1. How do the Caritas Processes manifest in this learning narrative?

2. Being alongside in her husband's dying, how did the author show up in authentic presence and hold space for self/other?

3. How does this narrative explore deep listening and the voice of the inner teacher?

REFLECTIVE QUESTIONS

1. You are invited to revisit and reflect on the Caritas Processes. Which one do you find most relevant to your work? Why?

2. Guided by the Caring Science touchstones described in this chapter, what self-care practices might be helpful to you?

3. How might the touchstones help you in being/becoming reflective in the moment?

4. How might being in authentic presence, holding space, and co-creating intentional listening support you in deepening your journey of self-reflection?

5. How can you grow and nurture a community of reflective learning?

REFERENCES

Anderson, J. (2018). Caritas coaching: An overview. In S. Horton-Deutsch & J. Anderson (Eds.), *Caritas coaching: A journey toward transpersonal caring for informed moral action in healthcare* (pp. 3–26). Sigma Theta Tau International.

Andrews, E. (2017). Holding space with women in the labyrinth. *Midwifery Today, 121,* 9–11.

Belenky, M. F., Clinchy, B. M., Goldberger, N. R., & Tarule, J. M. (1997). *Women's ways of knowing* (10th anniversary ed.). Perseus Books.

Biley, A. (2019a). *Birds hold our secrets: A Caritas story of grief and remembering.* Watson Caring Science Institute: Lotus Library.

Biley, A. (2019b). Remembering purpose: An autoethnography. In W. Rosa, S. Horton-Deutsch, & J. Watson (Eds.), *A handbook of caring science* (pp. 633–641). Springer.

Biley, F. C. (2010). In search of mindfulness. *International Journal of Healing and Caring, 10,* 1.

Blake, W. (1863). *Auguries of innocence.* CreateSpace Independent Publishing Platform.

Christopher, R., Tantillo, L. & Watson, J. (2020). Academic caring pedagogy, presence and communitas in nursing education in the COVID-19 pandemic. *Nursing Outlook, 68*(6), 822–829. https://doi.org/10.1016/j.outlook.2020.08.006

Cowling, W. R. (2012). Healing as appreciating wholeness. In W. K. Cody (Ed.), *Philosophical and theoretical perspectives for advanced nursing practice* (5th ed., pp. 119–137). Jones & Bartlett.

Critchley, S., & Bernasconi, R. (2002). *The Cambridge companion to Levinas.* Cambridge University Press.

Einion, A. (2022, February). Holding space. *Practicing Midwife, 10.*

Francis, S. (2018). *The courage way. Leading and living with integrity.* Berrett-Koehler.

Frank, A. W. (2013). *The wounded storyteller* (2nd ed.). University of Chicago Press.

Gibran, K. (1926/1991). *The prophet*. Pan Books.

Giovannoni, J. (2019). Holding sacred space for loving-kindness and equanimity for self/other. In W. Rosa, S. Horton-Deutsch, & J. Watson (Eds.), *A handbook of caring science* (pp. 355–371). Springer.

Halifax, J. (2008). *Being with dying*. Shambhala.

Halifax, J. (2015). *Standing at the edge*. Flatiron Books.

Horton-Deutsch, S., & Anderson, J. (2018). Introduction. In S. Horton-Deutsch & J. Anderson (Eds.), *Caritas coaching: A journey toward transpersonal caring for informed moral action in healthcare* (pp. xxxiii–xxxvi). Sigma Theta Tau International.

Horton-Deutsch, S., & Rosa, W. (2019). Caring science and reflective practice. In W. Rosa, S. Horton-Deutsch, & J. Watson (Eds.), *A handbook for caring science* (pp. 163–171). Springer.

Johns, C. (2022). *Becoming a reflective practitioner*. John Wiley & Sons, Ltd.

Julian of Norwich. (1998). *Revelations of divine love*. (Translated by Elizabeth Spearing). Penguin.

Kumar, S. (2013). *Soil, soul, society*. Leaping Hare Press.

Levine, S. (1986). *Who dies?* Gateway.

Lombard, K., & Horton-Deutsch, S. (2017). Creating space for reflection: The importance of presence in the teaching-learning process. In S. Horton-Deutsch & G. Sherwood, *Reflective practice: Transforming education and improving outcomes* (2nd ed., pp. 77–93.). Sigma Theta Tau International.

Lourie. (2020). Peace, compassion, love. [Facebook page] In J. Watson, *Caring science as sacred science* (Revised ed.). Watson Caring Science Institute: Lotus Library.

Maher, F. A., & Tetreault, M. K. (1996). Women's ways of knowing in women's studies, feminist pedagogies and feminist theory. In N. Goldberger, J. Tarule, B. Clinchy, & N. Belenky (Eds.), *Knowledge, difference and power* (pp. 148–174). Basic Books.

Nepo, M. (2020). *The book of awakening*. Red Wheel.

Newman, M. A. (2008). *Transforming presence*. F. A. Davis.

Perkins, J. B. (2019). Unitary Caring Science and multi-cultural perspectives. In W. Rosa, S. Horton-Deutsch, & J. Watson (Eds.), *A handbook of caring science* (pp. 539–554). Springer.

Phillips, J. (2017). New Rogerian theoretical thinking about Unitary Science. *Nursing Science Quarterly, 30*(3), 223–226. https://doi.org/10.1177/0894318417708411

Phillips, J. (2022a). The revelation of beauty in nursing. *Nursing Science Quarterly, 35*(1), 46–53. https://doi.org/10.1177/08943184211051362

Phillips, J. (2022b). Rogerian theoretical musings on well-becoming. *Nursing Science Quarterly, 35*(4), 475–476. https://doi.org/10.1177/08943184221115125

Phillips, L. K. (2020). Concept analysis: Presence. *I-manager's Journal on Nursing, 10*(3), 54–61. https://doi.org/10.26634/jnur.10.3.17349

Plett, H. (2020). *The art of holding space*. Page Two Books.

Rinpoche, S. (1992). *The Tibetan book of living and dying*. Rider.

Schön, D. A. (1987). *Educating the reflective practitioner: Toward a new design for teaching and learning in the professions*. Jossey-Bass.

Silva, C. G., Crossetti, M. G. O., & Giménez-Fernández, M. (2021). Nursing and "being with" in a world with COVID-19: An existentialist outlook. *Revista Gaúcha de Enfermagem, 42*(spe): e20200383. https://doi.org/10.1590/1983-1447.2021.20200383

Turkel, M. C., Ray, M. A., & Kornblatt, L. (2012). Instead of reconceptualizing the nursing process let's re-name it. *Nursing Science Quarterly, 25*(2), 194–198. https://doi.org/10.1177/0894318412437946

Warner, F. (2013). *The soul midwives' handbook.* Hay House.

Watson, J. (2005). *Caring science as sacred science.* F. A. Davis.

Watson, J. (2008). *The philosophy and science of caring* (Revised ed.). University Press of Colorado.

Watson, J. (2012). *Human caring science.* Jones & Bartlett.

Watson, J. (2018). *Unitary caring science.* University Press of Colorado.

Watson, J. (2021). *Caring science as sacred science* (Revised ed.). Watson Caring Science Institute: Lotus Library.

Wilber, K. (1993). *Grace and grit.* Shambhala.

Wright, S. G. (2017). *Burnout as a spiritual crisis. From stress to transformation.* Sacred Space Publications.

PART II
SELF-REFLECTION: BUILDING OUR CAPACITY FOR INTROSPECTION AND INTENTIONAL PRACTICE IN ACADEMIC AND CLINICAL SETTINGS

4   Self-Reflection Through the Lens of Unitary Caring
Science: Learning to Listen and Listening to Learn 67

5   Deepening Our Foundations: Reimagining Ourselves,
Reimagining Nursing Identity 89

6   The Role of Reflection in Guiding the Evolution of Care,
Compassion, and Social Change 115

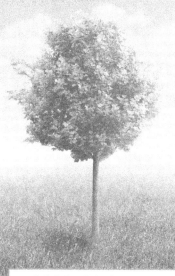

CHAPTER 4

SELF-REFLECTION THROUGH THE LENS OF UNITARY CARING SCIENCE: LEARNING TO LISTEN AND LISTENING TO LEARN

–Christine Griffin, PhD, RN, NPD-BC, CPN, Caritas Coach & Leader
Sara Horton-Deutsch, PhD, RN, FAAN, ANEF, SGAHN

LEARNING OBJECTIVES/SUBJECTIVES

- Describe theoretical frameworks that support listening as an essential element of reflection and nursing's philosophical, moral, and ethical values.

- Explore ways to listen more deeply and wisely with others.

- Engage in individual and relational listening micropractices that serve to build and deepen the aptitude for reflection.

- Apply intentional listening to enrich personal and professional growth, enhance communication with others, and build caring-healing relationships.

"The inner life of any great thing will be incomprehensible to me until I develop and deepen an inner life of my own."

–Palmer, 1983

OVERVIEW

Building on the previous chapter's exploration of the nature of presence and space for caring and reflective practice, this chapter focuses on developing the learner's capacity for intentional deep listening. By listening deeply to oneself and others, learners gain a better understanding of their own needs and the needs of those around them. This form of intentional listening fosters compassion and connection and creates a supportive environment for personal growth and healing.

This chapter is designed to give you the resources you need to gain a deeper understanding of self and a better understanding of the perspectives and experiences of others. More specifically, this chapter will explore the concept of listening and expanding the capacity for listening through the lens of Unitary Caring Science and in alignment with the new American Association of Colleges of Nursing (AACN) Essentials and the American Nurses Association (ANA) definition of nursing. The chapter draws on the expertise of reflective practitioners, providing a guide on how to evolve the capacity to listen to ourselves and others.

SUPPORTING THEORETICAL FRAMEWORKS AND EVIDENCE

Like early chapters, the fundamental underpinning of this chapter is Unitary Caring Science (Watson, 2018). This theory fosters a kindhearted and reflective practice that allows for exploring the depths of being and recognizes that human beings are not simply physical entities but complex beings with emotional, psychological, and spiritual dimensions. Unitary Caring Science and the 10 Caritas Processes are discussed more fully in Chapter 1.

Listening plays a significant role in Caring Science as it is an essential component of establishing authentic and compassionate connections with others. Listening in the context of Caring Science goes beyond simply hearing words. It involves being fully present and attentive to the person, creating a safe and supportive environment for them to express themselves. Listening fits within the framework of Caring Science and the 10 Caritas Processes via:

- **Caritas Process #2:** Authentic presence: When you truly listen to someone, you are fully present in the moment and attuned to their needs. This requires setting aside distractions, suspending judgment, and focusing on the person's experience. Being present and fully engaged shows that you care and respect the individual.

- **Caritas Process #4:** Building trusting caring relationships: Listening with empathy involves not only hearing what someone says but also trying to understand their emotions, values, and beliefs. It involves being sensitive to nonverbal cues and the underlying meaning behind their words. By authentically listening, caregivers can acknowledge and validate the person's experiences, enhancing their sense of being heard and understood. This is vital for building a trusting-caring relationship.

- **Caritas Process #5:** Allowing for the expression of positive and negative feelings: Authentically listening to another person's story provides a safe outlet for emotional release, enhances awareness, strengthens connections, and facilitates problem resolution and growth. Understanding another person's feelings helps to individualize the approach to care, provide meaningful support, and offer empathy through validation of their feelings.

- **Caritas Process # 7:** Engaging in transpersonal teaching and learning: Caring Science emphasizes the establishment of a transpersonal relationship, where the nurse or caregiver connects with the person at a deeper level. Listening attentively fosters trust and promotes a sense of safety, allowing the person to share their concerns, fears, and emotions more openly. Through active listening, healthcare providers can better understand the person's unique perspective and offer appropriate support and teaching by staying within the other person's frame of reference.

- **Caritas Process #8:** Co-creating healing environments: By being fully present, listening, and attending to the energy of self and other, the nurse co-creates healing environments that promote the well-being of individuals and facilitate their healing processes. Authentic listening helps caregivers gather information about a person's needs, preferences, and goals. This knowledge can then be used to co-create an environment that respects their autonomy and fosters their healing, thus enhancing the overall care experience.

Application of these processes aligns with the new AACN Essentials, particularly the domains of Knowledge for Nursing Practice; Person-Centered Care; Professionalism; and Personal, Professional, and Leadership Development (AACN, 2021). These processes are universal to the four spheres of care that encompass all delivery settings defined by AACN: disease prevention/promotion of health and well-being, chronic disease care, regenerative or restorative care, and hospice/palliative/supportive care.

The Knowledge for Nursing Practice domain stresses the significance of evidence-based practice and continuous learning in nursing to support high-quality patient care. Unitary Caring Science complements this domain by emphasizing the importance of self-reflection and ongoing learning in nursing practice. It expands the concept of evidence-based practice to include all forms of knowledge and invites consideration of caring literacies rather than just competencies. *Caring literacies* refer to ways of being and relating to others that nurses need to cultivate continually. Unitary Caring Science also supports person-centered care, which involves understanding each patient's unique needs and preferences, providing individualized care, and extending it to focus on transpersonal care reflecting the relationship between nurse and patient. Professionalism, defined by ethical behavior, accountability, and a commitment to excellence, is essential in nursing practice and is emphasized in Unitary Caring Science. Nurses who practice from this perspective act with integrity, take accountability for their actions, and strive for excellence in all aspects of their practice. Finally, the Personal, Professional, and Leadership Development domain highlights the importance of ongoing personal and professional growth in nursing. Unitary Caring Science recognizes this significance and encourages nurses to engage in self-reflection, personal and professional development, and continually evaluate their practice to provide the best possible care to their patients through an ever-evolving caring consciousness.

The ANA definition aligns well with the principles of Unitary Caring Science, which emphasize the art and science of care, facilitation of healing, compassionate presence, and recognition of connection of all humanity:

> Nursing integrates the art and science of care and focuses on the protection, promotion, and optimization of health and human functioning, prevention of illness and injury; facilitation of healing; and alleviation of suffering through compassionate presence. Nursing is the diagnosis and treatment of human responses to advocacy in the care of individuals, families, communities, and populations in recognition of the connection of all humanity. (ANA, 2021, p. 7)

The *art of nursing* refers to nursing practice's humanistic and empathetic aspects. It involves connecting with patients on a deep level, listening to their concerns, and providing compassionate care that addresses their unique needs and preferences. The art of nursing is closely connected to the principles of Unitary Caring Science, which emphasizes the importance of caring and compassion to the healing process and caring as a sacred act.

LEARNING TO LISTEN

In healthcare, listening is an essential act. When a nurse authentically listens to a patient, they build trust, facilitate accurate treatment, and lay a foundation for the patient and relationship-centered care. Unitary Caring Science invites a more expansive form of listening to help nurses and patients find meaning and purpose. This type of listening begins with the nurse's commitment to seeing each person's uniqueness, humanity, and wholeness. Through this lens, the nurse sees beyond what the patient says to hear what is being shared in the space between words. This form of deep listening allows the nurse to read the field and use their heart's intuitive intelligence and innate instinct for compassion to determine what is required in the moment (Watson & Browning, 2012, 2019). Without this awareness, Watson (2008) reminds us that we can "harden our self to the feelings of others and close down our hearts, making us insensitive and even cruel, just when others may be in most need of our loving-kindness" (p. 69).

Moments with patients that demonstrate care lay a foundation for developing trust. Trust is a basic need in a nurse/patient relationship, but nurses cannot assume it is given freely. Trust is negotiated through a series of moments when a vulnerable patient offers what they need and then waits for the nurse's response (Dinc & Gastmans, 2013). While trust is gained through listening, it can quickly be lost when rushed, stressed, or lost in "task mode," which is why Watson (2008) regards listening as a sacred act. This chapter will expand our collective understanding of listening as a sacred act by distinguishing the layers of listening from shallow to deep and offer practices for listening to self and others with intention and loving-kindness.

WAYS OF LISTENING

Nurses and other healthcare professionals are taught a variety of ways to listen and communicate. The healthcare field is inundated with communication tools and acronyms like SBAR, LAST, AIDET, Check Back, Time Out, and a variety of handoff tools. In addition, nurses learn crucial communication, verbal de-escalation, and emotional intelligence to master high-level responses when interacting with a patient and their families. While these tools and approaches serve a vital purpose, at the bedside, nurses readily recognize the limits of more structured scripts and the need for a deeper understanding and connection with the patient to create a calm, caring, and healing environment. This chapter poses the question: What if it is as much about my ability to be fully present and listen in the moment as it is about what I say?

Through Unitary Caring Science and the 10 Caritas Processes, nurses learn a more holistic way of listening by attending to how to be still, connect to their hearts, and listen to their intuition. They learn how to read the environment, bring forth a calming presence, and ultimately raise the collective consciousness. By listening from this philosophical lens and using this knowledge in moments of care, nurses build life-giving and life-receiving relationships with patients.

Healthcare settings and patient rooms within a hospital are typically fast-paced, inherently stressful, and often sterile, with noisy machines, bright lights, and intimidating medical equipment and supplies. The humans within these environments are influenced by the atmosphere and the emotions they are experiencing, most likely containing lower vibrational energy like fear, vulnerability, anger, and tension. How do nurses ensure the environment becomes a space where a patient can heal?

Watson (2018) contends creating a healing environment begins with an awareness that, through heart-centered practices and awareness, the nurse becomes the healing environment—an environment that offers dignity, respect, understanding, and empathy, combined with the keen ability to listen, tune in to what is held in the space, and pay attention to what is said beyond words. Becoming the healing environment means that each nurse brings what is needed, regardless of what the external environment offers. The potential to experience the dilemma from the patient's perspective lives and derives from a moment of presence. Disconnecting from the noise in the environment and connecting with the human behind all the machines creates a focal point, communicating to the patient they are not alone and are cared for. Watson describes the importance of this practice of being and becoming a Caritas consciousness:

> By being sensitive to our presence and Caritas Consciousness, not only are we able to offer and enable another to access his or her belief systems of faith-hope for the person healing, but we may be the one who makes the difference between hope and despair in a given moment. (Watson, 2008, p. 62)

Watson describes this connection created between a nurse and patient as a transpersonal caring moment. *Transpersonal care,* or the moments when an authentic connection between two individuals allows both to give and receive caring/healing attention simultaneously, is the cornerstone of Unitary Caring Science (Sitzman, 2007). It is the relational aspect of care that allows both the nurse and the patient to reach a higher level of consciousness and, therefore, a higher degree of harmony and healing. Watson (2008) describes a transpersonal moment as one that "invites full loving-kindness and equanimity of one's presence-in-the-moment, with an understanding that a significant caring moment can be a turning point in one's life. It affects both nurse and patient and radiates out beyond the moment" (p. 79).

OVERCOMING FRENZY

It is essential to pause and be open and honest about the barriers nurses face as they set intentions to create transpersonal caring moments. Formidable external pressures will test even the most seasoned and compassionate nurse. For example, there are often too many tasks to complete in a shift. The documentation demands alone draw nurse attention away from patients and their families. In addition, nurses are facing a remarkable increase in physical and verbal violence; thus, deciding how to enter a room is more challenging (Kafle et al., 2022). A typical nurse today grapples with the balance of needing more time or stamina to manage the demands. Consider the type of frenzy described here. It is hard to imagine any one person being able to shift these barriers toward something new.

To get in touch with this aspect of caring, recall a caring quality a person brought to you in a time of need. Was it a gentle touch that reminded you that you mattered? Was it someone who looked you in the eye and authentically asked you how you were? Maybe you hoped for a moment of levity to settle your mind and looked for an encouraging sign within the complexity of your situation. Each of these qualities happens within moments when we are focused less on what we are doing and can tune into how we are showing up moment-by-moment.

Transpersonal caring moments can happen unconsciously between a nurse and a patient. However, when we build them into a conscious practice of presence, every moment with a patient can be more meaningful, healing, and life-giving for the patient and the nurse. Being present in a moment is described as having the awareness and consciousness to be still and pay attention to the environment and all the people within it. Eckhart Tolle (2005) recognizes that choosing to be present with another is more powerful than anything a person (nurse) could do or say. As he describes: "In the stillness of presence you can sense the formless essence in yourself, and the other are one. Knowing the oneness of yourself and the other is… true care, true compassion" (p. 176).

Breaking down the moments of care into practices of awareness and openness does not disregard the complexities nurses face. Instead, it empowers the nurse to have ways to step into this work and own the parts of caring that external factors can't touch—to build a practice of being centered and finding a way to flow within the frenzy. Be in the storm but do not allow the storm to be within yourself. Unitary Caring Science offers practices that empower nurses to understand that the ability to be present with their patients lies solely within the nurse's consciousness.

No one can take away a nurse's choice to see beyond a diagnosis to the human behind the procedure or even beyond the behaviors they exhibit in their moment of need. No policies stop a nurse from pausing before entering a room to set an intention and let dignity be the objective of the encounter. A nurse can learn to own their practice so they are in touch with their authentic purpose and focus on the task at hand and how they will be aware and tuned into their patient's needs. The practices of Unitary Caring Science empower nurses to have the capacity within themselves to radically change a moment by practicing deep listening and loving-kindness for themselves and others. How do we prepare nurses for this form of deep listening?

LISTENING TO SELF

Before listening to others, a nurse must learn to listen to self—connecting and asking themselves who they are in their most authentic state, listening to what wholeness means to them as individuals with the same basic needs and desires as those they will help. For each nurse to meet their potential, they must first develop an evolved consciousness from within (Horton-Deutsch & Anderson, 2018). When we listen to self, we "seek a higher deeper source for inner wisdom and our truths...without attending to this aspect of caring we will have limited success in working with the humanity of others if we cannot accept and love self first" (Watson, 2008, p. 68).

Often this notion of seeing self first is uncomfortable for nurses who connect deeply to being in service of others. Nurses often miss the connection that being whole, or what Watson (2008) refers to as the right relationship with self and source, is directly correlated to their ability to be of service or in the right relation with another. One of the most important practices nurses can do for their patients is to focus on their being and becoming, as this increases their ability to meet their patients' physical, mental, emotional, and spiritual needs.

The duality of a transpersonal caring moment also honors what the nurse gives and receives. Often, a transpersonal caring moment is only possible because the nurse has enough within themselves to sustain both themselves and the other in that moment. This comes with a deepening understanding that by sustaining compassion for themselves, they are also able to sustain compassion for their patient. As they care for themselves, they have more capacity to care for others. As they learn to listen to themselves, they build the capacity to listen to another. This requires a sustained practice of meeting one's needs first and tangible ways of being and becoming more in the right relationship with self and source.

RIGHT RELATION WITH SELF

Being in the right relationship with self and source is a connection or quite often a reconnection to whom we are meant to be (Watson, 2008, 2018). Knowing our talents and gifts and being aligned with our core values help us to know our purpose—the unique reason we are here on earth at this time.

Connecting to purpose is tangled closely with the practice of listening to self. To know one's purpose, one must get in touch with something deeper, connecting an inner voice, a unique identity, or what some call the soul, the divine within, or the core of being. Whatever it is called, the practice of connecting with it often requires practice outside of normal day-to-day activities. To find a space to be still, ask the right questions and then listen. A quiet space with low stimuli and no distractions can let the mind quiet so the soul can catch up and be heard—one where the mind can quiet and the body can settle. Being in nature often helps to connect to something bigger than the self. Each person can discover what they need to be still, be quiet, feel safe, and reflect.

CARING SCIENCE CENTERING MICROPRACTICE

- *Find a quiet and comfortable place to sit or stand. Take a moment to ground yourself, placing your feet firmly on the ground and feeling the support of the earth beneath you.*

- *Take a deep breath through your nose, and slowly exhale through your mouth. As you exhale, release any tension or stress you may be holding in your body.*

- *Close your eyes or soften your gaze and recall a person or situation you care deeply about—a loved one, a patient, a friend, a pet, or a cause that you're passionate about.*

- *As you picture this person or situation, focus on sending them compassion, kindness, and love. Imagine wrapping them in a warm, comforting embrace and sending them positive energy and healing thoughts.*

- *As you continue sending compassion and love to this person or situation, extend these feelings to yourself. Know that caring for yourself is just as important as caring for others, and allow yourself to feel deserving of compassion and love.*

- *In this space of compassion for self and others, gently ask yourself, what gifts do I bring to this world? What can others depend on me for? What have others told me they are grateful to me for?*

- *As you breathe in your gifts, imagine how these gifts tie to your purpose. As a nurse, as a person, how do you want to live out this purpose?*

- *Take a few more deep breaths, and visualize yourself surrounded by love and care. See yourself living authentically to your unique purpose.*

- *When you feel ready, slowly open your eyes, and return to the present moment, carrying the feeling of love and care with you as you go about your day.*

As a nurse more profoundly understands and connects to their authentic self, they can begin to build more self-care practices that keep them in the right relation with whom they are meant to be. Unitary Caring Science offers a road map for practices for self-care within the 10 Caritas Processes. While often highlighted as ways of being and becoming in response to patient needs, when practiced with self first, the nurse naturally has the inclination and capacity to offer them to the patient (Watson, 2008, 2018).

LISTENING TO OTHER

The practice of attuning to the self first gives nurses the capacity they need in the moments they are called to listen to one another. It is within the same practices of getting in the right relation with self and source that we can now extend that practice to include being in the right relation with the other. This practice requires the nurse to intentionally begin and end each patient encounter with care, compassion, and dignity in which they see the whole person in front of them without reducing them to a set of tasks or asking that they arbitrarily conform to the system or standardized processes.

This does not mean that the nurse must give all of themselves away, either. It is in the practice of equanimity and loving-kindness for self and other that Unitary Caring Science describes the balance for maintaining the right relation. Unitary Caring Science reminds the nurses in these moments that being in right relations allows them to listen to both positive and negative expressions without taking them into their hearts. *Equanimity* is the practice of finding balance in a given moment, not getting stuck in negativity or, conversely, pretending everything is OK. Watson links this practice to her first Caritas process, practicing loving-kindness and equanimity for self and others within the context of caring consciousness (Watson, 2008). She states that equanimity is a "gentle acceptance of what is, without having to resist or avoid or alter what it is" (Watson, 2008, p. 53). It is like being in the storm but not allowing the storm to be in you. This is not to minimize the moment or give permission for its occurrence. It allows the nurse a vast amount of space to hold all the emotions in a moment. This way nurses remain present, read the environment, quickly decide what they need to hold onto, what is meant for them to own, and begin to let go of what is not serving themselves or others in the space.

Logstrup (1997), a Danish philosopher whom Watson draws upon to expand our ethical knowledge of caring for others, reminds us that if "we care beyond our limits we will lose our capacity to care and eventually violate those we intended to serve" (p. 47). Watson honors both the nurse and patient in the caring relationship in expressing the need to see both individuals' humanity in the moment:

We learn from one another how to be human by identifying our self with other and finding their dilemma in ourselves. What we all learn from this is self-knowledge. The self we learn about...is every self. It is the universal human self. We learn to recognize ourselves in others. It keeps alive our common humanity and avoids reducing self or other to the moral status of object. (Watson, 2008, p. 81)

HOLDING SPACE

The art of listening to others can be served by learning the practices of holding space for another. Watson (2018) speaks of holding space for another as a way of staying in awareness of the whole person in front of you—to see them as the whole and complete entity that they are and be able to mirror back to them their uniqueness and beauty. It requires us to pay attention to everything, especially paying attention to the parts of the other person that we cannot see. In this way, the small acts of kindness, compassion, and awareness become sacred acts for that other person.

The ability to hold space for a patient is often more complex based on the intensity of what they are medically dealing with. As their vulnerability increases, so might their need for the nurse to help sustain them. Plett (2020) describes this vulnerable place as a liminal space or a place of uncertainty and stress. The patient may feel insecure about the outcome they face, and holding space for them during that uncertainty includes helping them manage their anxiety, fear, tension, or sometimes anger. Plett (2020) describes what is needed in these moments:

> Holding Space is what we do when we walk alongside someone on a journey through liminal space. We do this without making them feel inadequate, without trying to fix them, and without trying to impact the outcome. We open our hearts, offer unconditional support, and let go of judgment and control. (p. 18)

Unitary Caring Science supports the nurse's ability to hold this space by offering a solid place for them to fall back on. A foundation of knowing themselves is complemented with the skills to hold space by setting a caring intention, by being present for whatever the patient needs and the knowledge that small, sacred acts of kindness and compassion are often enough to sustain the patient during this time.

DEEPLY LISTENING

Deeply listening to another offers the nurse an opportunity to connect with the other person at a heart-to-heart level beyond the need to fix or control an outcome and attune to dignity and care without judgment or to solely meet a goal. In clinical settings, nurses are often asked to put aside what their heart is telling them the patient needs and instead meet the demands of throughput, budget restraints, or decrease the length of stay. The COVID-19 pandemic highlighted the intense struggle that nurses endured when asked to go against their compassionate nature and meet the demands of the moment. Unitary Caring Science asks each nurse to critique these moments and build in a practice to pause for themselves and potentially the system to do better for their patients by shifting away from the pressure of doing and focusing on being.

DOING TO BEING

Listening to others from a lens of being rather than doing includes the practice of pausing and setting an intention. This offers the moment nurses may need for centering and readiness to be and become the healing environment for surrounding the patient. By setting down judgment and the need to control, the nurse can co-create transpersonal caring moments that are life-giving and life-receiving for both nurse and patient. Being fully present in the moment also allows the nurse to practice loving-kindness and equanimity for self and others and balance this with doing the required tasks. Unitary Caring Science also reminds each nurse that at any moment they are drawn away from being fully present they can simply pause and begin again.

LISTENING IN THE CLINICAL ENVIRONMENT

Practicing intentional listening to self and others requires developing self-care habits. This begins with being well-resourced when we arrive at work. Clinical environments are rarely positioned to ensure the nurse can prioritize healing environments and transpersonal caring moments. Finding space again requires us to look for the practices we have the capacity to manage. *Micropractices* are in-the-moment practices we can draw upon quickly to offer a reset or, Watson would say, let our souls catch up to us (Watson, 2008). In a clinical setting, we will offer these by looking at the moments that contain a shift and/or moments that complete an experience. For a shift, Watson offers touchstones that allow a nurse to build practices for caring for self and others at the beginning, in the middle, and at the end of a workday. Setting an intention, honoring the need to reset and renew, and caring for self at the end of the day offers the path nurses need to sustain themselves. These touchstones were introduced in Chapter 3.

Imagine if the nurse were to draw on these practices on an even smaller micro level and develop similar practices for each encounter. Each experience nurses have with a patient can be parceled into what we refer to as the sacred moments of care called to pause, presence, and peace (see Figure 4.1).

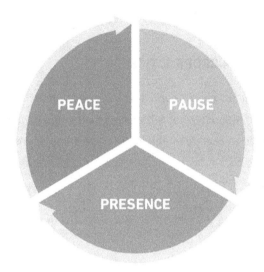

FIGURE 4.1.   Sacred moments of a patient encounter.

The pause occurs before entering someone else's environment and is used to slow down, check in with self, and set an intention for what will transpire next. Pausing in this way gives us the vital basic needs we forget to offer ourselves. It gives nurses a moment to breathe, settle, and ask what they need before they step in. While this process does not require much time, it does require a commitment to self-care and self-awareness as a practice.

The presence is the practice we fall back on when we are co-creating a moment with our patients. It draws on our knowledge of oneness, authenticity, and the consciousness of compassion and care we have known will be in service. As Jean Watson describes before, it is taking ourselves off autopilot and paying attention to what is happening right now. Authentic presence, much like listening, is a true gift nurses can give to their patients. In the middle of their vulnerability, having someone who not only is a witness to their experience but actively says I see your suffering—you are not alone, and I am here to help—can be a pillar when it is most needed.

Finally, peace is the reflective practice used after the experience to learn, grow, process, and set down what we can to move intentionally into the next moment, the next encounter. This is a personal practice that comes from understanding what you need to walk back toward your wholeness after giving yourself to someone else. At times it is as simple as an acknowledgment of the care provided. Other times it requires a moment of forgiveness for yourself or another who may have not shown up in the best way. For the experiences that linger, nurses may need to process them out loud with a peer or write out a narrative to allow the paper to hold the heaviness of the moment.

PAUSE, PRESENCE, PEACE MICROPRACTICE

- **Pause:** *Slow down, check in with yourself, and set an intention.*
- **Presence:** *Pay full attention to what is happening in the moment of care.*
- **Peace:** *Set down what you can to intentionally move to the next moment of care.*

Each of these practices is part of the process. Each holds significance, and each contributes to the other. When we rush, we forget to pause. When we get distracted, we forget to see the whole person in front of us and risk reducing them to the moral status of an object. When nurses don't take time to reflect, they risk stacking experience on top of experience until they have built a wall that is heavy, hard to carry, and difficult to break through to recover their authentic selves.

Hospitals that embrace these practices have shown practical and tangible ways to help support the nursing staff. One example highlights the use of touchpoints to invite staff to pause throughout their day. Signs on each patient door with a practice of pause to care remind staff to care for themselves before entering the patient's room. Signs above handwashing stations similarly offer a way to use the time to center and set an intention and cleanse both their hands and their minds. Other hospitals have created space on each unit where the staff can step away for a moment to care for themselves without having to leave the unit. These serenity rooms illustrate that the hospital cares about the nurses and is encouraging them to care for self as well (ANA, 2019; Crewe, 2016; Lee et al., 2020; Salmela et al., 2020; White, 2016).

Another Unitary Caring Science best practice comes from a hospital recognizing that building self-care practices occurs both within and outside of a shift. The Caritas Council at one organization decided to bring the practices of Unitary Caring Science to the nurses during work hours. The Caritas Coaches created Caritas Circles, a safe space for caregivers to come together and share the emotional facets of being a nurse. Over six months, the Caritas Circles convened and together learned about Unitary Caring Science, including the practices of pausing, being present, and finding peace, all while building a community of support. Measuring the results revealed the contribution these reflective practices have for nurses. The data demonstrated a significant increase in how participating nurses treated themselves with loving-kindness, practiced self-care as a means for meeting their own basic needs, created a caring environment that helped them flourish, and valued their own beliefs and faith, allowing for personal success (Griffin et al., 2021).

LISTENING IN THE LEARNING ENVIRONMENT

Extending the Caritas (Griffin et al., 2021) or Healing Circle (Baldwin & Linnea, 2010) format to educational settings provides a valuable tool for creating a safe space for learning. The primary difference between a Caritas and a Healing Circle is that the former is facilitated through the lens of Caring Science. The formats and intentions are the same. This type of format creates a restorative space that involves bringing learners together to share their thoughts and feelings in a respectful and nonjudgmental manner. Connecting in this manner helps build trust and foster a sense of community. In addition, it promotes emotional well-being by providing a space for learners to share their experiences. This can be particularly helpful for learners who may be struggling with personal or academic challenges. By practicing actively listening to and sharing with their peers, learners better understand one another's perspectives and experiences. This approach to teaching-learning creates a more inclusive and supportive learning environment, builds a sense of community, fosters a culture of respect and understanding, and creates an environment where learners are empowered to share their thoughts and ideas (White-Trevino et al., 2021). It creates a safe learning space as a foundation for brave learning spaces where learners engage in more complex, challenging, and controversial aspects of healthcare. Transitioning from safe to brave learning spaces is explored further in Chapter 6.

The format, shown in Figure 4.2, is conducive to building caring literacy, expanding ways of knowing and knowledge development, and practicing person-centered care, professionalism, and personal and professional development.

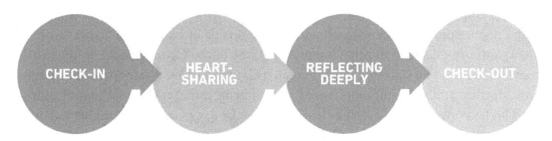

FIGURE 4.2 Healing Circles.

CHECK-IN

A learning environment that applies a circle format begins with a welcome and *check-in*, which allows educators to listen and assess the learner's state of being and mirrors how they approach interactions with patients. At the beginning of class, this involves the educator welcoming each learner. Once class begins, the educator genuinely expresses care by asking how they are, perhaps by asking what is on their heart or mind. This can be accomplished through direct questions such as "What is on your heart today?" or through a more artistic question such as "If you were a color, what would you be?" or "What is your weather report today?"

HEART-SHARING

The next component of the circle is *heart-sharing.* Applied to the learning environment, it is an opportunity for learners to share their thoughts, feelings, and experiences. This is typically done in a semi-structured format, with each learner given a set amount of time to share their perspective. During heart-sharing, learners are encouraged to listen to each other, offering support and validation as needed. The focus is on creating a safe and supportive space where participants can speak openly and honestly about their thoughts and feelings without fear of judgment or criticism. The educator may provide prompts or questions to help guide the sharing, but ultimately it is up to each learner to decide what they want to share. This can include personal experiences, insights, struggles, hopes, or anything else that feels relevant or meaningful to them. The goal is to create a space for authentic and vulnerable sharing, promoting emotional healing, self-reflection, and personal and professional growth. By sharing their experiences, participants can gain new perspectives and deepen their connections, compassion, and understanding.

Importantly, this approach supports the neuroscience of learning, recognizing that our brains use existing neural connections to process and store new information effectively. It also supports the development of personal, experiential, and ethical knowledge, which needs to be addressed in deference to empirical knowledge alone. When learners share based on their knowledge and experience, their brains can use existing neural connections to process and store the new information more effectively. This is because the new information can be integrated into existing schemas or mental frameworks that learners already have in place (Bresciani Ludvik, 2016).

REFLECTING DEEPLY

The third component of a circle learning format is *reflecting deeply* or harvesting. In the circle learning format, this is the process of reflecting on and synthesizing the insights, understandings, and experiences that have emerged during the class related to a topic or theme. Reflecting deeply or harvesting typically involves a group discussion, during which participants share their thoughts, feelings, and insights. The educator naturally asks open-ended questions or provides prompts to encourage participants to reflect on their experiences and connect them to readings and broader themes or issues. The goal is to help learners better understand themselves and their relationships and incorporate new knowledge and the broader social and cultural contexts in which they live. It is also intended to help develop strategies for applying the insights and learnings gained to their lives outside the class.

CHECK-OUT

The final component of a circle format is *check-out*. It is a time for learners to reflect on their experience and offer any final thoughts, insights, or takeaways. It is an integral part of learning, as it provides closure and an opportunity to share what they learned, why it matters, and how they plan to apply it. The educator may also ask for feedback, including what worked well and what could be improved. Like the check-in, check-out is typically done in a structured format, with each participant given a set amount of time to share their perspective. The educator may also offer closing words or a reflection before class ends. It can also be one word where learners express gratitude, offer support, and deepen their connections with each other. By reflecting on the course and sharing their thoughts and feelings, participants can leave the space feeling more connected, supported, and empowered.

REFLECTIVE SUMMARY

This chapter provided a deep exploration of presence and space in caring as the foundation for becoming a deep listener and reflective practitioner. It focused on intentional deep listening practices to expand caring consciousness for self and others. This form of listening allows us to understand both our own needs and the needs of those for whom we care, promoting personal and professional growth and healing. The lens of Unitary Caring Science demonstrates how listening and reflecting through the 10 Caritas Processes is a guide for developing caring literacy. Caring Science and caring literacy demonstrate living the AACN Essentials domains of Knowledge Development; Person-Centered Care; Professionalism; and Personal, Professional, and Leadership Development; and abiding by the latest ANA definition of nursing. Drawing from the knowledge and experiences of reflective practitioners, this chapter guides and enhances the capacity for listening to self and others in academic and practice settings.

LEARNING NARRATIVE

A new nurse, Maria, sees the call light go off in a patient's room and gets up to respond. This patient, Victor, was traveling from South Africa to find a medical solution for an ongoing and debilitating health crisis. It is just he and his mother who made the journey because of finances. Another nurse on the unit remarks, "Beware. I just saw the patient's mom enter the room. You know what happened last time she was here." Maria enters the room to find the mother of her 25-year-old patient standing next to the enteral feeding pump and bag. Before Maria can say anything, the mother, who understands English but speaks with a deep accent, begins to yell that she has found some dirt on the inside of the feeding bag. She yells that Maria is incompetent and is trying to harm her son. She demands to see the manager of the unit and wants to fire Maria immediately. Maria knows that what appears to be dirt inside the bag is a new ferrous sulfate supplement ordered this morning and added to the feeding before the family had arrived. Maria quickly explains this to the mother, but her anger doesn't subside; it only heightens her resolve to explain that the bag is dirty and that no one cares that her son is receiving dirty food, that this is not the first time she has complained about the food, and how no one on this unit cares about her son until she gets angry and demands it. After several minutes of hearing insults and shouldering all the anger, Maria decides to leave the room. She finds the charge nurse to explain that the mother would like a different nurse. The charge nurse explains that it is not possible to change assignments at the moment, but when she has time, she will go into the room and talk with the patient and family to try and smooth things out. Twenty minutes later, the call light goes off again, and the mother demands to see Maria immediately. Maria is standing outside of the room, knowing that the charge nurse has not been in yet, and is trying to find the courage to open the door.

1. Imagine what would be running through your mind if you are in this nurse's shoes. What is your intention when you enter this room for the second time, carrying with

you the first experience? How deep does the hurt go for you? How do you prepare yourself to open the door?

2. Notice if your first thoughts are to be able to explain, rationalize, or set the record straight with the mother. Are there parts of you that want to be heard? Do you want to convince the mother that you and the other nurses care about all the patients? Does letting this moment go unresolved diminish you in any way or affect your ability to care authentically?

Now imagine using the practices we reviewed in this chapter to inform and repattern the potential outcomes of this scenario. Notice we say *potential outcomes* because even when we show up as the best versions of ourselves, we cannot control the response of others. The practices of Unitary Caring Science help us understand that when the best version of ourselves show up, the outcome is secondary. What matters is authentically living out who we are meant to be, making the unique difference we are called to make, and having peace within knowing that we did not contribute to reducing another human being in any way. No simple ask, especially when you are asked to do this while others may fail. This is why nursing is not just a profession; it is a calling. It is why Jean Watson says nursing sustains another until they can do it for themselves.

1. Apply the practices of pause, presence, and peace to repattern this experience.

2. What is a meaningful pause you can take before entering a patient room that could be filled with tension? Think about what you might need to do first to care for yourself. Perhaps take a breath, talk it over with a fellow nurse, get a drink of water, or let them know you will be in in a few minutes so you can gather your thoughts.

3. What intention do you want to set before entering this room? Perhaps it is the ability to listen deeply without needing to correct what is said. Perhaps it is a practice of equanimity, where you set an intention not to own any negativity and keep an internal boundary of what you accept as fact vs. perception. Perhaps you intend to infuse the environment with dignity for everyone, including yourself, so that you know when it is time to listen, respond, and step away if necessary.

4. What will you need to stay present with the patient and the mother? Is there a practice you know that can help you settle in? Does it help to ask them to sit down with you? Do you need permission to take notes, so you capture everything? What will you do if you find you are distracted? How will you reset or re-center yourself?

5. How will you work to find the peace you need after this experience? Will you take a few moments to process this? Will you find another nurse and ask them to listen to

you? Will you allow yourself space in the moment to set it down and set an intention to talk it out or write about it later?

Now imagine a Unitary Caring Science approach to this scenario.

As Maria stands at the door, she takes a moment to pause and take a deep breath. She reflects on the words the mother had said about her son's food being dirty and wonders what that meant to this mother. She imagines that if she walked into a room of a loved one and assumed the care was subpar, how vulnerable, guilty, and out of control that would make her feel. She looks beyond the words and imagines what it would be like to be in a foreign place with language and cultural differences and tries to imagine being trusting and at ease within those barriers. Maria sets an intention of listening to this mother with the only intention of helping her suffer less at this moment—to ease her burden and make sure the mother can feel this nurse's authentic presence and care.

As she opens the door, the mother points to the pump and remarks coldly that it was beeping and that maybe Maria can at least manage that. She then asks when another nurse will take over her son's care. Maria notices that she needs to reset after hearing this remark and takes a nice slow breath to remember her intention. She asks the mom if this was an OK time for them to talk and invites her to sit down with her in the window seating area. Reluctantly, the mother joins her. Maria praises the mother for fighting so hard for her son's care and tells her she admires how much she loves him. Then she asks if she could help her understand what she meant when she said that her son was receiving dirty food. This gives the mother permission to explain that in their home, they could not always afford the best food for their large family. They often had to resort to buying food that wasn't fresh or past the expiration, sometimes even using the scraps of other people's meals to feed themselves. She said that she believes this is why her son is having so many difficulties and blames herself for his poor health. Within minutes, Maria can now see a bigger picture of pain, guilt, and the redemption this mother needs. While not excusing the behavior, it gives a new lens to process it through. Maria then asks the mother what she needs to trust the nurses taking care of her son. The patient's mother shares that the food is always prepared outside the room, so she never sees the packages or process, and she imagines that because they are from another country, they are not getting the same as other patients. Maria shows the mother where the food is stored, how new feeding bags are opened, and what safeguards are in place to ensure the enteral food was prepared to the highest of standards. The mother had no idea how many steps had happened before the pump was brought into the room.

After the shift, Maria sits quietly in her car before driving home. She allows herself to reflect on all the events of the day and her experiences within them. With just one patient, she felt a continuum of emotions from frustration and fear to compassion and understanding. Each emotion required something from her, and she notices that she was physically and emotionally drained. She then reflects on the ways she showed up that she was proud of and the real moments when her ego and survival brain took over. Overall, she is proud of herself for the courage she found to go back into the patient's room and the new perspective she learned by setting the intention of dignity. She does a practice to set down the shift and, as usual, turns on some loud music to sing her way home and let go of being a nurse so she could also be human. The next shift, Maria notices that she has this patient again and finds herself looking forward to seeing the patient, Victor, and his fierce mother.

REFLECTIVE QUESTIONS

1. How well do I listen to others? Assess your listening skills and attention to the other's words, tone, and body language.

2. How do I process and reflect on what I hear from others? Examine an interaction to assess how you take time to pause and reflect on what was said or quickly move on to the next topic. What steps can I take to deepen my reflective practice and become a more intentional listener?

3. Recall an encounter. What are my assumptions about the person I am listening to, and how might these assumptions impact my ability to hear and understand what they are truly saying?

4. How do I respond to difficult or uncomfortable conversations? How do I stay present and engaged, even when the conversation is challenging?

5. How can the 10 Caritas Processes guide me in listening and responding?

6. What micropractices can I use to improve my listening skills and stay fully present in conversations? How can I practice listening to others in more mindful, attentive, aware, and empathetic ways?

REFERENCES

American Association of Colleges of Nursing. (2021). *The essentials: Core competencies for professional nursing education.* https://www.aacnnursing.org/Portals/42/AcademicNursing/pdf/Essentials-2021.pdf

American Nurses Association. (2021). *Nursing: Scope and standards of practice* (4th ed.).

Baldwin, C., & Linnea, A. (2010). *The circle way: A leader in every chair.* Berrett-Koehler.

Bresciani Ludvik, M. (2016). *The neuroscience of learning and development: Enhancing creativity, critical thinking, and peace in higher education.* Stylus Publishing.

Crewe, C. D. (2016). *The Watson Room: Managing compassion fatigue in clinical nurses on the front line*. https://scholarworks.waldenu.edu/dissertations/2531/.

Dinc, L., & Gastmans, C. (2013). Trust in nurse-patient relationships: A literature review. *Nursing Ethics, 20*(5), 501–516. https://doi.org/10.1177/0969733012468463

Griffin, C., Oman, K. S., Ziniel, S. I., Kight, S., Jacobs-Lowry, S., & Givens, P. (2021). Increasing the capacity to provide compassionate care by expanding knowledge of caring science practices at a pediatric hospital. *Archives of Psychiatric Nursing, 35*(1), 34–41. https://doi.org/10.1016/j.apnu.2020.10.019

Horton-Deutsch, S., & Anderson, J. (2018). *Caritas coaching: A journey toward transpersonal caring for informed moral action in healthcare*. Sigma Theta Tau International.

Kafle, S., Paudel, S., Thapaliya, A., & Acharya, R. (2022). Workplace violence against nurses: A narrative review. *Journal of Clinical Translational Research, 8*(5), 421–424.

Lee, D., Batra, C., & Knutson, M. (2020). *Evaluation of a renewal room for nurses*. DNP Project.

Logstrup, K. (1997). *The ethical demand*. University of Notre Dame Press.

Palmer, P. (1993). *To know as we are known: Education as a spiritual journey*. Harper.

Plett, H. (2020). *The art of holding space: A practice of love, liberation, and leadership*. Friesens.

Salmela, L., Woehrle, T., Marleau, E., & Kitch, L. (2020). Implementation of a "serenity room": Promoting resiliency in the ED. *Nursing Management, 50*(10), 58–63. https://doi.org/10.1097/01.NURSE.0000697160.77297.06

Sitzman, K. (2007). Teaching-learning professional learning based on Jean Watson's Theory of Human Caring. *International Journal of Human Caring, 11*(4), 16–18. https://doi.org/10.20467/1091-5710.11.4.8

Tolle, E. (2005). *A new earth: Awakening to your life's purpose*. Penguin Books.

Watson, J. (2003). Love and caring: Ethics of face and hand—An invitation to return to the heart and soul of nursing and our deep humanity. *Nursing Administration, 18*(18), 197–202.

Watson, J. (2008). *Nursing: The philosophy and science of caring* (Rev. ed.). University of Colorado Press.

Watson, J. (2018). *Unitary caring science: The philosophy and praxis of nursing*. University of Colorado Press.

Watson, J., & Browning, R. (2012, August 11). Caring science meets heart science: A guide to authentic caring practice. *American Nurse*. https://www.myamericannurse.com/viewpoint-caring-science-meets-heart-science-a-guide-to-authentic-caring-practice/

Watson, J., & Browning, R. (2019). Caring science and heart science: A guide to heart-centered praxis. In W. Rosa, S. Horton-Deutsch, & J. Watson (Eds.), *A handbook for caring science* (pp. 119–131). Springer.

Watson, J., & Smith, M. C. (2002). Caring science and the science of unitary human beings: A trans-theoretical discourse for nursing knowledge development. *Journal of Advanced Nursing, 37*(5), 452–461. https://doi.org/10.1046/j.1365-2648.2002.02112.x

White, J. (2016). *'Renewal rooms' fight nurse burnout and stress*. http://www.healthcarebusinesstech.com/nurses-renewal-rooms

White-Trevino, K., Blackburn, A., Amin, R., & Rosa, V. (2021). Culture of care in a school of nursing: Faculty embark on a quality improvement plan. *International Journal of Human Caring, 26*(4), 1–11.

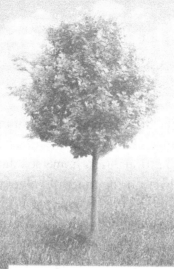

CHAPTER 5

DEEPENING OUR FOUNDATIONS: REIMAGINING OURSELVES, REIMAGINING NURSING IDENTITY

–*Gwen Sherwood, PhD, RN, FAAN, ANEF*
Meg Moorman, PhD, RN, CNE, ANEF
Crystal Morales, MS, BSN, RN

LEARNING OBJECTIVES/SUBJECTIVES

- Develop reflective practices for attending to self as nurse for increasing self-awareness.

- Cultivate strategies for renewal in contributing to healthy work environments that promote well-being.

- Catalyze development of organizational well-being programs to reimagine emotional and organizational support in managing the intensity of nurses' work.

- Reimagine nurses' education and development based on Unitary Caring Science for sustaining well-being and growth over their professional career.

- Foster well-being for thriving in post-pandemic healing.

OVERVIEW

Nursing is the care of people in all the dimensions of being human. Nursing is more than a rational practice based on exploding scientific evidence; it carries an emotional labor as well, melding affective and empirical rationalities. Immersed daily in the drama and nuances of human lives, nurses intervene in lives during times of vulnerability. As nurses internally process events in their work, sustaining their own capacity for care, compassion, love, listening, acting, and responding is challenging while also continually building their own personal and professional development. As essential healthcare team members in the COVID pandemic, nurses' personal and professional reservoirs of strength and sustenance have been tested. It is timely to reconceptualize nursing's value proposition to realize the full potential of what it is to be a nurse, to care for and to be cared for (Porter-O'Grady & Pappas, 2022).

Reconnecting to our disciplinary roots through Unitary Caring Science provides a moral-philosophical-theoretical foundation and a meaningful way to thrive as a discipline. Grounded in the consciousness and clarity of Unitary Caring Science, a relational ontology of connectedness and belonging of all living things, moves humanity closer to a moral community where we care for self and others. A singular focus on biomedical-technical science with a separatist worldview focuses on task orientation and fails to capture the human element of nursing and healthcare, which exacts an emotional and physical toll on nurses (Watson, 2016). Integrating Unitary Caring Science as the foundation for the discipline of nursing provides a road map for interpersonal practice where there is both being and doing, transforming healthcare with a relational way of being that sustains our shared humanity.

This chapter is theoretically guided by the concepts and practices of Unitary Caring Science in exploring work environments for creating and sustaining nurses' well-being through "attention to self as nurse." Caring for self is a way of finding restoration from the heavy work demands situated in a complex environment and systematically working to make sense of practice events in sustainable ways across one's professional journey. The chapter provides resources for reimagining self as nurse through reflective practices derived from narrative inquiry, mindful practice, and appreciative inquiry in developing emotional intelligence and an array of reflective practices applied to self-care that cultivate relationships for improving how we work and grow together. Micropractices describe well-being strategies for individual and organizational models to help nurses apply reflective practices to make sense of the complexities of their work.

SUPPORTING EVIDENCE AND THEORETICAL FRAMEWORKS

Professional practice is based on melding multiple types of knowledge and multiple applications in practice. The complexity manifests in the need to adapt to evolving situations, participate in interprofessional teams, and work with patients and families from multiple cultures with differing health beliefs and values. Theory-based nursing practice provides structure for knowledge development, acquisition, and application. Unitary Caring Science helps inform transformational education, utilizing reflective practices to promote well-being and practice development.

UNITARY CARING SCIENCE: DEVELOPING CARING PRACTICES

Nursing is a complex set of interactions with patients, families, and other members of the caregiving team. Nursing is characterized as a caring practice that is based on science but guided by the moral art and ethics of care and responsibility. Empirical knowledge alone cannot answer certain questions about humanity (people, families, communities) and what it means to care, to be human. Conventional science is designed for providing empirical evidence and less about specific individual responses that offer insights into the depth of human experiences such as pain, joy, suffering, fear, forgiveness, or love. Other ways of knowing provide an "in-depth exploration of humanity learned through self-knowledge, self-discovery, and shared human experiences, combined with the study of human emotions and relations that mirror our shared humanity" (Watson, 2008, p. 20).

Unitary Caring Science emphasizes a set of universal values including kindness, concern, and love for self and others (Watson, 2016). As nurses mature through reflective and mindful practices, they are able to cultivate an awareness and intentionality to sustain a guided vision for life and work. The practice of loving-kindness toward self and others honors the gift of being able to give and receive with a capacity to love and appreciate all of life's diversity and the individuality of each person. These emotions and experiences are the essence of what makes us human and deepens our humanity and connection with the human spirit. This awareness connects us to our source, breath, the gift of life, and where we access energy and creativity for living and being. Through this process, we let go of the ego-self and recognize that we all belong to the universe of humanity and all living things. The relationship-centered moral and ethical view of nursing recognizes the "privilege place of nursing," in contrast with the biomedical view, which concentrates on the science that often dominates education and practice.

DEVELOPING PROFESSIONAL IDENTITY: MAKING SENSE OF PRACTICE

Nursing is a complicated and multifaceted profession that sets high demands in preparing learners for the profession. Education has often overemphasized knowledge and skills with less emphasis on understanding human sciences and how to use that knowledge in person-centered care. Nurses are taught ideal practice during their academic preparation, but they may not have adequate preparation in coping with realities of practice that often do not match the textbook portrayal. Making sense of contradictions in practice often creates *cognitive dissonance,* an unsettling of the mind deriving from conflicting values, beliefs, or events. Making moral and ethical choices in the midst of real-world complexities is not simply an objective, detached exercise. Nurses call on multiple ways of knowing how to tailor care—within both objective science undergirding evidence of care standards and individualized care for a particular patient and family—a critical-thinking process that is part of forming professional identity (Sandvik & Hilli, 2023).

Caring theory provides a foundation for developing professional identity formation so that learners see themselves within a broader perspective, with mutual support in the professional formation of becoming a caring nurse. Through an exploratory study, Jaastad and colleagues (2022) identified essential elements for learners in developing professional identity using reflective practices. Written reflections were analyzed to understand how reflection grounded in caring theory deepened the students' understanding of caring and their professional formation of becoming a caring nurse. Three themes emerged: understanding of caring by developing a language for caring; an understanding of seeing the person behind the illness; and increasing self-understanding and awareness of oneself as a caring nurse. Instruction in caring theories and participation in reflection groups, with reflection grounded in caring theory, has a key function in facilitating students' development of a language for caring in nursing and appropriation of caring theory.

A study by Sandvik and Hilli (2023) found that instead of focusing on reinforcing particular skills, clinical nursing education should focus on learning reflective, critical thinking and the ways of being and becoming a nurse to better prepare nurses for real-world practice. In the rapidly changing world of the 21st century, an understanding-based education is needed as a more meaningful and authentic approach. Therefore, an ontological turn in nursing education, towards both doing and being, is the best education for a practice-based discipline:

> Professional identity is developed through a self-understanding as a nurse along with experience in clinical practice and understanding of practice roles. Personal and professional factors can influence its development, the self, the role itself, and the context of practice. (Rasmussen et al., 2021, p. 7)

Nurses learn and grow throughout their careers as a mark of professionalism. The shock of transitioning to practice is lessened through professional identity formation developed as part of their formal education. Habits of questioning help nurses continually examine and develop insights into the real-world nurse role and ease the transition to practice. Content-based formal learning helps develop knowledge and skills, but nurses still must assimilate the norms, values, and attitudes that guide "thinking like a nurse" and help make sense of practice, and simultaneously develop their own self-care practices.

Nurses' development follows a continuum from novice to expert as they develop higher levels of comprehension of the complexities of practice. Novice nurses often feel disconnected or out of place because they do not yet fully understand the scope of their work with real patients. Novice nurses feel pressed to demonstrate their skill know-how as a way to demonstrate their competence to feel comfortable in the work environment and gain acceptance as team members; confidence comes with competence as part of professional identity and working in a supportive environment. As nurses gain experience, they begin to develop *practical* or *tacit knowledge*—learning from everyday experience—that allows continuous adjustment and refinement of textbook knowledge.

KNOWING AND NAVIGATING THE CONTEXT OF WORK ENVIRONMENTS

Understanding and developing professional identity while adjusting to the context of nurses' work environments can be disorienting. The increasingly complex practice environment requires evidence-based decisions to manage care, but uncertainty in applying what one knows, how to speak up, and ways to be a part of the care team creates tension in the transition to practice. While nurses have a compelling need for an empirical knowledge base for practice, content overload in many curricula suppresses the opportunity to develop reflective and critical-thinking skills to balance evidence with person-centered care sensitivity. Reflection can be the first step in the evidence-based nursing process for weighing the evidence itself, making the crucial decision to honor patients' values and beliefs even in the light of evidence, or allowing answerable questions to surface to improve care (Johnson, 2022). To develop learners who become users of all forms of evidence, nurse educators must nurture habits of the mind that cultivate reflection in and on a person-centered practice framework.

Finding a balance of rational thinking with caring ideals in the real world of practice is critical to avoid burnout, a common cause of nurse turnover. Dissatisfaction often results from working in controlling environments that stifle questioning and limit the ability to find the balance within the rational and affective dimensions, to learn coping skills to make sense of the intensity of working with human beings, and to resolve frustrations from the gap between theory and actual practice. Registered nurse turnover is a serious economic issue in the healthcare industry in almost every country (International Council of Nurses, 2022). Economics are only one side of the issue; the loss of human capacity through emotional drain cannot be measured in economic terms.

The context in which practice takes place is multifaceted, complex, and often contradictory. Making sense of practice is a critical element in how nurses process their work, find meaning and purpose, and feel a sense of belonging that leads to satisfaction in work. The nursing practice environment has a social embeddedness expressed in the unit culture and work routines in the formal and informal way that work gets completed (Sherwood, 2003). New nurses on the unit find it confounding to absorb both the social and political contexts to integrate into a practice framework that makes sense to them (Scheel et al., 2021). To instill the habit of inquiry, having nurses continually questioning through reflection-on-action (see Chapter 2) can help them determine outcomes of work events by asking questions such as the following:

- What did I do?

- What should I have done that I did not do?

- How would I act differently? What could I do next time?

Dearmin (2000) includes an exemplar on the value of reflection to make sense of practice and to handle the stress of a particularly difficult day at work. Nurses can use reflection to sort out "the good and the bad bits of the day and the whole situation" (p. 163) and to integrate the evidence derived from research on which to base interventions. "Rather than just do things," it is "integrating research, theory and practice. If I am not happy about a certain way of doing something, I'll go read about it, get the research, talk to people and question things rather [than just do it without a reason]. It [reflection] was helpful because it proved to me that I did know what I was doing and I did have the skills and knowledge to handle the situation" (Dearmin, 2000, p. 163).

The high stakes of nursing results in high stress that, if not managed, risks emotional fatigue that affects nurses, organizations, and patients (Xie et al., 2021). Nurses who feel respected and supported by their management team and colleagues experience feelings of compassion satisfaction, leading to greater engagement and care towards their patients. Compassionate care is fundamental to nurses' identity and nursing care (Younas & Maddigan, 2019). Caring educators and clinical leaders help remove organizational barriers that limit compassionate care delivery. Systematically addressing nurses' needs to successfully balance physical care with compassionate nursing care contributes to nurses' well-being (Patrician et al., 2022) and improves the patient experience (Jakimowicz et al., 2018).

> Well-being at work refers to a nurse's positive assessment of oneself and their contribution to nursing work, operating at their best self with ability to adapt and overcome adversity and relates to both individual and organizational well-being. (Patrician et al., 2022, p. 7)

The increased stress induced by the COVID-19 pandemic on nursing and midwifery students was mitigated by social support and resilience in controlling their negative emotions, reducing emotional fatigue, and increasing their well-being. Well-developed resilience can reduce compassion fatigue (Li et al., 2023). Accordingly, resilience-based interventions should be developed to reduce compassion fatigue.

Reflection is essential for students to learn and understand caring as core for their formation as human and caring beings and meeting patients in a caring way. Learning support focused on understanding caring and becoming caring nurses facilitates nursing students' development into caring professionals. Instruction in caring theories, participation in reflection groups with reflection grounded in caring theory, and caring role models guide learners' development in caring literacies. Appropriation of caring theory helps nurses see themselves within a broader perspective of meaning and purpose and provides mutual support for becoming a caring nurse.

ATTENDING TO SELF AS NURSE

Nursing is a value-laden profession. Working in congruence with values leads to inner reward and meaning, giving purpose to life. The dissonance that comes when work is incongruent with values robs the joy of meaningful work, diminishing emotional energy. Nurses are humans as well, so making sense of practice is guided by how well we attend to ourselves as person and nurse. Our actions are guided by our internal compass (Freshwater, 2008). Self-development to stay true to our internal compass helps manage the emotional work inherent in nursing. Engaging in reflective practice promotes self-care, develops leadership capacity, improves responses through emotional intelligence, and develops mindfulness to engage in work activities, factors that contribute to safe, quality patient care (Horton-Deutsch, 2016).

DEVELOPING SELF-AWARENESS AND MINDFUL PRACTICE

Reflective practice skills to make sense of practice take time to develop, and still nurses must develop confidence in the technical aspects of care to begin to feel competent to meld objective and subjective knowing to understand the context of the patient's illness experience and develop trust in their decision-making. Reflective practice is a growth strategy inherent in developing professional identity. Figure 5.1 presents a framework for reflecting to enhance personal and professional growth as adapted from Patel and Metersky (2021).

Reflection is an asset in the sense-making process and in approaching patient care with a sense of what is right and honoring the "privilege place of nursing." Willis and Sheehan (2019) added spiritual knowing as an important means of patient and clinician well-being and feeling whole. *Spiritual knowing* refers to human beings' perceiving and appreciating nonmaterial spiritual qualities and experiences that provide meaning and purpose, awareness of a greater reality, and uplifting of the human spirit. Nonmaterial spiritual qualities and experiences foster a sense of well-being. Spiritual knowing incorporates patience, compassion, hope, forgiveness, humility, gratitude, unity, love, and connection to the sacred/divine as individually defined in ways that uplift the spiritual consciousness of humans, promoting a sense of well-being.

Contreras et al. (2020) reported self-reflective practices have positive effects on academic learners in decreasing stress and anxiety and increasing learning, competency, and self-awareness of nursing practice using written and verbal reflections and other forms. Chang and Chen (2020) reported the effects of integrating a strategy using reflective assessment, engagement, and action-reflection to develop health promotion among nursing students.

Hagerman et al. (2020) reported a link of self-compassion to providing compassionate care, personal well-being, resilience, and emotional intelligence while supporting indicators of academic success. A key recommendation is to include compassion literacy, mindfulness training, and experiential exercises into nursing curricula to enhance compassion in nursing students for self and others, applied within a supportive organizational environment.

Younas and Maddigan (2019) call for academic nursing and professional practice settings to foster students' compassion and to build environments cultivating a compassionate care culture. Reflective practice is an effective professional development tool used in clinical practice for learners and nurses. Educators and employers are encouraged to provide space and opportunities to instill multiple strategies for developing professional practice, including open-ended questions, reflecting privately and with others for peer support, responding to case studies or unit discussion of cases, and journaling (Scheel et al., 2021).

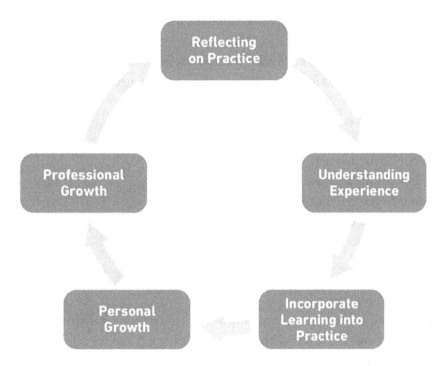

FIGURE 5.1. Reflecting for personal and professional growth.
Source: Adapted from Patel and Metersky (2021)

Reflection helps develop self-awareness, an essential aspect of emotional intelligence (Horton-Deutsch & Sherwood, 2008; Sherwood & Horton-Deutsch, 2008). Reflection provides insights into behavior and responses and contributes to self-management and self-improvement by examining relationships with self and others. Importantly, it encourages the spirit of inquiry as an important link to quality care.

EMOTIONAL INTELLIGENCE

Emotional intelligence is the ability to monitor our own and others' feelings and emotions, to discriminate among them, and to use this information to guide thinking and actions.

Mindfulness is the basic social process for working through difficult situations (Horton-Deutsch & Horton, 2003). Mindfulness allows individuals to become fully aware of perceptual experiences (O'Haver Day & Horton-Deutsch, 2004). Becoming fully engaged through mindful presence allows one to think through with reflective responses rather than lapsing into habitual behaviors that might perpetuate and intensify situations. Habits developed from the processes of emotional intelligence—self-awareness, awareness of others, empathy, motivation—can guide one in reflective response (Horton-Deutsch & Sherwood, 2008). With openness and curiosity about our experiences, mindfulness leads to greater awareness and insight. Reflection-in-action involves paying attention to the moment-to-moment experience and exploring thoughts, feelings, bodily sensations, and critical judgments. Reflection-in-action and mindfulness help nurses develop insight into how perceptions shape actions, identify and understand other people's viewpoints, and incorporate this knowledge into more deliberate and effective responses. Chapter 2 describes the different phases of reflection in more depth.

REFLECTIVE MINDFUL PRACTICES

Reflective mindful practices guide personal and professional growth through consciously caring for self while simultaneously pursuing professional goals; it becomes a way of being.

RELATING TO OTHERS

Personal development is the basis of transformative leadership. Transformative leaders influence the connection of the self with others. Reflection provides a mirror to the self by helping to confront and work to resolve actual and desired work practices. To understand the work environment, leaders call upon their emotional intelligence to manage responses by considering the impact of three facets of the workplace environment: consciousness of context, self, and others, as illustrated in Figure 5.2 (Shankman & Allen, 2008).

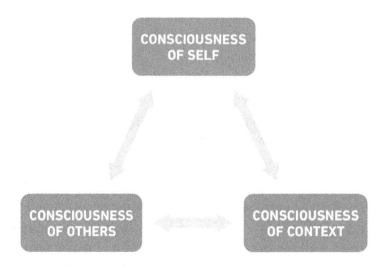

FIGURE 5.2. Three facets of leadership to develop emotional intelligence to manage the work environment.

Source: Shankman & Allen, 2008

- **Context:** The work environment combines setting and situation. Setting is the structure of the organization. Situation includes the many different forces of a particular time and place, such as individual personalities, organizational politics, and tensions or challenges within the setting. Changing context relies on unique sets of knowledge, skills, and attitudes for situational awareness.

  - *Reflection:* What are the informal traditions and values of the group? Does your style of leadership and practice fit within the culture?

- **Self:** Self is knowing who you are, what you stand for, your strengths and limitations, and how your responses and actions impact others. Emotional self-perception, honest self-understanding, healthy self-esteem, emotional self-control, authenticity, flexibility, achievement, optimism, and initiative are facets of self.

  - *Reflection:* What knowledge, skills, and attitudes do you bring to the organization or activity? What would others say are your strengths and weaknesses?

- **Others:** Consciousness of others is awareness of coworkers and how relationships are working. The facets include empathy, citizenship, inspiration, influence, coaching, change agents, conflict management, relationships, teamwork, and capitalizing on differences.

  - *Reflection:* How does consciousness of others impact each of these facets of the work environment: leadership styles, teamwork, and the unit culture?

REFLECTIVE NARRATIVES: REIMAGINING SELF AND NURSING

Studies validate how learners and nurses use narratives in developing professional identity and enhance knowledge development. Increasing use of narratives can help educators observe how learners address challenges in practice and develop decision-making as they develop their professional practice (Alteren, 2019). Choperena et al. (2019) described three areas for narrative development: looking back to past experiences, creating space for dialogue, and bridging theory and practice. Chapter 7 includes a more detailed exploration of narratives, visual thinking, and reflection.

LEARNING FROM NARRATIVES

Rasmussen et al. (2021) encourage critical thinking through telling and interpreting stories to make sense of and explain what they see in practice, thus interpreting concerns, intents, and motives. Narrative reasoning creates deep understanding of the patient as both a patient and a person. Narrative is an important tool of reflection. It supports exploration of the context of caring, which fosters caring knowledge and skills in all situations (Choperena et al., 2019). Sharing stories of experiences helps turn the experience into practical knowledge and a deeper understanding of events, which forms a basis for future meaningful responses (Alteren, 2019).

Appreciative inquiry is a positive change process to consider how to work with others by thinking of times that have worked well. Narrative approaches fit well with appreciative inquiry guided by the following set of reflective questions:

- What happened?

- How do I make sense of the situation?

- What was meaningful?

- What questions did I ask, and how did I ask them in a patient-centered way?

- When and how did I know I had connected with the other person?

- How can I do it again to make it an integral part of my practice?

Processes for developing reflection-on-action are virtually unlimited. *The Scholarship of Reflective Practice* position paper (Sherwood et al., 2005) provides international perspectives for incorporating reflective learning both for self-development and educational programs, with details on using a myriad of reflective strategies. Narratives associated with aesthetics (such as drawing, painting, montage, poetry, a literature vignette, role-playing, or other creative endeavors) are innovative possibilities.

Sherwood (1997) described using movies as a narrative device examining and understanding the human condition. Analyzing a movie or story using a structured reflective format for examining the central characters, the underlying motivations, and how each character responded helps develop capacity for working with others. Movie nights provide an opportunity to enhance teamwork while having a focused discussion to analyze the meaning of the storyline within the context of the ethical and spiritual dimensions of the plot to gain human understanding applicable in practice.

These narrative devices offer another language through which we can connect to another. Sharing aesthetic ways of knowing helps us reach into our innermost thoughts and feelings to surface values and attitudes that are so much a part of how we respond to others. By reflecting on the meaning found in the language of poetry, the message conveyed in a painting, or the human narrative in stories or movies, we can better appreciate how others respond to contextual and interpersonal cues, experiencing renewal in our professional dimensions. Thus, we can mindfully embrace the development of our emotional intelligence as we seek self-awareness, self-regulation, self-motivation, and empathy through various aesthetic approaches individually or collectively.

WRITING TO LEARN

Evidence shows that recording meaningful events in reflective journals can be an effective way to evaluate the experience and promote learning (Choperena et al., 2019; Scheel et al., 2021). Learning through reflective journaling helps to stimulate learning through analysis, discussion, and documentation of critical incidents. Journaling helps the learner's personal growth through increasing self-awareness for interacting with others as described in Chapter 9. Writing can help separate oneself from the experience to be able to see it through a new lens. Having a systematic approach to guide the stories within the journal establishes clear aims and purpose. Reflective writing leads to deeper thinking, a way of speaking in one's own voice. Writing preserves one's thoughts about events that are lost during life and helps plot developmental processes, as both an assessment and evaluation that is consistent with principles of adult education (Cranton, 2006).

In addition to reflective journals, written critical incidents, narratives of work encounters, or case study analysis, learners can audiotape stories from practice as an alternative to writing and use a reflective guide as they listen to the story (Patel & Matersky, 2019). These written accounts are different from a clinical log, which is merely the recording of actions without including reflection on the experience.

VISUAL THINKING STRATEGIES

Visual arts or paintings provide a way for nurses to connect and share aesthetic knowing. Art can transform people and encourage them to think in different ways. Exposing nurses to art can allow them to engage in deep, meaningful discussions and practice discussions and debate. It also allows them the opportunity to develop critical thinking and reasoning. Museums offer safe learning environments free from hierarchy and status, providing a place to employ reflection and discussion. Visual Thinking Strategies (VTS) is a teaching tool developed to engage art museum visitors to discuss art. *Visual literacy* is the ability to understand and use images as representations for thinking and learning (Fransecky & Debes, 1972), and, through VTS, participants can practice expressing their observations to others.

Educational theorist Lev Vygotsky developed the socio-cultural theory of learning supporting the concept of *scaffolding,* or supporting learning based on each other's ideas and knowledge evident in VTS. The concept of thinking out loud, purported by Vygotsky, involves verbalizing one's thoughts and rationale for an idea or interpretation, which can inform others who can listen and learn from others' thought processes (Vygotsky, 1971). VTS helps develop problem-solving and observational skills, regulate one's own thinking process, and listen to other viewpoints. The act of thinking out loud and reflecting on artwork are powerful social interactions that demonstrate critical thinking and reasoning.

Abigail Housen and Phillip Yenawine created VTS as a teaching technique based on three questions posed by a VTS facilitator regarding a work of art:

- What is going on in this piece?

- What are you seeing that makes you say that?

- What more can we find?

USING VISUAL THINKING STRATEGIES FOR REFLECTIVE LEARNING

To provide space for nurses to openly talk about the artwork, choose pieces that reflect diverse content. A painting that reflects cultural differences or racial issues can represent situations that nurses may need to talk about or reflect on. Using a VTS facilitator, have nurses gather and take a few moments to look at the work of art. Then, the facilitator will ask the group, "What is going on in this painting?" As a person responds, the facilitator will ask, "What are you seeing that makes you say that?" After responding, the facilitator will paraphrase back what the participant said, then ask the group, "What else can we find?" After each person in the group has responded, the facilitator can ask, "What were the three questions I posed?" What did you notice about what the facilitator did with each person's response? What was the correct answer? (Groups will note that there is no one right answer and that each person's interpretation is honored and respected.) How can you use this in your nursing? What did you notice about how the group responded? These questions allow the group to interact and think out loud about a situation and draw conclusions about the process. This debriefing can inform the group and help to identify cultural differences noted in the painting and allow nurses to discuss a cultural scenario together. The practice of gathering and working on interpretations together allows the nurses to listen to each other and work to understand cultural differences and similarities. Many art museums have VTS training and offer docents with experience in VTS discussions.

Art museums provide safe places to explore and learn because there is no hierarchy, and nurses can be in serene spaces away from the chaos of a bustling unit where hierarchy and critical decisions abound. Analyzing artwork through VTS develops reasoning and lets nurses practice expression, share their opinions, and develop insight and interpretation. Because interpretations can be so varied, nurses can explore meanings of works of art and disagree or agree based on visual evidence and discussion. The act of holding disparate beliefs or interpretations is critical in today's world and important as nurses face patients who hold differing political and healthcare beliefs. Art affords nurses the opportunity to consider others' viewpoints without judging or disparaging those whose beliefs are different (Moorman et al., 2017).

RETHINKING SELF-CARE TOWARDS WELL-BEING

Nurses are often challenged in balancing their own personal health and well-being with their dedication, commitment, and passion for improving the lives of others. Distress, depression, and burnout often result from the work environment and culture, as well as challenges with prioritizing self-care. Distress and burnout among nurses have been associated with compassion fatigue, poor sleep quality, trouble concentrating, limitations in performing mental or interpersonal tasks, time-management challenges, workplace bullying, lower productivity, absenteeism, increased turnover, and compromised quality of care provision and quality of life (Della Bella et al., 2022; Melnyk, 2022). Evidence demonstrates that *modifiable factors* associated with increased burnout include negative perceptions of support and value in the workplace, inadequate academic preparedness to meet professional challenges, inadequate coping skills, and interactions with coworkers who are experiencing significant emotional demands (Melnyk, 2022).

Nurses and other healthcare providers experienced extreme stress as the COVID-19 pandemic swept across the world. Even prior to the pandemic, nurses were experiencing emotional fatigue, absenteeism, and high turnover (Melnyk, 2022). Investing in work environments to improve organizational well-being directly impacts nurses' engagement in their work (Della Bella et al., 2022). Organizations need a paradigm shift to demonstrate support for nurse well-being by integrating well-being into every facet of the organization from mission and vision, work policies, safety metrics, and attending to broken systems and processes. Leaders help create and sustain well-being cultures when they role-model health and well-being, communicate clearly, cultivate caring and connections, and provide easily accessible well-being programs.

Patrician et al. (2022) also reported that nurses' well-being is affected by a complex interaction of the contextual components of the work environment and personal life environment. Chung et al. (2021) developed the Well-being Health-Promoting Lifestyle and Work Environment Satisfaction model with three fundamental elements: well-being, a health-promoting lifestyle, and work environment satisfaction. Well-being is a multi-dimensional subjective concept that leads to life satisfaction associated with healthy lifestyle and job satisfaction and may be measured by feelings of contentment and joyfulness.

Stress is a part of life that wears at one's sense of well-being. Five types of harmful stress can be summarized as traumatic, grief, moral, wear and rear, and self-doubt, shown in Figure 5.3.

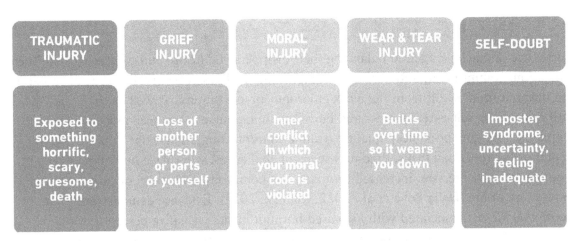

FIGURE 5.3 Five types of stress injury.

Hope is an essential aspect of recovery from stress injury. Five essential factors can promote recovery from adversity and stress: a sense of safety, calming, connection with others, self-efficacy, and hope. These can be developed through the activities in the sidebars.

HOPE

Feeling a sense of being able to overcome and something to look forward to enhances the capacity to recover from stress and trauma.

MICROPRACTICE: STRATEGIES FOR CREATING WELL-BEING

Challenges are a universal experience. To manage stress for daily renewal and well-being, everyone needs habits of self-care, covering a range of activities:

- *Set boundaries and realize that "No" is a complete sentence!*
- *Take care of the physical self through exercise, nutrition, relaxation techniques, and sleep hygiene.*
- *Use attitude adjustment strategies such as spiritual care practices, social encounters, positive self-talk, or connecting with people who encourage healthy habits and positive attitudes.*
- *Maintain a gratitude journal to promote a positive attitude; use reflective prompts such as recording three good things that happened on your shift, or three things you are grateful for today. Reflect on the balance of satisfaction of fulfilling work duties and the personal cost to be able to make changes as appropriate.*
- *Appreciate your strengths by reducing negative self-talk, instead talking to yourself as you would to someone you love.*
- *Normalize responses to difficult situations.*
- *Recognize and seek what you truly need to be effective in your work.*
- *Reduce guilt and let go of the "tyranny of the shoulds." When you feel the "should" creeping in, ask yourself:*
    - *Does this really matter to me?*
    - *Do I have the energy for this right now?*
- *Focus your energy on things you have control over, provide input where you have influence, and learn to ignore and accept that there are things that you can neither control nor influence.*
- *Be a part of creating a supportive, caring work environment by providing social support to coworkers.*

MICROPRACTICE: PEER SUPPORT GROUPS

Offering one-on-one peer support during high-stress times or scheduling group debriefings using a common process to guide discussion in productive communication can reduce whining or gripe sessions.

- *Peer support may include statements such as:*
  - *"I will sit here with you."*
  - *"Can I call someone for you?"*
  - *"You don't have to do this alone."*
- *Reassuring statements may include:*
  - *"You are not alone."*
  - *"I understand why you might feel that way."*
  - *"You are going to get through this, but it will take time."*

Peer support also means there are things not to say! Do not be overly reassuring or dismissive of someone's dissonance.

- *Do not use platitudes such as:*
  - *"These things happen."*
  - *"It could always be worse."*
  - *"You know this always happens in this place."*

MICROPRACTICE: FISHBOWL CHECK-IN—GROUP DEBRIEFING OF AN EXPERIENCE

- *Critical incidents record snapshots of the daily work of nurses, providing a lens for examining opinions, personal actions, judgments, and beliefs. Select events in which the intervention made a difference, went well, captured the essence of nursing, was particularly demanding or satisfying, or could have been handled differently.*

Reflect on a work event where you were personally distressed by an unanticipated patient outcome or an event that created distress among your team. Elements to include in the narrative can also provide a basis for discussion similar to Morbidity and Mortality (M and M) rounds:

- *The context of where and when it happened*
- *What happened*
- *Why it was significant*
- *What concerns there were at the time*
- *What you were thinking about and feeling at the time and afterward*
- *What choices did you make and why? What else could have happened if other choices had been made?*
- *Understand the WHYs not the WHOs*

CREATING CULTURES OF WELL-BEING

Many workplaces are now focusing on strategies to improve quality of life among nurses through workplace well-being and mindfulness-based strategies to enhance coping and self-care. Participating in well-being activities, such as mindfulness-based stress reduction, is associated with reduction in stress, improved coping, and better empathy among nurses and nursing students (Della Bella et al., 2022). More specifically, nurses and nursing students who participated in mindfulness courses reported improvements in well-being, relaxation, life and job satisfaction, feelings of personal accomplishment and coping skills, and reductions in anxiety, stress, perceptions of time pressure, emotional exhaustion, and burnout symptoms (Della Bella et al., 2022).

Innovative initiatives are transforming nursing work environments. For example, planned naps are being tested at several hospitals, primarily for nurses working 12-hour night shifts as part of a diffusion of innovation; research is needed to measure effectiveness and application in other shifts (Drake & Malcuit 2021).

INSTITUTIONAL WELL-BEING PROGRAM

One school of nursing created a well-being program with a mission to promote quality of life, workplace well-being, and overall well-being among students, faculty, and staff (Giscombe, 2017). The goal is to facilitate a sustainable culture of well-being within the school, model ongoing reflective practices, and help nurses develop self-care practices for all stages of career development. Creating habits of ongoing reflective practice is the foundation for developing practice, expanding professional expertise, and encouraging attention to wholeness of mind, body, heart, and spirit. Learners experiencing role-modeling during their academic programs can adopt these habits for lifelong well-being practices. Nurses' commitment to caring for patients often overshadows the imperative for attention to self, contributing to stress, burnout, and compromised health. The model is adaptable in all settings for transforming practice to a culture of balancing caring for others with caring for self. Examples of activities include:

- *An annual Nursing Well-being and Quality of Life workshop including clinical partners and campus community.*
- *Nursing Well-being and Quality of Life content integrated into core courses in academic programs, particularly in courses focusing on population health, professional development, and role development.*
- *"Morning Mindfulness" sessions for faculty, students, staff, nurses from clinical partners, and others.*
- *Chair massages in collaboration with local massage therapy school available for students, faculty, and staff.*
- *Partner with campus recreation programs to provide fitness and health-promoting initiatives in the school of nursing including yoga sessions, healthy eating socials, and well-being workshops.*
- *Cultivate an ambiance of tranquility and well-being through posters, bulletin boards, and video messaging.*
- *Teach and model "well-being language" to replace "martyr language" among nurses, students, faculty, and staff. For example, replace "I only slept four hours last night" or "I did not use the bathroom for four hours" with "I make sure that I take a mobility break each day to stand or walk for 15 to 30 minutes" or "I took a nap for 10 minutes in the break room to refresh to be ready for afternoon tasks!" or "I scheduled a walking meeting to break traditional meeting habits and encourage creative thinking."*
- *Well-being competitions challenging physical fitness or well-being activities such as comparing steps per day or stairs climbed each week.*

APPLICATION FOR PERSONAL AND PROFESSIONAL DEVELOPMENT

Reflection builds emotional intelligence to monitor feelings, to discriminate among emotional reactions, and to use the information to guide future responses and actions. Debriefing with colleagues after a stressful situation can help put events in perspective and build reflective capacity. By remaining open to their experiences, clinicians develop expertise when they test and refine propositions, hypotheses, and principle-based expectations in actual practice situations. Experience, therefore, can provide career and personal development. The link between reflection and confidence acknowledges the synergy between competence, confidence, experience, and reflection (Dearmin, 2000).

Johns (1995) developed a model of structured learning to account for multiple ways of learning. He offers reflective questions as cues to guide learning based on aesthetic, personal, ethical, empirical, and reflexive ways of knowing. Nurses can use these questions along with reflective narratives such as journaling, critical incident reports, or aesthetic experiences. A model such as Johns' (see Table 5.1) can serve as a guide to multiple ways of knowing and facilitate ongoing professional development.

TABLE 5.1 REFLECTIVE QUESTIONS: MAKING SENSE OF PRACTICE	
FRAMEWORK OF KNOWING	**REFLECTIVE QUESTIONS**
Aesthetic	What was I trying to achieve?
	Why did I respond as I did?
	What were the consequences to others and how did they feel?
Personal	How did I feel?
	How was I influenced by my internal beliefs and values?
Ethical	How did my actions match my values and beliefs?
	What influenced me to act incongruently with my beliefs and values?
Empirical	What evidence informed how I acted?
	Did I ignore evidence that should have guided my actions?
Reflexivity	How are my actions in this situation connected with previous behaviors?
	How can I handle future situations better?
	How can I anticipate the consequences to others if I change how I act in the future?
	How has this changed my ways of knowing?

Source: Adapted from Johns' (1995) Model of Structured Learning Using Ways of Knowing

REFLECTIVE SUMMARY

Reflective practice is an important self-development strategy for continuing growth, making sense of our work, and applying innovative change methods. Reflection provides a systematic way of thinking about our actions and responses to change future actions and responses. Reflective practice guides our learning from experience by considering what we know, believe, and value within the context of an event. Systematic analysis through reflection contributes to sense-making to see the whole; the continuing journey helps us evaluate our contributions, leading to greater satisfaction and sense of purpose in our work. Developing reflective practice is a lifelong journey that supports and sustains career development. Reflection helps clarify how we work according to our sense of mission and purpose and as such guides us in developing the spiritual resources for managing and balancing our personal and professional lives.

LEARNING NARRATIVE

Attending to self: Using the art of clay to deepen our foundation (adapted from Parker, 1994).

Purpose: Practice mindfulness through stillness as a personal growth strategy to focus on self in wholeness, who you are as person and nurse, to support and encourage reflection on values, attitudes, beliefs, and renew your state of being.

Premise: Aesthetic expression leads us into "inner knowing places," into our creative connection within our self, and expands our situational awareness.

Method: Alone or with participants, sit quietly with soft, unobtrusive music in the background. Hold a piece of clay in your hands and begin to warm it to a softened state. Then work with the clay in any way you want—kneading it, opening, circling, pinching, or pounding—simply be in the moment. Clear any preconceived notions or barriers about creating art. Shaping the clay is getting in touch with yourself working from inside out. Breathe slowly, in and out, using principles of reflection, and go into a place within yourself where you reach beyond to transcend to your undiscovered affective dimensions, often crowded by the rational self.

Reflection: The aliveness of clay as an organic, natural matter emerges into a form; meaning emerges into consciousness. Listen to your inner voice as you come out of the shaping experience. What is surfacing from your soul? Share with others in the group; write your experience as a critical reflection, a poem, or other narration to enhance the feelings of renewal and self-awareness, better able to meet realities around you.

REFLECTIVE QUESTIONS

1. What are ways you commit to cultivating renewal for self-care?

2. What are three ways your workplace can offer peer-to-peer support?

3. How can you help catalyze development of a well-being focus on your work environment?

4. How can organizations offer support for new graduates transitioning to practice, facilitating first-year integration to reduce turnover?

5. What are steps in designing a group session for debriefing critical incidents useful as part of a unit well-being initiative?

REFERENCES

Alteren, J. (2019). Narratives in student nurses' knowledge development: A hermeneutical research study. *Nurse Education Today, 76,* 51–55. https://doi.org/10.1016/j.nedt.2019.01.015

Chang, Y.-Y., & Chen, M.-C. (2020). Using reflective teaching program to explore health-promoting behaviors in nursing students. *The Journal of Nursing Research: JNR, 28*(3), e86. https://doi.org/10.1097/jnr.0000000000000358

Choperena, A., Oroviogoicoechea, C., Zaragoza Salcedo, A., Olza Moreno, I., & Jones, D. (2019). Nursing narratives and reflective practice: A theoretical review. *Journal of Advanced Nursing, 75*(8), 1637–1647. https://doi.org/10.1111/jan.13955

Chung, H.-C., Chen, Y.-C., Chang, S.-C., Hsu, W.-L., & Hsieh, T.-C. (2021). Development and validation of nurses' well-being and caring nurse–patient interaction model: A psychometric study. *International Journal of Environmental Research and Public Health, 18*(15), 7750. https://doi.org/10.3390/ijerph18157750

Contreras, J. A., Edwards-Maddox, S., Hall, A., & Lee, M. A. (2020). Effects of reflective practice on baccalaureate nursing students' stress, anxiety and competency: An integrative review. *Worldviews on Evidence-Based Nursing, 17*(3), 239–245. https://doi.org/10.1111/wvn.12438

Cranton, P. (2006). *Understanding and promoting transformative learning: A guide for educators of adults.* Jossey-Bass.

Dearmin, N. (2000). The legacy of reflective practice. In S. Burns & C. Bulman (Eds.) *Reflective practice in nursing: The growth of the professional practitioner* (2nd ed., pp. 156–172). Blackwell Science.

Della Bella, V., Fiorini, J., Gioiello, G., Zaghini, F., & Sili, A. (2022). Towards a new conceptual model for nurses' organizational well-being: An integrative review. *Journal of Nursing Management, 30*(7), 2833–2844. https://doi.org/10.1111/jonm.13750

Drake, D.. & Malcuit, M. (2021). To nap or not to nap? *American Nurse, 16*(10), 92–94.

Fransecky, R. B., & Debes, J. L. (1972). *Visual literacy: A way to learn—A way to teach.* Association for Educational Communications and Technology.

Freshwater, D. (2008). Reflective practice: The state of the art. In D. Freshwater, B. J. Taylor, & G. Sherwood (Eds.), *International textbook of reflective practice in nursing* (pp. 1–18). Blackwell Science.

Giscombe, C. (2017). Textbox 11.1. In S. Horton-Deutsch & G. Sherwood (Eds.), *Reflective practice: Transforming education and improving outcomes* (2nd ed.). Sigma Theta Tau International.

Hagerman, L. A., Manankil-Rankin, L., & Schwind, J. K. (2020). Self-compassion in undergraduate nursing: An integrative review. *International Journal of Nursing Education Scholarship, 17*(1). https://doi.org/10.1515/ijnes-2020-0021

Horton-Deutsch, S. (2016). Open and visionary: Remaining open to the possibilities of nursing praxis. In W. Rosa (Ed.), *Nurse leaders: Evolutionary visions of leadership*; pp. 311–322. Springer Publishing Company.

Horton-Deutsch, S. L., & Horton, J. M. (2003). Mindfulness: Overcoming conflict. *Archives of Psychiatric Nursing, 17*(4), 186–193.

Horton-Deutsch, S., & Sherwood, G. (2008). Reflection: An educational strategy to develop emotionally competent nurse leaders. *Journal of Nursing Management, 16*(8), 946–954. https://doi.org/10.1111/j.1365-2834.2008.00957.x

International Council of Nurses. (2022). *The global nursing shortage and nurse retention*. Author.

Jaastad, T. Ueland, V., & Koskinen, C. (2022). The meaning of reflection for understanding caring and becoming a caring nurse. *Scandinavian Journal of Caring Sciences, 36*(4), 1180–1188. https://doi.org/10.1111/scs.13080

Jakimowicz, S., Perry, L., & Lewis, J. (2018). Insights on compassion and patient-centred nursing in intensive care: A constructivist grounded theory. *Journal of Clinical Nursing, 27*(7–8), 1599–1611. https://doi.org/10.1111/jocn.14231

Johns, C. (1995). Framing learning through reflection within Carper's fundamental ways of knowing in nursing. *Journal of Advanced Nursing, 22*(2), 226–234. https://doi.org/10.1046/j.1365-2648.1995.22020226.x

Johnson, J. (2022). Quality improvement. In G. Sherwood & J. Barnsteiner (Eds.), *Quality and safety in nursing: A competency approach to improving outcomes* (3rd ed., pp. 155–184). Wiley-Blackwell.

Klugman, C. M., Peel, J., & Beckmann-Mendez, D. (2011). Art rounds: Teaching interprofessional students visual thinking strategies at one school. *Academic Medicine, 86*(10), 1266–1271. http://dx.doi.org/10.1097/ACM.0b013e31822c1427

Li, J.-N., Jiang, X.-M., Zheng, Q.-X., Lin, F., Chen, X.-Q., Pan, Y.-Q., Zhu, Y., Liu, R.-L., & Huang, L. (2023). Mediating effect of resilience between social support and compassion fatigue among intern nursing and midwifery students during COVID-19: A cross-sectional study. *BMC Nursing, 22*(1), 42. https://doi.org/10.1186/s12912-023-01185-0

Melnyk, B. M. (2022). Shifting from burnout cultures to wellbeing cultures to improve nurse/clinician well-being and healthcare safety: Evidence to guide change. *Worldviews on Evidence-Based Nursing, 19*(2), 84–85. https://doi.org/10.1111/wvn.12575

Moorman, M. (2017). The use of visual thinking strategies and art to help nurses find their voices. *Creative Nursing, 23*(3), 167–171. https://doi.org/10.1891/1078-4535.23.3.167

Moorman, M., Hensel, D., Decker, K. A., & Busby, K. (2017). Learning outcomes with visual thinking strategies in nursing education. *Nurse Education Today, 51*, 127–129. https://doi.org/10.1016/j.nedt.2016.08.020

O'Haver Day, P., & Horton-Deutsch, S. (2004). Utilizing mindfulness-based therapeutic interventions in psychiatric nursing practice—Part II: Mindfulness-based approaches for all phases of psychotherapy. *Archives of Psychiatric Nursing, 18*(5), 170–177. https://doi.org/10.1016/j.apnu.2004.07.004

Parker, M. (1994). The healing art of clay: A workshop for remembering wholeness. In D. A. Gaut & A. Boykin (Eds.), *Caring as healing: Renewal through hope* (pp. 35–145). National League for Nursing Press.

Patel, K. M., & Metersky, K. (2021). Reflective practice in nursing: A concept analysis. *International Journal of Nursing Knowledge, 33*(3), 180–187. https://doi.org/10.1111/2047-3095.12350

Patrician, P. A., Bakerjian, D., Billings, R., Chenot, T., Hooper, V., Johnson, C. S., & Sables-Baus, S. (2022). Nurse well-being: A concept analysis. *Nursing Outlook, 70*(4), 639–650. https://doi.org/10.1016/j.outlook.2022.03.014

Porter-O'Grady, T., & Pappas, S. (2022). Affirming nurses' value. *Nursing Outlook, 70*(3), 361–364. https://doi.org/10.1016/j.outlook.2022.03.006

Rasmussen, P., Henderson, A., McCallum, J., & Andrew, N. (2021). Professional identity in nursing: A mixed method research study. *Nurse Education in Practice, 52*, 103039. https://doi.org/10.1016/j.nepr.2021.103039

Sandvik, A.-H., & Hilli, Y. (2023). Understanding and formation—A process of becoming a nurse. *Nursing Philosophy: An International Journal for Healthcare Professionals, 24*(1), e12387. https://doi.org/10.1111/nup.12387

Scheel, L. S., Bydam, J., & Peters, M. D. J. (2021). Reflection as a learning strategy for the training of nurses in clinical practice setting: A scoping review. *JBI Evidence Synthesis, 19*(12), 3268–3300. https://doi.org/10.11124/JBIES-21-00005

Shankman, M. L., & Allen, S. J. (2008). *Emotionally intelligent leadership: A guide for college students.* Jossey-Bass.

Sherwood, G. (1997). Developing spiritual care: The search for self. In M. S. Roach (Ed.), *Caring from the heart* (pp. 196–211). Paulist Press.

Sherwood, G. (2003). Leadership for a healthy work environment: Caring for the human spirit. *Nurse Leader, 1*(5), 36–40. https://doi.org/10.1067/S1541-4612(03)00107-1

Sherwood, G., Freshwater, D., Taylor, B., & Horton-Deutsch, S. (2005). *The scholarship of reflective practice* [Position paper]. Sigma Theta Tau International. http://www.nursingsociety.org/docs/default-source/position-papers/resource_reflective.pdf?sfvrsn=4.

Sherwood, G., & Horton-Deutsch, S. (2008). Reflective practice: The route to nursing leadership? In D. Freshwater, B. Taylor, & G. Sherwood (Eds.), *International textbook of reflective practice in nursing* (pp. 157–176). Oxford, England: Blackwell Publishing & Sigma Theta Tau International.

Vygotsky, L. (1971). *The psychology of art.* MIT Press. (Original work published 1925).

Watson, J. (2008). *Nursing: The philosophy and science of caring* (Rev. ed.). University of Colorado Press.

Watson, J. (2016). Human caring literacy. In S. Lee, P. Palmieri, & J. Watson (Eds.), *Global advances in human caring literacy* (pp. 3–11). Springer Publishing Company.

Willis, D., & Sheehan, D. (2019). Spiritual knowing: Another pattern of knowing in the discipline. *Advances in Nursing Science, 42*(1), 58–68. https://doi.org/10.1097/ANS.0000000000000236

Xie, W., Chen, L., Feng, F., Okoli, C. T. C., Tang, P., Zeng, L., Jin, M., Zhang, Y., & Wang, J. (2021). The prevalence of compassion satisfaction and compassion fatigue among nurses: A systematic review and meta-analysis. *International Journal of Nursing Studies, 120*, 103973. https://doi.org/10.1016/j.ijnurstu.2021.103973

Younas, A., & Maddigan, J. (2019). Proposing a policy framework for nursing education for fostering compassion in nursing students: A critical review. *Journal of Advanced Nursing, 75*(8), 1621–1636. https://doi.org/10.1111/jan.13946

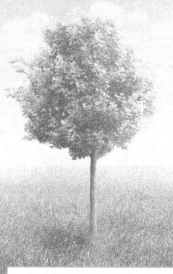

CHAPTER 6

THE ROLE OF REFLECTION IN GUIDING THE EVOLUTION OF CARE, COMPASSION, AND SOCIAL CHANGE

–Erica Hooper, DNP, RN, CNL, CNS, PHN
Sara Horton-Deutsch, PhD, RN, FAAN, ANEF, SGAHN

LEARNING OBJECTIVES/SUBJECTIVES

- Examine reflective practice skills and strategies for expanding the capacity for compassionate care for self and others.

- Explore theoretical frameworks that guide care and compassion for self, others, community, and society.

- Demonstrate the value of personal experiences and stories as an inner teacher for guiding personal and professional development.

- Prioritize habits of self-care and self-compassion as the foundation to authentically care for others.

- Recognize the necessity of creating safe learning spaces as the foundation for brave learning spaces central to social change.

OVERVIEW

Care and compassion are widely acknowledged as crucial components of nursing education and practice, forming the core of nursing as a practice-based discipline (Raustøl & Tveit, 2023). The nursing profession places great emphasis on nurturing these qualities in aspiring nurses and cultivating their ability to reflect on their care for others. However, the systems and structures of education and healthcare frequently impede the development and implementation of caring and compassionate practices, which are fundamental to the discipline of nursing.

Reflective practice has been identified as a key tool for promoting compassionate care and improving the systems that hinder such practices (Horton-Deutsch & Sherwood, 2017). However, the demands of nursing combined with institutional and societal barriers, biases, and burnout limit time for reflection. Institutional support is critical to social changes promoting a culture of caring and compassion that would also fulfill the Institute for Healthcare Improvement Quadruple Aim (Arnetz et al., 2020), adding improving the caregiver work experience as equally important to other quality measures.

In this chapter, we explore the evidence supporting reflective practices and their potential to guide the evolution of care, compassion, and social change impacting nursing. By prioritizing reflective practices and recognizing their crucial role in promoting compassionate care, we can help ensure that nursing remains a profession that places care and compassion at the forefront of its practice, elevating the experience of both the care receiver and the caregiver.

REFLECTION AS A CENTRAL COMPONENT OF NURSING PRACTICE

Recent initiatives in nursing education speak to the importance of reflective practice as a method for guiding the evolution of care, compassion, and social change within the nursing profession. As a prominent nursing organization, the International Council of Nurses (2021) recognizes care and compassion as central to the practice of nursing. According to the American Association of Colleges of Nursing (AACN) Essentials (2021), all nursing education programs at any level must incorporate compassionate person-centered care, self-reflection, and self-care into curricula. Historically, however, many educational programs largely focus on skills-based learning and test-taking preparation, limiting opportunities for students to practice compassionate care for themselves and others in school and throughout their careers (Hooper & Horton-Deutsch, 2023; Mårtensson et al., 2022). Coffey et al. (2019) identified compassion and care as the two key components needed by healthcare delivery systems to provide quality healthcare. Integrating self-compassion and compassionate care into nursing education programs is essential for offering reflective, sustainable, and empathetic nursing practice (Mårtensson et al., 2022).

Reflection is an essential component of nursing practice that allows nurses to critically evaluate their actions and experiences to improve their care practices. Reflecting on clinical experiences is the basis for nursing students to develop competency and professional growth (Alsalamah et al., 2022). Through reflection, nurses gain insights into their values, biases, and assumptions that may impact how they care for patients. Reflection also helps nurses identify areas where they need to develop further skills and knowledge to provide the best care possible. Clinical supervision, in the form of reflective practice groups, can help nurses realize new perspectives of their work that can improve engagement, increase nursing work satisfaction, and counteract burnout (Sundgreen et al., 2020).

Reflection is a critical tool for improving the quality of nursing care and advancing the nursing profession toward compassionate care (Johns, 2022). Reflective practice contributes to the evolution of compassionate care and social change by encouraging nurses to challenge the status quo and advocate for policies and practices that prioritize patient-centered care. To reinforce learning across the professional continuum, incorporating reflective practice into nursing education and continuing education programs, nurses can develop reflective skills for examining their experiences, facilitating growth as compassionate and caring healthcare professionals. Nursing is a high-stress profession operating in ever-changing healthcare environments. Reflection is foundational as nursing students develop their professional practice. Learning reflective skills improves self-awareness, enhances well-being, and develops resilience.

SUPPORTING THEORETICAL FRAMEWORKS AND OTHER EVIDENCE

Four scholars—Watson, Neff, Noddings, and hooks—have been instrumental in challenging the traditional notions of education by developing more caring, compassionate, inclusive, and empowering approaches that value inclusivity, diversity, creativity, and critical thinking.

Caring Science and the 10 Caritas Processes focus on developing a caring relationship and being compassionate (Watson, 2018). By promoting self-care and growth, authentic presence, allowing for the expression of positive and negative feelings, creative problem-solving, creating a healing environment, assisting with basic needs, engaging in spiritual practices, using reflective practice, and honoring the unique individuality of each patient, nurses expand their capacity for compassionate care. Implementing these processes with intention and authenticity enhances the patient's overall well-being and promotes a sense of healing and wholeness in both the patient and the nurse.

Dr. Kristen Neff is a leading influence in developing self-compassion. Neff emphasizes the importance of treating ourselves with kindness, care, and understanding. Self-compassion involves three main components: mindfulness, common humanity, and self-kindness. *Mindfulness* means being aware of our thoughts and feelings without judgment or criticism, while *common humanity* recognizes that all human beings experience suffering and struggle in life. Self-kindness involves treating ourselves with warmth, empathy, and forgiveness rather than harsh self-criticism. Practicing self-compassion can lead to greater emotional resilience, increased well-being, and stronger relationships with others (Neff, 2011).

Building care and compassion within academic and practice settings demonstrates the importance of relationships. Nel Noddings (2013), an educational philosopher, made significant contributions to curriculum design, particularly in the caring curriculum. Traditional curricula overly focused on intellectual development and neglected education's emotional and ethical ways of knowing. Noddings' caring curriculum emphasizes the importance of relationships and the development of empathy, compassion, and responsibility in students. Curricula centered on caring involves emotional and intellectual engagement with the subject matter and the people involved.

The writer, educator, and social activist bell hooks (1994) emphasizes the importance of education as a tool for social change and liberation. hooks developed critical pedagogy, which seeks to empower students to think critically about their experiences and the world around them, similar to both transformative education and emancipatory learning discussed elsewhere in this book.

Stressing the need for education to be more than just the acquisition of knowledge and skills, critical pedagogy involves a critical examination of the social and cultural systems that shape our lives, leading to a process of self-discovery and personal transformation (Van Schalkwyk et al., 2019). By encouraging students to challenge the status quo and think critically about their experience, education can be a powerful tool for social justice and empowerment.

THE VALUE OF PERSONAL EXPERIENCE AND STORIES

Personal experiences and stories are valuable tools applied in reflective learning in a meaningful context for the promotion of care and compassion. Listening to stories allows learners to relate to the experiences of others, empathize with their struggles, and gain insight into different perspectives and ways of thinking; learning becomes more engaging and memorable for future recall and application of their value. Stories help make abstract concepts more concrete and easier to understand by providing a vivid and relatable illustration of how concepts work in practice. Personal experiences and stories create a sense of community and belonging in the learning environment. By sharing their stories with others, individuals can create connections and build trust with their peers, which helps create a supportive and collaborative learning environment.

Murray and Tuqiri (2020) describe the value of storytelling for nurses and midwives for person-centered compassionate care and the development of the Heart of Caring framework incorporating four themes: connecting human to human, engaging as a team, fostering self-care and well-being, and creating positive workplace cultures. Roddy et al. (2021) explore storytelling to support practice innovation and discuss how storytelling can help practitioners deepen understanding and curiosity in a way that inspires change in practice.

Storytelling is a tool used within appreciative inquiry to help people develop a shared understanding that promotes community and sustainable change. *Appreciative inquiry* is an example of an organizational framework that is strength-based and focuses on what is going well within an organization through the phases of discovery, dream, design, and destiny to encourage practice improvement, effective collaboration, cultural transformation, and innovative change (Naca-Abell, 2020). Appreciative inquiry as a reflective approach to working with others is explored in Chapter 15.

Hooper and Horton-Deutsch (2023) scaffold a personal experience/storytelling paper in their wellness course to evaluate health professions students' personal/professional development and mastery of course content. The critical reflection paper invites learners to share their personal/professional experiences through the Describe, Examine, and Articulate Learning (DEAL) model (Ash & Clayton, 2009). DEAL asks learners to describe a personal or professional experience with a rich description of the story. Next, they are given specific reflection questions in the "Examine" section to facilitate the exploration of multiple perspectives and biases that may be present. After completing the "Examine" section, "Articulate Learning" questions are responded to in the final section of the paper to prompt deeper reflection and articulations of new understandings, enhanced communications, and critical thinking. The DEAL assignment can be used in multiple ways—for personal/professional development, civic engagement, or academic advancement—and has established psychometrics and a rubric. For the authors' purposes, students write the Describe at the beginning of the semester and complete the Examine and Articulate Learning at the end of the semester where they have the opportunity to incorporate course readings and insights gained throughout the semester. The DEAL sidebar explains this model further.

DEAL

DEAL (Describe, Examine, and Articulate Learning) is different from your typical academic paper. It should be written in the first person. It is an opportunity to tell your story. You will write the Describe for this assignment and the Examine and Articulate Learning at the end of the semester. Using APA format (include a cover page), write a three to four page paper in response to the following:

I. DESCRIBE: Think of a time when you, a friend, a family member, or a patient you cared for were ill and how caring influenced healing. Write the narrative/story of the experience. *This should be a three to four page thick description of the experience. You might read a thick description in a novel where the author provides details that connect you to your senses. Note: This is your story... once you start writing, it will flow, just like you are telling your friend the details of an event. This should not take much time... we want this to come from your heart.*

Now give the experience a name. The name should reflect the experience.

Name of the experience_____.

For example, Jane might name her story of using Reiki to care for her chronic pain The Power of Energy Healing.

During the final week of the semester, you will add three to four pages to the original paper through the addition of Examine and Articulate Learning sections. Begin by rereading your original paper. Now write a response using the following prompts as your inspiration (be sure to reference your two textbooks and at least one additional reading and add a reference page for the paper).

II. EXAMINE (to look closely for the purpose of learning) in fair detail the following questions. *Where you see a blank, insert the name you gave the experience. The purpose of this is to externalize the experience for examination purposes as well as deconstruct (critique dominant understandings of a particular topic—in this example, we are looking at illness).*

If _____ could talk to me, what would it say to me? For example: What would it say if The Power of Energy Healing could talk to me?

What are the main themes related to _____ embedded in the narrative?

What does _____ have you thinking about wellness practices to support healing?

What does _____ have you doing about wellness practices?

Does _____ encourage ethics/values about wellness practices?

Now, reflect on your answers and write a reflective summary statement.

III. ARTICULATE LEARNING: Respond to the following questions.

What did I learn? About myself? Healing? What I thought I thought? Etc.

How did I learn it? (Be specific. It is not sufficient to merely state what you reflected or wrote.)

Think about what it was regarding the assignment, afterward conversation, reflection, etc. that prompted your learning.

Why does it matter (personally and professionally)?

What will I do in the future, in light of it (personally and professionally)?

When you've completed your assignment, attach your Word doc for review.

REFLEXIVE PEDAGOGIES FOR GUIDING THE DEVELOPMENT OF CARE AND COMPASSION

Nursing school can be demanding through constant pressure to perform well both from didactic and workplace learning, often contributing to performance anxiety in students. Learners' responsibilities and expectations to excel in various areas, including exams, skill demonstrations, and clinical practice, can lead to stress and self-doubt. Learners worry about their ability to meet the myriad expectations of nursing school and the expectation to apply theoretical learning in both simulated practice situations and with real patients.

From the authors' experiences, learners are often hard on themselves and push themselves to be the best, causing them to strengthen their inner critic. Self-criticism can be especially damaging when combined with the stress and pressure of nursing school, as student performance and overall well-being can be impacted by negative self-talk and self-doubt. These negative habits can carry over into the nursing profession if students are not prepared to better manage their stress. To maximize positive transition, nursing students need to recognize when their inner critic is being overly harsh and develop strategies to pause, reflect, and manage their stress and anxiety.

Some ways to lessen the effects of performance anxiety in nursing school include self-care, time management, support from peers, setting realistic goals, positive self-talk, and getting support from mental health professionals (Sherwood, 2022). Focusing on one's strengths and accomplishments as well as using positive affirmations can benefit students by counteracting negative self-talk and building self-confidence. Nursing students who understand that making mistakes is a normal part of the learning process are more readily able to be kind and compassionate towards themselves as they navigate the challenges of nursing school. Introducing and guiding learners in self-care and compassion is a useful way to model the importance of improving self-care and weakening the inner critic to reduce stress and anxiety while in school and across their professional careers. During their wellness course, the authors introduce and allow students to complete a self-care plan to emphasize that care and compassion for self are the foundation for caring for others (Hooper & Horton-Deutsch, 2023). See the "Self-Care Plan" sidebar.

SELF-CARE PLAN

In the boxes below, write your self-care goals in support of the wellness of your mind, body, and spirit. Write your goals using the S.M.A.R.T. (specific, measurable, attainable, realistic, and time-oriented) format. An example would be: Starting this Sunday I will walk in the park for 30 minutes every day of the week.

My goal to support my physical wellness is

My goal to support my mental wellness is

My goal to support my spiritual wellness is

It is important to identify what may be helpful and what may be a challenge to the attainment of your goals so that you may be more focused on what you need to do to meet your goals.

The following are barriers to achieving my self-care goals (e.g., being tired at the end of the day):

1.

2.

3.

The following are helpful to achieving my self-care goals (e.g., going to the gym with a friend):

1.

2.

3.

By meeting my self-care goals, I hope to_____ (e.g., feel more peaceful):

1.

2.

3.

Nurses begin formulating their personal professional identity as they begin their academic studies. Nurses' professional identity formation is characterized by a sense of oneself in relationship with others and enacted within the norms of nursing practice (Godfrey & Young, 2020). Professional identity formation begins by developing therapeutic relationships expressed in empathy, care, and compassion. Academic nursing programs have a responsibility to model a culture of care and compassion for their learners as they grow in professional identity and professionalism (AACN, 2021). Programs can model a culture of care by emphasizing compassionate care for self and others, basing learning activities on real-world situations (Noddings, 2013), and advancing their understanding of nursing through reflective practices (Percy & Richardson, 2018). Compassion is a cognitive emotion central to nursing that is learned from role models and deepened through reflective practices (Raustøl & Tveit, 2023) and can be emphasized in simulated case studies and reinforced in debriefing.

Hooper and Horton-Deutsch (2023) provide a wellness course example of integrating the concepts of care and compassion and applying reflective practice into the educational preparation of nurses and other health professionals. The wellness course has a strong emphasis on the value of caring for self and self-compassion as essential in maintaining well-being in professional practice. Learners participate in storytelling through the DEAL assignment described earlier in this chapter, complete readings and discussions in Caring Science and self-compassion, and apply the 10 Caritas Processes to their interactions with self and in dialogue with others. Learners are assigned multiple group discussions to engage in deep listening and reflecting on the learning community. They explore concepts such as forgiveness, surrender, curiosity, gratitude, courage, and empowerment. These discussions serve to soften the inner critic and expand care and compassion for self and other. See Table 6.1 for a list of assignments students must complete in the course and Table 6.2 for learner examples of completed course assignments highlighting reflections on compassion for self and others.

TABLE 6.1 WELLNESS COURSE REFLECTION EXAMPLES FOR UNDERGRADUATE HEALTH PROFESSIONS STUDENTS	
ASSIGNMENT	**REFLECTION QUESTIONS**
DEAL (Describe, Examine, and Articulate Learning) Experience Reflection Paper	At start of course: Think of a time when you or a friend, family member, or patient you cared for were ill and how caring influenced healing. Write the narrative/story of the experience. • What is your story and why did you select this particular story? • How does this story impact your journey into the health professions? At end of course: • What does _____ have you thinking about wellness practices to support healing? • What will you do in the future (personally and professionally), in light of it?
Self-Care Practice Plan	Complete a self-care plan for yourself. • What is your current self-care practice? • What do you plan to add to your self-care practice this semester?
Caritas Group Discussion	Read and reflect on the Caritas Processes and how they appear in the health professions. Choose one Caritas Process and share an example of how it *was or was not* reflected in your clinical, work experience, or personal experience in a healthcare setting. Provide as much description as possible to explain in 250 words or less how the example relates to the Caritas Process chosen and post an image that captures the feeling of your experience.

continues

TABLE 6.1 WELLNESS COURSE REFLECTION EXAMPLES FOR UNDERGRADUATE HEALTH PROFESSIONS STUDENTS (CONT.)

ASSIGNMENT	REFLECTION QUESTIONS
Self-Compassion and Self-Care Group Discussion	Reflect on the concepts of self-compassion and self-care, and post a discussion about what they mean in your own life. Include an aesthetic representation (poem, quote picture, song, etc.) that sums up your post (approx. 250 words). Use the following questions as a guide for your post: 1. In what ways are you developing self-compassion and self-care in your own life? 2. From an intellectual/mental perspective, what makes practicing self-compassion and self-care challenging for you? 3. How do self-compassion and self-care benefit you and others, particularly those for whom you provide care?
Caring Moment Exemplars Group Discussion	• What are examples of caring moments you have witnessed, and how were others impacted? • How do you plan to create caring moments in your own practice as a health professional? • How does this practice relate to the Jesuit value of *cura personalis* (caring for the whole person)?
Commitment to Change Paper	Write a two to three page single-spaced paper (double space between paragraphs) identifying two to three possible changes you will make in your current or future professional role, identifying your level of commitment to making these changes as well as your resistance to change. Use the following questions to frame your analysis: 1. What will be your obstacles to making these changes? 2. What will be the value of making these changes? 3. How can these values help you work toward achieving this change?
Health Professional as Healing Environment Group Discussion	Reflect on your thoughts of the practice of health professionals being the healing environment. • What does this mean to you, and how can you put this into practice?

Short Video Reflections

At start of course:

- What prompted you to enroll in this course?
- What do you hope to take away from the course?

At end of course:

- What has been the greatest learning for you throughout this course?
- How has this course most impacted how you care for yourself and others?
- In what ways do you plan to continue your work in this course throughout the remainder of school and/ or into the profession?

Healing Circle Prompts

- What is on your heart today?
- How has this course influenced your development as a healthcare professional?
- Describe what it is like for you to be deeply listened to and to deeply listen to another?
- Were you able to express what is truly on your heart right now during this round?
- What deeper truth did you uncover?
- Was there something else that started to arise from your listening to yourself?
- As new beginnings call out to you, what do they say and see?
- What is holding you in this community, and how does this community support new beginnings?

REFLECTIVE QUESTIONS

1. How can you integrate the theoretical frameworks explored in this chapter into your practice as a guide for care and compassion for yourself, others, communities, and society?

2. In what ways do you incorporate self-care and self-compassion into your life? Is there more you can do?

3. Explore how your unique life experience(s) serve as a guide for professional practice.

4. What approaches do you utilize to reflect on your practice as a means for professional development?

5. In what ways can you proactively create a safe learning space that fosters vulnerability, inclusivity, and trust, and thereby supports brave conversations and actions for social change?

TABLE 6.2 STUDENT WELLNESS COURSE REFLECTION EXAMPLES	
COURSE ASSIGNMENT	**STUDENT REFLECTIONS**
Journal #1	"After completing exercise one, I noticed that I am very negative when it comes to my self-talk. I constantly call myself a 'fool' or say 'I'm so stupid' when I make a simple mistake. This exercise made me realize the consequences of talking to myself in this manner. It isn't productive at all and if anything, it puts me in more of a depressive state. I am currently on antidepressants, so doing this exercise was helpful in a way because it allowed me to identify behavior that was contributing to my depression. As a nursing student, I find myself feeling as though I have to be perfect and get straight As. I also have the bad habit of comparing myself to my peers, and feeling miserable when they do better than me on tests/assignments. This exercise showed me that I need to be nicer to myself, because negative self-talk is only doing harm to my mental health and my self-esteem."
	"Thinking through things as the self-critic reminded me of how I tend to initially be harsh on myself and cause myself to feel angry and upset. Then, thinking through things as the criticized aspect of myself makes me reevaluate the truthfulness of my judgment and criticism. Are the things I said about myself true? Did the way I criticize and judge myself align with the reality of my actions? Lastly, putting myself as the compassionate observer helped me be honest with myself and understand my emotions better. It put me in a position where I could be honest about myself in a way that was positive, open, and accepting of all the 'good' and 'bad' I often categorize myself as. I was able to take things as a whole and give myself the opportunity to be supportive of myself. Overall, both of those exercises helped me change my perspective on how I should treat and talk to myself. Being a mother, nursing student, and having other life responsibilities has caused me to develop a harsh, critical connection with myself, so this exercise allowed me to think better about myself and open up about how much good I do."

| DEAL Paper #1 | "My grandpa is a very stubborn person, which at times is one of his best qualities. When it comes to some of his treatments, however, it can make things more complicated. Caring looks different for everyone, and some people require more than others. The important thing to do is to recognize what every individual needs and meet them where they are. My grandpa requires more passive care that allows him to decide. In this way, it is very important to ensure that he keeps his independence while still making sure that he is safe and secure." |
| | "As a future nurse, I really value my experience of being injured and needing to rely on the care of another person. I got a glimpse of what it feels like to not be able to independently perform ADLs, and the feelings of embarrassment and stress that can arise from that. I will always remember that a kind and helpful caretaker allows a person to focus on healing, and to feel dignified even when they are not at their best." |

In addition, learners are introduced to presencing exercises to help provide space for them to begin undoing the "go-go-go" mentality and to start practicing "being." This exercise is a valuable aid in reducing stress, improving focus, increasing self-awareness, and ultimately, improving their ability to provide compassionate care. Each week learners are provided with a centering exercise to help them stay grounded and develop resilience for navigating life's challenges in school and beyond in their profession (see Table 6.3). One example of a centering exercise is a YouTube video (The Whole MD, 2018) that teaches students how to practice heart-focused breathing. This and similar presencing exercises give students useful self-care strategies to incorporate into their wellness routines as they continue their journey in the profession of nursing. Cultivating healthy self-care habits during their education helps nurses develop the necessary tools to take care of themselves while caring for others. It allows them to recognize the warning signs of compassion fatigue and burnout and to take proactive measures to prevent and manage these conditions. Additionally, practicing self-care helps nurses maintain their physical, emotional, and mental well-being, which ultimately leads to better patient outcomes, increased job satisfaction, and reduced turnover rates in the nursing profession.

TABLE 6.3 EXAMPLES OF REFLECTIVE PRACTICES	
METHOD	**PRACTICE**
Sacred Pause	Stop and ask yourself at any moment: 1. What do I need? 2. What am I holding onto? 3. What do I need to let go of?
Mindfulness	Come into the moment by increasing awareness of your senses through reflecting on the following: 1. What can I see? 2. What do I feel? 3. What can I hear? 4. What do I taste? 5. What do I smell?
Deep Breathing	Focus on breathing deeply in and out of the abdomen and/or heart area.
Journaling	Write your feelings down in a journal without stopping for a minimum of five minutes.
Deep Listening	Ask someone to just listen to you without responding for a minimum of two minutes and reflect on what you discover about yourself.
Centering	Start work meetings with a centering moment, such as an example of caring for someone with compassion.
Healing Circle	Hold safe space for healing and reflection guided by a host and a guardian in a structured format while promoting care and compassion among participants.
Storytelling	Write a story about an example of caring and compassion you witnessed in the clinical setting.
Critique	Read a story describing a caring moment and analyze how the delivery of care and compassion could be improved.

MOVING FROM SAFE TO BRAVE LEARNING SPACES TO GUIDE SOCIAL CHANGE

Creating safe learning spaces is crucial for learners to feel comfortable and supported while they are learning. When individuals feel safe, they are more likely to engage in the learning process and take risks in professional and personal growth. Safe learning spaces help foster a sense of community among learners and encourage them to collaborate and share ideas. Moving from safe to brave learning spaces involves creating an environment that not only provides a sense of physical and emotional safety but also encourages learners to take risks, challenge their assumptions, and confront their biases (Plett, 2020). It requires a shift from a culture of compliance to a culture of creativity, innovation, and experimentation.

Some ways to move from safe to brave learning spaces include:

- **Foster a culture of trust.** Establish a culture of trust where learners feel free to express themselves and share their ideas without fear of judgment or ridicule. Encourage learners to take risks and make mistakes as part of the learning process.

- **Encourage critical thinking.** Encourage learners to challenge their assumptions, ask difficult questions, and engage in critical thinking. This will help learners develop a deeper understanding of the subject matter and develop their own perspectives.

- **Sit with discomfort.** It is important for learners to notice when they are inclined to run. Encourage them to sit with discomfort and inquire further into it. Why is this feeling surfacing? What can they learn from it? What hidden aspect of themselves might it reveal? What growth opportunity is being presented?

- **Emphasize collaboration.** Encourage learners to collaborate and work together on projects and assignments. This will help them develop teamwork and communication skills while also learning from one another.

- **Encourage bravery.** Encourage learners to challenge themselves and move forward toward growth versus remaining stagnant and complacent.

According to WikiEducator (2012, para. 1.3), "reflexive pedagogy means strategically supporting and enabling professional learners with the knowledge and skills to change their thinking and actions in the social context in which they learn and do their work to overcome barriers and improve outcomes." The reciprocity generated by creating a culture of learning that is well-versed in reflexive pedagogy as well as caring for nurses within the profession is one where nurses will naturally lean into social change and compassion for others. Nurses have the potential to become exceptional caregivers and leaders when the systems they work, learn, and progress in prioritize listening to their voices, comprehending their needs, and providing support. Spaces for healing, learning, and reflection, such as healing circles, wellness courses, and mindfulness classes, are valuable contributors to social change and the evolution of care and compassion within the nursing profession.

One prominent example of the profession of nursing utilizing the power of reflection is the American Nurses Association Racial Reckoning Statement (2021), which acknowledges the suffering of Black and other nurses of color due to racism in the profession both from the past and present day. Through reflection, nursing was able to recognize the need for a statement to create a platform for healing, listening, forgiveness, and the restoration of harm from racism. Through the journey of racial reconciliation, deep listening is essential to those harmed to be heard and to build trust. It is important that nurses use this statement to reflect on the current profession of nursing to help influence actions necessary for changing the cycle of perpetuated systemic racism. Ask these reflective questions:

- In what ways do I contribute to and/or not contribute to perpetuating the cycle of racism in nursing?

- How can I heal the impact of racism in nursing on myself and others?

- How can caring for myself support me to hold space for listening to others share their experiences of racism in nursing?

Tutu and Tutu (2014) and hooks (1994) highlight the importance of creating brave spaces for social change. They argue that a foundation occurs through safe and inclusive learning environments that encourage open and honest dialogue and respect for diverse perspectives. Through time these conversations evolve into braver spaces where learners are prepared to challenge systemic inequalities and promote social justice and transformative change. Learners who practice this form of critical reflection and dialogue are prepared to confront uncomfortable truths and take action to address systemic oppression and injustices. Creating brave spaces requires a willingness to be vulnerable, empathetic, and courageous, demonstrating commitment to ongoing learning and growth.

APPLICATION FOR PERSONAL AND PROFESSIONAL PRACTICE

Nurses are an essential pillar of healthcare, serving as the largest and most trusted profession. Their vital role in delivering compassionate care is the cornerstone of the patient experience as defined in the Quadruple Aim (Bodenheimer & Sinsky, 2014). However, despite the love and appreciation expressed by the public, unprecedented numbers of nurses are expressing dissatisfaction, prematurely leaving the profession, retiring early, and in the most tragic cases, committing suicide. This is due to a range of complex factors, including poor management, incivility, insufficient staffing, burnout, low wages, and feeling undervalued (Shah et al., 2021). It is therefore imperative that education and healthcare systems collaborate in modeling a culture of caring and providing ongoing professional development opportunities to promote nurses' well-being amid the growing epidemic of burnout.

There is also an urgent and increasing need for nurses to give one another permission to care for themselves both personally and professionally. Indeed, nurses must recognize that self-care is not just an option but a necessity for their physical, emotional, and mental well-being. By giving each other permission to prioritize self-care, nurses create a culture that values self-compassion and self-preservation. This, in turn, enables nurses to better care for their patients and sustain their professional careers in the long term. Nurses are consistently exposed to traumatic events and emotional stressors, making it crucial that they take active steps to prevent compassion fatigue and burnout by engaging in self-care practices such as exercise, meditation, spending time with loved ones, or taking a break from work when needed. When nurses support each other in these efforts, it strengthens the entire nursing community and fosters a positive work environment that values well-being, kindness, and respect. Ultimately, promoting self-care and compassion among nurses benefits the individuals themselves and leverages a positive impact on patient outcomes, enhancing the nursing profession as a whole.

The promotion of a nursing culture that prioritizes self-care and compassion involves a multifaceted implementation of innovative and creative strategies. The social norms of nursing emphasize task orientation, efficiency, and real-time critical thinking that foster a nonstop mentality. Transitioning from a *doing* mode into a *being* mode requires intentional effort from individuals and educational and healthcare systems. Even when faced with challenging and emotionally taxing situations, nurses are socialized to prioritize their patients' needs over their own, and while this is a critical aspect of nursing care, it can lead to neglect of one's health and well-being.

Nurses who give precedence to self-care and self-compassion become more resilient and better equipped to manage the demands of nursing. This involves accepting and acknowledging one's imperfections and limitations and treating oneself with the same care and compassion that one would give to a patient. Some examples of nurses caring for themselves are taking regular work breaks, using the restroom as needed, asking for help, using sick time when not feeling well, and getting adequate sleep and exercise. Some examples of self-compassion are positive self-talk, giving oneself a hug when having a bad day, saying daily positive affirmations, writing love letters to oneself, keeping a gratitude journal, and not feeling guilty for not doing everything perfectly. By shifting the nursing culture and systems to model the value of self-care and self-compassion, the overall health and well-being of the nursing workforce will be improved, ultimately positively impacting the quality of care provided to patients.

REFLECTIVE SUMMARY

Nurses play a critical role in providing care and compassion to a world in dire need of it. To foster a culture of care and compassion, educational institutions and healthcare systems must not only develop policies and organizational structures that support nurses but also provide them with opportunities to reflect on their well-being and that of their patients. This includes promoting self-care and compassion towards themselves and those they serve. By creating an environment that values the physical, emotional, and mental well-being of nurses, organizations ensure they are better equipped to provide high-quality care to patients and sustain the professional careers of nurses.

The ever-evolving nature of the healthcare system highlights the crucial need for nurses to receive adequate resources, preparation, and support to deliver compassionate care effectively. To achieve this, it is imperative to foster a supportive nursing academic and work culture that values caring and compassion. When nurses work collaboratively in such a culture, they can provide high-quality care that contributes to optimal health outcomes and positive social change, benefiting themselves and the nursing profession. This, in turn, requires a shift in societal attitudes towards advocacy for nurses, recognizing that, as the most trusted profession, nurses can only care for others to the degree they can provide care and compassion for themselves (Watson, 2018). Nurses, like all health professionals, benefit from a social contract that ensures the well-being of everyone in the institution and society (Ginwright, 2022). By prioritizing the well-being of nurses, healthcare organizations can create an environment that promotes excellence in patient care while also supporting the professional growth and sustainability of nurses.

LEARNING NARRATIVE

Jackie is a 20-year-old BSN nursing student who has recently started the fourth year of her program. She is one month into her semester and already feeling sleep deprived, malnourished, stressed, and anxious. This semester Jackie is pleased to be taking a wellness course designed to support her learning to develop self-compassion and to take better care of herself. These concepts are new to Jackie; many of the reflective course assignments feel foreign. However, Jackie realizes she needs to change her habits and begins to incorporate new methods for thriving in school.

Jackie is relieved that her course faculty have given her permission to care for herself, as she has been so focused throughout school on caring for others, learning new skills, and passing her exams. In her wellness course she has completed a few reflection assignments emphasizing care and compassion, and she is feeling both intrigued and curious. For the first time, Jackie has become self-aware of her inner critic that often insults her worth and makes her feel bad when she doesn't get the perfect grade. She has just been given an assignment to develop a self-care plan for how she is going to care for her mind, body, and spirit over the rest of the semester. She is not sure where to begin but knows she needs to make a change to be more caring and compassionate with herself.

REFLECTIVE QUESTIONS

1. In what ways does the practice of self-care and self-compassion allow one to better care for others?

2. How does reflective practice serve as a guide for care and compassion in one's personal and professional life?

3. What do students need to learn in nursing educational programs about reflection, self-care, and self-compassion as a means for social change in nursing?

REFERENCES

Alsalamah, Y., Albagawi, B., Babkair, L., Alsalamah, F., Itani, M. S., Tassi, A., & Fawaz, M. (2022). Perspectives of nursing students on promoting reflection in the clinical setting: A qualitative study. *Nursing Reports, 12*(3), 545–555. https://doi.org/10.3390/nurserep12030053

American Association of Colleges of Nursing. (2021). *The essentials: Core competencies for professional nursing education.* https://www.aacnnursing.org/Portals/42/AcademicNursing/pdf/Essentials-2021.pdf

American Nurses Association. (2021, June 11). *Journey of racial reconciliation: Racial reckoning statement.* https://www.nursingworld.org/practice-policy/workforce/racism-in-nursing/RacialReckoningStatement/journey-of-racial-reconciliation-toolkit/

Arnetz, B. B., Goetz, C. M., Arnetz, J. E., Sudan, S., vanSchagen, J., Piersma, K., & Reyelts, F. (2020). Enhancing healthcare efficiency to achieve the Quadruple Aim: An exploratory study. *BMC Research Notes, 13*(1), 362. https://doi.org/10.1186/s13104-020-05199-8

Ash, S & Clayton, P. (2009). Generating, deepening and documenting learning: The power of critical reflection in applied learning. *Journal of Applied Learning in Higher Education,* fall, 25–48.

Bodenheimer, T. & Sinsky, C. (2014). From triple to quadruple aim: Care of the patient requires care of the provider. *Annuals of Family Medicine, 12*(6), 573–576. https://doi.org/10.1370/afm.1713

Coffey, A. , Saab, M., Landers, M. M., Cornally, N., Hegarty, J., Drennan, J., Lunn, C., & Savage, E. (2019). The impact of compassionate care education on nurses: A mixed-method systemic review. *Journal of Advanced Nursing, 75*(11), 2340–2351. https://doi.org/10.1111/jan.14088

Doran, D., Phillips, J., & Board, M. (2018). Compassionate care in the community: Reflections of a student nurse. *British Journal of Community Nursing, 25*(1). https://doi.org/10.12968/bjcn.2020.25.1.16

Ginwright, S. (2022). *The four pivots: Reimagining justice, reimagining ourselves.* North Atlantic Books.

Godfrey, N., & Young, E. (2021). Professional identity. In J. Giddens (Ed.), *Concepts of nursing practice* (3rd ed., 379–389). Elsevier.

hooks, bell. (1994). *Teaching to transgress: Education as the practice of freedom.* Routledge.

Hooper, E., & Horton-Deutsch, S. (2023). Integrating compassion and theoretical premises of Caring Science into undergraduate health professions education. *Creative Nursing, 29*(1), 1–10.

Horton, A. G., Gibson, K. B., and Curington, A. M. (2021). Exploring reflective journaling as a learning tool: An interdisciplinary approach. *Archives of Psychiatric Nursing, 35*(2), 195–199. https://doi.org/10.1016/j.apnu.2020.09.009

Horton-Deutsch, S., & Sherwood. (2017). *Reflective practice: Transforming education and improving outcomes* (2nd ed.). Sigma Theta Tau International.

International Council of Nurses. (2021). *The ICN code of ethics for nursing.*

Johns, C. (2022). *Becoming a reflective practitioner* (6th ed.). Wiley Blackwell.

Mårtensson, S. K., Knutsson, S., Hodges, E. A., Sherwood, G., Broström, A., & Björk, M. (2022). Undergraduate nursing students' experiences of learning caring using a variety of learning didactics. *International Journal for Human Caring, 37*(1), 271–281. https://doi.org/10.1111/scs.13077

Murray, S. J., & Tuqiri, K. A. (2020). The heart of caring—Understanding compassionate care through storytelling. *International Practice Development Journal, 10*(1). https://doi.org/10/19043/ipdj.101.004

Naca-Abell, K. J. (2020, October 19). Appreciative inquiry: Building teamwork and leadership. *American Nurse Journal.* https://www.myamericannurse.com/appreciative-inquiry-building-teamwork-and-leadership/

Neff, K. (2011). *The proven power of being kind to yourself: Self-compassion.* HarperCollins.

Noddings, N. (2013). *Caring: A relational approach to ethics and moral education.* University of California Press.

Percy, M., & Richardson, C. (2018). Introducing nursing practice to student nurses: How can we promote care compassion and empathy. *Nurse Education in Practice, 29,* 200–205. https://doi.org/10.1016/j.nepr.2018.01.008

Plett, H. (2020). *The art of holding space: A practice of love, liberation, and leadership.* Page Two.

Raustøl, A., & Tveit, B. (2023). Compassion, emotions, and cognition: Implications for nursing education. *Nursing Ethics, 30*(1), 145–154. https://doi.org/10.1177/09697330221128903

Roddy, E., MacBride, T., Coburn, A., Jack-Waugh, A., & Dewar, B. (2021). Moving stories: Exploring the LIFE session storytelling method as a way of enhancing innovative, generative outcomes in practice. *International Practice Development Journal, 11*(1). https://doi.org/10.19043/ipdj.111.006

Shah, M. K., Gandrakota, N., Cimiotti, J. P., Ghose, N., Moore, M., & Ali, M. K. (2021). Prevalence of and factors associated with nurse burnout in the US. *JAMA Network Open, 4*(2). https://doi.org/10.1001/jamanetworkopen.2020.36469

Sherwood, G. (2022). Resilience and self-care in nursing. In. C. Huston (Ed.), *Professional nursing issues* (6th ed., pp. 229–245). Wolters Kluwer.

Sundgreen, M. KM., Millear, P. M., Dawber, C., & Medoro, L. (2020). Reflective practice groups and nurse professional quality of life. *Australian Journal of Advanced Nursing, 38*(4).

Swenson, M., Sims, S., & McCandles, K. (2017). Reflective ways of working together: Using liberating structures. In S. Horton-Deutsch & Sherwood (Eds.), *Reflective practice: Transforming education and improving outcomes* (2nd ed., pp. 291–311). Sigma Theta Tau International.

Tutu, D., & Tutu, M. (2014). *The book of forgiving: The fourfold path to healing ourselves and our world.* Harper One.

Van Schalkwyk, S. C., Hafler, J., Brewer, T. F., Maley, M. A., Margolis, C., McNamee, L., Meyer, I., Peluso, M. J., Schmutz, A. M., Spak, J. M., Davies, D., & Bellagio Global Health Education Initiative. (2019). Transformative learning as pedagogy for the health professions: A scoping review. *Medical Education, 53*(6), 547–558. https://doi.org/10.1111/medu.13804

Walter, R. (2017). Emancipatory nursing praxis: Becoming a social justice ally. In G. D. Sherwood & S. Horton-Deutsch (Eds.), *Reflective practice: Transforming education and improving outcomes* (2nd ed., pp. 355–378). Sigma Theta Tau International.

Watson, J. (2018, Supplement). Social justice and human caring: A model of Caring Science as a hopeful paradigm for moral justice for humanity. *Creative Nursing, 24*(1), 1–8. https://doi.org/10.1891/1078-4535.14.2.54

The Whole MD. (2018, January 6). *The science of heart-focused breathing* (with quick demo) [Video]. YouTube. https://www.youtube.com/watch?v=JxNjw3bcfVo&t=7s

WikiEducator. (2012, February 8). *3-Os/reflexive pedagogy.* https://wikieducator.org/3-Os/Reflexive_Pedagogy

PART III

REFLECTING WITH OTHERS

7   Sharing Our Stories: Co-Creating Learning Through
    Narrative Pedagogy, Silence, and Listening 141

8   Reimagining Practicing Together: Reflection in
    Simulation-Based Learning 161

9   Reflective Learning: Recalibrating Collaboration and
    Evaluation for Safety and Quality Competencies 179

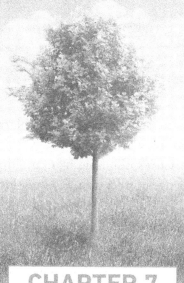

CHAPTER 7

SHARING OUR STORIES: CO-CREATING LEARNING THROUGH NARRATIVE PEDAGOGY, SILENCE, AND LISTENING

–Carole Hemmelgarn, MS
Gail Armstrong, PhD, DNP, RN, ACNS-BC, CNE, FAAN
Gwen Sherwood, PhD, RN, FAAN, ANEF

LEARNING OBJECTIVES/SUBJECTIVES

- Describe theoretical models for implementing various forms of narrative pedagogy.
- Demonstrate reflective practices guiding the healthcare team in learning from narratives and developing self-awareness.
- Examine the power of stories in co-creating person-centered care.
- Explore reflective practices in building authentic connections using the dynamics of listening and silence.

OVERVIEW

Stories as a form of narrative are a powerful learning tool. Narrative pedagogy provides learners and clinicians with methods for co-creating new ways of learning and developing their practice by reflecting on experiences, thinking from multiple perspectives, questioning assumptions, and exploring knowledge application. Co-creating experiences in which educators and learners think together and seek new ways to understand their experiences extends and enhances conventional pedagogy.

Stories have immense power to change mindsets, behaviors, and actions. Educators across the globe can use the power of stories to inspire change in behaviors to advance practice and renew the image of nursing. As pedagogy, stories personalize knowledge application, which enhances knowledge retention for future use (Armstrong et al, 2021). Reflection on stories uncovers meaning from multiple perspectives. Stories encourage learners and practitioners to explore different views of participants, as demonstrated in stories revealing myriad experiences during the COVID-19 pandemic. Reflection through stories allows learners to explore their emotional experiences to co-create new knowledge.

Reflection on a story is valuable in developing critical thinking, where context matters. Story-based learning touches people where they are, promoting change. Stories can imbed information, emphasizing deeper learning beyond memorization and surface learning, promoting knowledge retention and recall with higher accuracy. Recent research indicates that "critical incident narratives" remain with clinicians for the entirety of their practice career (Sandhu et al., 2023).

Because story explores both antagonists and advocates, it raises preconceived biases, shakes up old ways of thinking, and strengthens empathy. Story-based learning explores and shapes culture, behavior norms, beliefs, and values. Stories present an opportunity for learners to make sense of life situations through personal reflection and critical reflection with others. Stories are dynamic, with the power to engage learners emotionally and transform perspectives that lead to action in practice. Story-based learning can change traditional classrooms into deeper interactive learning, whether in an academic or clinical setting, to inspire new generations of nurses prepared for today's complex practice environments.

In this chapter, we explore ways to use narrative pedagogy to co-create, facilitate, and coach learners in developing and using stories also presented in case studies. Corollary concepts of self-awareness, listening, and silence are explored as effective phenomena that can enhance reflective teaching and learning with narrative pedagogy. Learners apply reflective practice skills for questioning inherited practices and processes in nursing, interpreting experiences, developing new ways of thinking informed by multiple perspectives, and engaging in authentic connections using the dynamics of listening and silence.

SUPPORTING THEORETICAL FRAMEWORKS AND EVIDENCE

Co-creating narrative pedagogy begins when educators, learners, and clinicians share their experiences from practice, life, or educational programs. Co-creation is significant to communally bear witness to the experience in ways that allow learners to question the prevailing interpretation and to elicit thinking from multiple perspectives and thus arrive at deeper understanding and comprehension. Applying reflective practices in nursing narratives derives from looking back at past experiences, creating spaces for dialogue, and bridging theory and practice (Choperena et al., 2019).

NARRATIVE PEDAGOGY

Narrative is a potent reflexive model used for developing reflective healthcare practitioners. Narrative pedagogies maximize learning when properly facilitated in nursing education. Patients share narratives with nurses and nurses share narratives with other nurses, creating reflective ways of learning. Learners hold stories of patients and in turn share aspects of these narratives in their own learning space. Accounts of illness expose not only disruptions in a patient's sense of self, but patients often experience narration as an important means of connection, a way to make sense of their illness, and a path to restoring their personhood (Sakalys, 2003).

Narrative can be healing for those telling the story and for those holding the story. "The witnessing and helping to order illness narratives can be a caring/healing nursing practice modality with significant healing potential" (Sakalys, 2003, p. 228). One may even consider the stories that nurses are privileged to hear as a unique form of nursing knowledge (Boykin & Schoenhofer, 1991).

Narrative pedagogies are closely linked to transformative and emancipatory learning theories explained in Chapter 2. Narratives can help propel action, behavior change, and shifts in attitudes, or they can dispel assumptions in telling nuances of events that touch and inspire the listener. Stories, as narratives, inspire questions; asking questions that lead to sense-making is integral to narrative pedagogies. Through an attitude of inquiry, educators and learners explore surfacing questions as they collectively seek to make sense of and find meaning in an experience.

Situated in experience, stories reveal ambiguity, uncertainty, limits, and disruptions inherent in day-to-day nursing practice (Ironside et al., 2017). By contrast, in educator-centered pedagogies, the educator pre-plans the content, issues, and questions for discussion. In learner-centered pedagogies, educators are part of the conversation with learners to understand the experience in new, different, or more complex and nuanced ways. The learning encounter is about not only the acquisition of content knowledge or skill proficiency but also co-creating how they understand and experience the client's situation. Learners are not focused on discovering what the educator has already determined is important but on exploring with educators. For example, the experience being shared is not "an example" of diabetes or heart failure. The experiences are not directed merely to point out particular content knowledge in the situation (e.g., "This is a good example of why delegation is important"). Rather, the experience itself is a call to thinking about everything present and absent in the experience from multiple perspectives, with the only end in view being that educators and learners actively engage in reflecting on, thinking through, and questioning these experiences so that questions arise in the process rather than a priori.

In narrative pedagogy, questions may have more than one right or "best" answer, and rarely is the complexity of the practice encounter preserved in the question (Ironside, 2016; Ironside et al., 2017). Learners sift through their memory for the required piece of information (e.g., the side effects of medication being administered or the injection sites for appropriate administration; Ironside & Hayden-Miles, 2017).

Because the use of narrative pedagogy is contextual, the complexity of the story or patient situation is central to the dialogue. Indeed, without understanding the context of the experience, the experience cannot be understood at all. Narrative pedagogy enables educators and learners to co-create learning encounters to collectively explore, critique, and question their nursing knowledge and their understanding of the situations they encounter. Learners are encouraged to challenge assumptions and critique prevailing perspectives and the limits of current knowledge while exploring the meaning and significance of their interpretations as part of their emerging practice (Ironside et al., 2017). This kind of critical thinking is not separated from content knowledge as it is in conventional pedagogy, in which content on a particular condition is presented by a teacher prior to the interpretive encounter. Rather, when learners and educators co-create learning encounters using narrative pedagogy, they bring their current knowledge and questions to the conversation and, through dialogue with others, the gaps, oversights, and misunderstandings are explored co-equally with new knowledge, insights, and "aha" moments (Ironside & Hayden-Miles, 2017).

REFLECTIVE PRACTICE INFORMING NARRATIVE PEDAGOGIES

Reflective pedagogies are essential in implementing person-centered, relationship-based caregiving. Reflecting on experience allows one to debrief for growth, personal knowing, mindfulness, and cultivating human connections (Pitzl, 2017). Reflective narratives are a form of knowledge development. A study in Norway demonstrated how nursing learners used reflection to learn from their experiences caring for patients in community health settings (Alteren, 2019). Mæland et al. (2021) applied narrative learning to new graduates managing moral distress in transitioning into practice. A review of using reflective practice with baccalaureate nursing learners consistently provided notable benefits for learners, including decreasing stress and anxiety and increasing learning, competency development, and enhancing self-awareness of nursing practice (Contreras et al., 2020). Reflection as lived experience helped nurses navigate personally and professionally through storytelling during COVID-19 (Graham, 2022). Chapter 6 examines how learners sharing their personal experiences (DEAL) creates a basis for gaining knowledge and paying attention to themselves and a foundation for listening to the perspectives of others.

Using story, unfolding case studies, and other narrative devices, educators engage learners in understanding a situation, the assumptions they are making about it, and what might be wrong with the typical or habitual way of responding. For example, how do patients experience this medication regimen? How might this patient's experience facilitate or inhibit their willingness to take this medication as prescribed? How is this patient's response like, or different from, others with whom you have worked? The context defining the narrative guides the questions asked and the options for care that are relevant, safe, appropriate, or desirable in a specific situation or across several situations (Ironside & Hayden-Miles, 2017).

The model for working narratives in didactic or workplace learning shown in Figure 7.1 provides a structure for meaningful discussion.

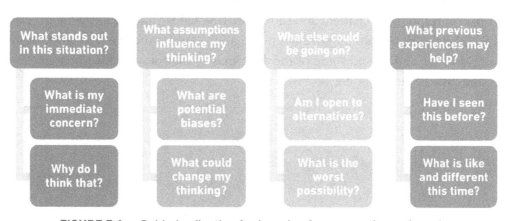

FIGURE 7.1   Guided reflection for learning from narrative pedagogies.

MICROPRACTICE: CO-CREATING SAFE LEARNING SPACES

The basic process of narrative pedagogy is a part of how we express caring as nurses. Patients have stories to share, and we *listen* differently when we approach taking a health history as hearing the patient's story. The experience that a patient has in co-creating a self-story with a nurse can be healing; as the self-story is heard by a caring person, memories are understood in fresh ways and the self-story is both affirmed and recreated (Gaydos, 2005).

Co-creating learning experiences with learners requires that educators create safe learning spaces by sharing with learners what they collectively intend in creating the course and why it is a part of becoming a nurse. Educators share the importance of creating fair, safe, and respectful learning spaces where everyone's voice is heard and respected. Confidentiality and trust between educators and learners and among learners are crucial in creating a community (how to create safe and brave learning spaces is explored in detail in Chapter 6). Learners are then poised to reflect on the narratives explored in the course, connect with other learners, and together share their perspectives. Shared reflections provide a rich context for dialogue and deeper reflective analysis, listening to each other, and thinking and learning in new ways (Betha, 2021).

Educators and mentors cultivate learners' and nurses' ability to reflect by asking them to share previous effective teaching practices, discuss among other learners, and identify best practices. For example, learners might respond to a prompt such as "The thing I have liked most about this school of nursing is . . ." or "Since I've been a nursing student, I've learned the most important way for teachers to help me learn is . . ." The educator or mentor does the assignment too, responding to similar prompts: "The thing I have liked most about this school of nursing is . . ." or "Since I've been a nurse, I've learned the most important way others can help me be the best nurse I can be is . . ."

Communally discussing patient stories promotes *community* as learners and nurses realize common responses to patient situations. Sharing helps validate authentic responses; learners feel their responses are important and begin to understand the true work of nursing. Learners also better understand some of the dilemmas of the role of educator, mentor, or manager and how others respond.

MICROPRACTICE: LEARNING COMMUNICATION THROUGH LISTENING

One nurse working with learners preparing for their first real-world clinical experience asked them to reflect on: "The thing I worry most about in coming to nursing school is . . ." and "The worst thing that could happen to me as a nurse learner is . . ." She finds that spending time reflecting on and discussing these issues creates a meaningful way for her to know and connect with learners and for learners to begin knowing and connecting within a shared paradigm of learning as common themes emerge. Sharing their emotions and concerns served to lessen the mystery of the real world of nursing and helped them to find effective ways to approach workplace learning.

MICROPRACTICE: JOURNALING ABOUT COMMUNICATION—STORIES FROM MULTIPLE PERSPECTIVES

Write about an experience that has meaning for you, describing a time when you and another person communicated well (or didn't communicate well). Try to tell the story in as much detail as possible so that as you read it to others, they can see and hear the situation. It might be helpful to think about the following as you get started:

- *What was going on at the time? (Time of day, setting, individuals involved, etc.)*
- *How did you know the communication was going well or not going well? What did you see or hear that told you this?*
- *What were you concerned about at the time?*
- *What was going through your head as the situation unfolded?*
- *What were you feeling during and after the experience?*
- *Did anything surprise you in the experience?*

When you have finished writing your story, write a second story from the perspective of another person who shared this same experience. Again, try to include as much detail as possible, and describe as clearly as you can what the situation looked like to that other person. What were that person's concerns? What do you suppose was running through their head as the situation unfolded?

(continues)

(continued)

Here is how one pre-clinical learner responded to these prompts:

While I was working as an assistant at a gym, a man who was severely hearing-impaired tried to speak with me using hand signals. When I did not understand him, he began to gesture more quickly and tensely, making things even worse. I could see the frustration and tension on his face. I felt completely helpless and tried to imagine how a patient would feel if he couldn't communicate his needs to his nurse. I knew I had to find a way to help him, and I remembered some signs from my high school American Sign Language class. I signed "hello" and the man completely relaxed, a big smile coming across his face. He signed that he spoke Spanish and knew little English—another challenge! I had also taken high school Spanish, and slowly, we found a way to communicate, which gave me a great sense of satisfaction. Each time he returned to the gym, he looked for me. I learned from that experience that sometimes just trying to help people communicates caring and makes a big difference in a person's life.

NARRATIVE PEDAGOGY: RECREATING NURSING EDUCATION

Educators using narrative pedagogy notice changes in learners' abilities to reflect on their experiences, think from multiple perspectives, question assumptions, and explore new possibilities for nursing education and practice. Yet these changes aren't readily captured in conventional assessment strategies like forced-choice exams. Pedagogically consistent evaluation mechanisms are addressed in Chapter 9.

To help learners develop habits of reflective practice, educators, speakers at education sessions, mentors, or nurse managers can encourage reflection by using focused prompts. Learners can write one-minute papers, nurses can put their responses on a notecard to post on the unit bulletin board, or managers can lead a discussion at the close of a team meeting.

- One thing I learned today that I did not know before is . . .
- One thing I knew before but now understand in a different way is . . .
- I still have questions or concerns about . . .

These prompts invite learners and nurses to reflect on what they have learned and the questions that remain for them before the session ends or make sense of a confusing work shift. Asking these questions provides an important opportunity for thinking through and articulating what they have learned—for themselves and the educator or leader—and to evaluate their own learning and needs for further study. These are important skills that can be cultivated through these seemingly simple strategies and can spark dialogue among educators, learners, nurses, managers, and mentors, creating further opportunities for learning. It can become a habit of self-assessment for continuous improvement and can make evaluation a shared responsibility in which educators or managers work together with learners or nurses to evaluate accomplishments and plan the next steps to accomplish further learning. In addition, by reading all learners' responses, the educator or manager is better able to intentionally expand on particular issues, respond to misunderstandings, or direct learners to further areas for discussion or study as the course progresses.

MICROPRACTICE: ONE THING I LEARNED TODAY THAT I DID NOT KNOW BEFORE IS . . .

Today I learned how critical it is to consider multiple perspectives. The patient's plan of care can't be decided on just one factor. There are many variables that have to be taken into account to formulate the best possible interventions. I also learned how vital it is to monitor the plan of care as it is being applied. For example, is it effective? What can we do to make it more effective?

MICROPRACTICE: ONE THING I KNEW BEFORE BUT NOW UNDERSTAND IN A DIFFERENT WAY IS . . .

Today I learned different aspects of critical thinking. Through everyone's stories, I was able to identify certain traits and skills required for critical thinking. First, critical thinking grows with experience. Also, nurses not only need to think clearly and plan the best care but be able to put thoughts into action and accomplish a goal. They need to think and communicate effectively but understand effectively as well. If nurses don't know how to interpret information properly, they won't be able to provide the best care.

NARRATIVE MEDICINE: STORIES IMPROVING PRACTICE

Dr. Rita Charon, a well-known researcher in narrative medicine, identifies the need for "narrative competence" for physicians, which is applicable to all healthcare professionals. This aptitude includes the ability to acknowledge, absorb, interpret, and act on the stories and plights of others (Charon, 2001). Similar to nursing theorists who acknowledge that nurses simultaneously hold and share stories, Charon identifies four situations where healthcare providers hold and share narratives: provider and patient, provider and self, provider and colleagues, and provider and society (Charon, 2001). When effectively integrated into health professions education, narrative medicine bridges separations that often occur between providers and patients, themselves, colleagues, and society, thereby offering restorative opportunities for empathetic and nourishing healthcare (Charon, 2001). A recent systematic review of the use of narrative medicine suggests that narrative medicine is a clear, replicable pedagogic tool and positively impacts learners' growing knowledge, skills, and attitudes specific to interacting with patients and families (Milota et al., 2019).

THE POWER OF STORIES

"Story, as it turns out was crucial to our evolution—more so than opposable thumbs. Opposable thumbs let us hang on; story told us what to hang on to."

–Lisa Cron

Stories have been in existence for thousands of years. Storytelling originated with visual stories found in cave dwellings and art and through body movement and dance. Today, we are most familiar with the written or oral formats of stories. Storytelling has power because it is one of the few universal traits connecting humanity (Wilson, 2013). Stories exist in every culture and are a mode of connection that children spontaneously learn at an early age. The beauty of storytelling is that everyone can tell a story, listen to a story, and understand a story. Stories are not linear. They weave, ebb, and flow and are created with a myriad of emotions. Stories captivate, influence, and transform conscious facets in our minds (Hall, 2019).

The most common form of storytelling is narration. It is how we explain our past, present, and future. It is how patients and families share their healthcare narratives of aches, pains, and improvements. Patient and family stories are more than the string of words they parse together; it is about the tone, rhythm, silence, facial expressions, and body movements.

Charon (2004, p. 862) has honed the art of teaching medical learners how to listen to a patient's narrative:

> I listen not only for the content of his narrative, but for its form—its temporal course, its images, its associated subplots, its silences, where he chooses to begin in telling of himself, how he sequences symptoms with other life events. I pay attention to the narrative's performance—the patient's gestures, expressions, body positions, tones of voice. After a few minutes, he stops talking and begins to weep. I ask him why he cries. He says, 'No one has ever let me do this before.'

THE SIGNIFICANCE OF THE PATIENT AND FAMILY NARRATIVE

"There is no agony like bearing an untold story inside you."

–Maya Angelou

Stories are how patients and families convey their healthcare concerns. They talk of their weekend warrior softball game: "I was rounding first base and had to slide into second to avoid getting out and collided with the second baseman...I heard this pop and tried to walk on my leg and my knee felt funny...now it is swollen the size of a grapefruit and hard to put weight on." They narrate the tale of a failing mother: "She is repeating the same story over and over again within a 20-minute period, and just last week she got lost driving to my home, a place she has been coming to for over 20 years."

The stories patients and families share are data with a soul (Brown, 2010). It helps to keep humanity front and center and not dehumanize people through lab values, disease, and illness. Hydén offers that patients' narratives provide a voice to suffering in a way that is outside of the familiar biomedical voice in medicine (Hydén, 1997). Patients and families know their bodies best, and while they may not use healthcare vernacular, if they are heard, they can potentially help with the diagnosis and treatment options in their own care. As patients and families tell their stories, the listener will start to fill in a narrative based on their experiences, sometimes blurring the lines between the message from the sender to the recipient. This muddling is a natural human response because stories elicit the need to forge bonds and create trust between people (Hall, 2019). This is also an aspect of narrative medicine where learners and practitioners connect with their patients and illness, recognize their own journey through medicine, form a kindship, and cultivate the relationship through reflective practice (Charon, 2001). Healthcare has embraced the power of stories by creating podcasts around storytelling and having dedicated sections in journals to connect the heart and the head and honor the moment, as outlined in Table 7.1.

TABLE 7.1	RESOURCES RELATED TO NARRATIVE	
PRINT RESOURCES FOR NARRATIVE STORY		
JAMA	**A Piece of My Mind**: Series devoted to telling stories about the joys, challenges, and hidden truths of practicing medicine in the modern era.	https://jamanetwork.com/collections/44046/a-piece-of-my-mind
NEJM	**Perspective**: This essay collection covers timely, relevant topics in healthcare and medicine in a brief, accessible style.	https://www.nejm.org/perspective-collections
Health Affairs	**Narrative Matters**: Essays with a compelling healthcare story.	https://www.healthaffairs.org/topic/narrativematters
AUDIO RESOURCES FOR NARRATIVE STORY		
TED Health	Podcasts for self-care and healthy lifestyles.	https://www.ted.com/podcasts/ted-health
Bedside Rounds	Podcast about narrative medicine, focusing on fascinating stories in clinical medicine.	http://bedside-rounds.org/category/podcasts/
The Healing Power of Narrative Medicine	Dr. Rita Charon speaks with Sydney Finkelstein on *The Sydcast*.	https://podcasts.apple.com/us/podcast/dr-rita-charon-the-healing-power-of-narrative-medicine/id1453232081?i=1000477966650
The Story Project Podcast	Podcast associated with the University of Arizona's Program for Narrative Medicine and Health Humanities.	https://www.narrativemedphx.com/story-project
VIDEO RESOURCES FOR NARRATIVE STORY		
Jack Gentry	The story shows compassion after medical error and taking care of the patient and family physically, emotionally, and financially.	https://psmf.org/story/jack-gentry

Lewis Blackman	Helen Haskell, Lewis's mom, tells the story of losing her son and how she made change through legislation.	https://psmf.org/story/lewis-blackman/
Shalynne McKinney	Shalynne was a young woman of color who died from medical errors and multiple biases in healthcare.	https://psmf.org/story/shalynne-mckinney/
Josie King	Sorel King, Josie's mom, talks about medical errors that happen every day in healthcare.	https://www.youtube.com/watch?v=MmeUSy-1Uxw
Alyssa Hemmelgarn	Carole Hemmelgarn shares the story of how her daughter Alyssa died and the importance of including patients and families in the learning process after medical errors.	https://psmf.org/story/alyssa-hemmelgarn/

LISTENING: A FORM OF CARING

"Hearing is listening to what is said. Listening is hearing what isn't said."
–Simon Sinek

Although they are often used interchangeably, listening and hearing are not the same. Listening is about being mentally attentive, present in the moment, and nonjudgmental (Low & Sonntag, 2013). Listening is dynamic and inclusive of an individual and shared process. It is about relating, belonging, and building trust. One of the greatest gifts we can give is presence. To be present, one needs to be relating to what is happening now—in the current state, situation, and with the person (Campbell, 2001). Recent research suggests that one of the most effective practices supporting relational care of older adult patients at the organizational and unit levels is effective listening when feedback is being offered (Dickson et al., 2017).

Listening is not an easy skill. Our brains work so fast and are constantly ready to respond, especially in a world where there is little silence and so much noise. Emotions play into our ability to listen, and this complexity can create an inverse relationship regarding what we hear. Both positive and negative emotions—like being excited, angry, upset, or fearful—impact the ability to listen. Sometimes we can pause, reset our emotions, and regain the ability to listen. Other times it is best to stop the conversation and come back to it when emotions have calmed.

At times it may appear we are listening, but instead another dialogue is playing in our heads. Effective listening is a conscious act (Caspersz & Stasinska, 2015). It requires us to be attentive, responsive, and active listeners.

Ulrich (2018) asks clinicians to question their intentions when they ask a patient, "How are you?" yet do not allow a response before interrupting to move on to their hurried agenda. Is the question a way of saying hello, a required task, or do you think you already know the answer? What nonverbal cues are sent to indicate you are no longer hearing the other? Listening has two parts: being in range to hear the response and hearing to comprehend. Interruptions assert dominance and erode trust and respect.

Ulrich (2018) suggests working with an accountability partner to practice listening:

1. Be present, and practice mindfulness.

2. Listen to hear rather than planning your response or next action.

3. Hold on problem-solving until you hear the story.

4. Use reflective practice by repeating back what you heard.

5. Apologize when you interrupt.

6. If time is limited, arrange a follow-up, and do it.

THE POWER OF SILENCE

"There are times when silence has the loudest voice."

–Leroy Brownlow

Silence is like white space on a piece of paper. There are times when it is a welcome friend and appreciated and other times when it harms and causes pain. To communicate authentically depends as much on silence as it does on words. We need silent moments between the words we speak and the pause and reflection after we have spoken (Campbell, 2001). Silence allows the words to sink in. Reflection creates the space to digest them. An ED nurse, Jonathan Bartels, introduced what he calls "The Pause" as a team ritual whenever there is a death in the ED. A purposeful, intentional pause honors those lives that do not get saved and gives the team a moment to contemplate the passage and bring the sacred into what is often an irreverent environment (Bartels, 2014).

Deep truths can arise from the spaces in between words, the void where thoughts are absent (Campbell, 2001). When there is silence, it creates space for new ideas and feelings to gestate and take form. The pauses and silences between words help us become more present and create deeper levels of truth to emerge from the subconscious. Clinicians who are effective listeners in complex clinical situations offer specific listening strategies for health professional learners. Clinicians who practice in pediatric oncology, where communication is often complex and difficult, offer effective approaches for the integration of silence. Opportunities for teaching the use of profound and stacked silences (series of silences interspersed with dialogue) with intention during difficult conversations is a fundamental aspect of communication (Rockwell et al., 2022).

Embracing silence gives you a chance to fully experience what you feel and to take in what you are hearing. It provides the time to process the words and emotions being exchanged. Silence gives rise to a sense of connection. Hill states, "It is the stillness of listening to humanity" (2018, p. 285).

Silence is fundamental in how human beings experience and create meaning in life (Røgild-Müller, 2022). As a culture, we feel uncomfortable and awkward when there is silence. Yet it can be a powerful tool to honor the moment, create an impactful learning opportunity, or sit with emotion.

APPLICATION FOR PERSONAL AND PROFESSIONAL PRACTICE

"Story is the language of the brain."

–Lisa Cron

Stories and storytelling are not exclusive to patients and families. Every day in healthcare, learners and practitioners are conversing through stories. Morning rounds, family meetings, handoffs, and morbidity and mortality conferences all use a story format. There is a subject or subjects, a plot, and typically a beginning, a middle, and an end. Communication tools like SBAR (situation, background, assessment, and recommendation) have a storytelling structure (Yeh et al., 2019).

Innovative health professions education acknowledges the power of the voices of patients and families, learners, and practitioners that inform teaching and the co-production process (Hawthornthwaite et al., 2018). Having the self-knowledge and awareness to recognize there is always more than one story happening means understanding that at the root of all great storytelling is simultaneous listening and appreciating all the voices. Stories are a vital source for co-production in healthcare processes. Healthcare is a co-production between patients and the healthcare team. Recognizing the essential co-productive character of healthcare grounds practitioners in listening to and respecting the expertise of the patient and family (Batalden et al., 2016).

A guided reflection for listening and learning from stories provides structure. The questions in Table 7.2 can guide a discussion, dissect a case study, or analyze a story

TABLE 7.2 GUIDED REFLECTION FOR LEARNING FROM STORIES	
REFLECTION	**QUESTION**
Critically consider beliefs or knowledge	What values guided the actions taken?
Bridge actual and desired practice/actions	What goals were evident?
Monitor reactions for intentional, conscious, deliberate actions	What reactions were evident?
Learn from experience, make sense of events	What happens in the future situations?

Narrative pedagogy, honoring and holding stories, learning to listen, and effective use of silence are complex interpersonal tools. Narrative competence in practice enhances clinicians' and patients' experience of care. Utilization of recurring learning strategies can help educators and learners appreciate their integration of these essential skills over time. Reflection papers are discussed in Chapter 9 as an effective, iterative approach to unfolding dialogue over time. Similarly, 6-word and 55-word stories, found in the Learning Narrative section, can help learners and clinicians realize their growing skill set in narrative competence in their practice.

REFLECTIVE SUMMARY

Narrative pedagogy provides a research-based approach for educators and mentors to enhance reflective practice learning experiences with learners and nurses. By focusing on developing and practicing learners' interpretive skills (reflecting on experiences, thinking in new ways and from multiple perspectives, and questioning their typical or inherited way of listening and responding to the situations they encounter), educators and learners can envision and enact new possibilities for understanding and working with each other and those for whom they care. Integration of the appreciation of story-honed listening skills and intentional silence are beneficial skills that further enhance both learning and the provision of care. In the context of these conversations, learners and educators often both say, "I never thought of it that way before," and become adept at asking, "Is there another way to think about this situation?" Given the complexity of the current healthcare environment and the challenges of preparing the future workforce, narrative pedagogy challenges the ubiquitous teacher-centered approaches to nursing education and opens new possibilities for dialogue among educators and learners toward improving nursing practice and education.

LEARNING NARRATIVE

Educators and facilitators can use a reflective writing technique based on two literary formats: the 6-word and 55-word story. Reflection rather than writing is the primary purpose. Reflecting helps choose words carefully to stay within 6 words. From the 6 words, participants expand their reflection to 55 words, remaining focused on clarity and message.

Implementing the 6-word reflection (see Figure 7.2 for examples):

* Make a list of three or four memorable experiences participants have participated in.

* Write the memories or experiences into a 6-word reflection (story).

* Choose words wisely, recognizing the power in words, and use only 6.

* Focus on clarity and completeness to accurately encompass the impression of the event with a short phrase.

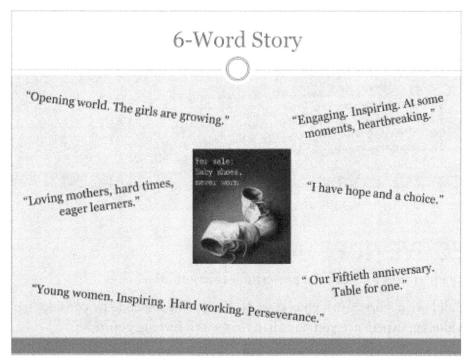

FIGURE 7.2. Examples of 6-word stories.

After completing the 6-word reflection, continue reflecting to extend it into a 55-word story to establish additional detail. The rules for 55-word stories (see Figure 7.3 for examples):

- The reflection must be exactly 55 words; it should tell a story and be reflective of the experience.

- Start by writing phrases and words and reflections of important images.

- Edit once completed to trim to 55 words.

- Focus on clarity and the power of the words selected. Consider the narrative elements that make this story significant or special.

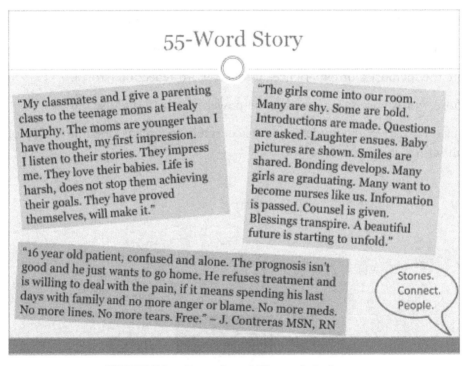

FIGURE 7.3. Examples of 55-word stories.

REFLECTIVE QUESTIONS

1. Why are stories considered a powerful learning tool?

2. We all have a story. Craft your story to share with someone by considering: What is a life-altering experience you have had that was a turning point?

   a. What values and intentions guided your actions?

   b. How have you responded to similar situations in light of this story?

3. Practice silence by remaining quiet for one minute. What did you hear? What were you thinking and feeling?

4. How can you cultivate active listening? Recall an incident today when you had to listen to another. How would you rate your listening skills?

5. Reflect on the intersection of story generation and the diagnostic process.

    a. How do assumptions influence how we first view another person?

    b. How can we as nurses hear the patient's full story to help the entire team in making care recommendations?

REFERENCES

Alteren, J. (2019). Narratives in learner nurses' knowledge development: A hermeneutical research study. *Nurse Education Today, 76,* 51–55. https://doi.org/10.1016/j.nedt.2019.01.015

Armstrong, G.. Sherwood, G., Ironside, P., Cerbie Brown, E., & Wonder, A. H. (2022). Reflective practice: Using narrative pedagogy to foster quality and safety. In G. Sherwood & J. Barnsteiner (Eds.), *Quality and safety in nursing: A competency approach to improving outcomes* (3rd ed., pp. 301–320). Wiley.

Bartels, J. B. (2014). The pause. *Critical Care Nurse, 34*(1), 74–75. https://doi.org/10.4037/ccn2014962

Batalden, M., Batalden, P., Margolis, P., Seid, M., Armstrong, G., Opipari-Arrigan, L., & Hartung, H. (2016). Coproduction of healthcare service. *BMJ Quality & Safety, 25*(7), 509–517. https://doi.org/10.1136/bmjqs-2015-004315

Botha, S. (2021). REFLECTION. Reimagining listening in clinical practice. *Australian Nursing & Midwifery Journal, 27*(4), 24–25.

Boykin, A., & Schoenhofer, S. O. (1991). Story as link between nursing practice, ontology, epistemology. *The Journal of Nursing Scholarship, 23*(4), 245–248. https://doi.org/10.1111/j.1547-5069.1991.tb00680.x

Brown, B. (2010, June). *The power of vulnerability.* TED Talk. https://www.youtube.com/watch?v=X4Qm9cGRub0

Campbell, S. (2001). *Getting real.* An H J Kramer Book published in a joint venture with New World Library.

Caspersz, D., & Stasinska, A. (2015). Can we teach effective listening? An exploratory study. *Journal of University Teaching & Learning Practice, 12*(4). https://ro.uow.edu.au/jutlp/vol12/iss4/2

Charon, R. (2001). Narrative medicine: A model for empathy, reflection, profession, and trust. *JAMA, 286*(15), 1897–1902. https://doi.org/10.1001/jama.286.15.1897

Charon, R. (2004). Narrative and medicine. *The New England Journal of Medicine, 350*(9), 862–864. https://doi.org/10.1056/NEJMp038249

Choperena, A., Oroviogoicoechea, C., Zaragoza Salcedo, A., Olza Moreno, I., & Jones, D. (2019). Nursing narratives and reflective practice: A theoretical review. *Journal of Advanced Nursing, 75*(8), 1637–1647. https://doi.org/10.1111/jan.13955

Contreras, J. A., Edwards-Maddox, S., Hall, A., & Lee, M. A. (2020). Effects of reflective practice on baccalaureate nursing learners' stress, anxiety and competency: An integrative review. *Worldviews on Evidence-Based Nursing, 17*(3), 239–245. https://doi.org/10.1111/wvn.12438

Dickson, M., Riddell, H., Gilmour, F., & McCormack, B. (2017). Delivering dignified care: A realist synthesis of evidence that promotes effective listening to and learning from older people's feedback in acute care settings. *Journal of Clinical Nursing, 26*(23–24), 4028–4038. https://doi.org/10.1111/jocn.13856

Gaydos, H. L. (2005). Understanding personal narratives: An approach to practice. *Journal of Advanced Nursing, 49*(3), 254–259. https://doi.org/10.1111/j.1365-2648.2004.03284.x

Graham, M. M. (2022). Navigating professional and personal knowing through reflective storytelling amidst Covid-19. *Journal of Holistic Nursing, 40*(4), 372–382. https://doi.org/10.1177/08980101211072289

Hall, E. A. (2019). *Stories that stick*. Harper Collins.

Hawthornthwaite, L., Roebotham, T., Lee, L., O'Dowda, M., & Lingard, L. (2018). Three sides to every story: Preparing patient and family storytellers, facilitators, and audiences. *The Permanente Journal, 22*(2), 117–119. https://doi.org/10.7812/TPP/17-119

Hill, S. (2018). 'Sacred silence'—The stillness of listening to humanity. *The Kyoto Manifesto for Global Economics: The Platform of Community, Humanity, and Spirituality*, 285–307. https://doi.org/10.1007/978-981-10-6478-4_17

Hydén, L. C. (1997). Illness and narrative. *Sociology of Health and Illness, 19*(1), 48–69. https://doi.org/10.1111/j.1467-9566.1997.tb00015.x

Ironside, P. M. (2016). Narrative pedagogy: Transforming nursing education through 15 years of research in nursing education. *Nursing Education Perspectives, 36*(2), 83–88.

Ironside, P. M., Brown, E. C., & Wonder, A. H. (2017). Using narrative pedagogy to foster quality and safety. In G. Sherwood & J. Barnsteiner (Eds.), *Quality and safety in nursing: A competency approach to improving outcomes* (2nd ed., pp. 221–232). Wiley-Blackwell.

Ironside, P. M., & Hayden-Miles, M. (2017) Narrative pedagogy: Co-creating engaging learning experiences with students. In G. Sherwood and S. Horton-Deutsch (Eds.), *Reflective practice: Transforming education and improving outcomes* (2nd ed., pp. 135–148). Sigma Theta Tau International.

Low, B. E., & Sonntag, E. (2013). Towards a pedagogy of listening: Teaching and learning from life stories of human rights violations. *Journal of Curriculum Studies, 45*(6), 768–789. https://doi.org/10.1080/00220272.2013.808379

Mæland, M. K., Tingvatn, B. S., Rykkje, L., & Drageset, S. (2021). Nursing education: Learners' narratives of moral distress in clinical practice. *Nursing Reports (Pavia, Italy), 11*(2), 291–300. https://doi.org/10.3390/nursrep11020028

Milota, M. M., van Thiel, G. J. M. W., & van Delden, J. J. M. (2019). Narrative medicine as a medical education tool: A systematic review. *Medical Teacher, 41*(7), 802–810. https://doi.org/10.1080/0142159X.2019.1584274

Pitzl, K. (2017). Reflective pedagogies in integrative nursing. *Master of Arts/Science in Nursing Scholarly Projects, 101*. https://sophia.stkate.edu/ma_nursing/101

Rockwell, S. L., Woods, C. L., Lemmon, M. E., Baker, J. N., Mack, J. W., Andes, K. L., & Kaye, E. C. (2022). Silence in conversations about advancing pediatric cancer. *Frontiers in Oncology, 12*, 894586. https://doi.org/10.3389/fonc.2022.894586

Røgild-Müller, L. (2022). SILENCE: Capturing the feeling of inner quietude. *Integrative Psychological & Behavioral Science, 56*(1), 133–162. https://doi.org/10.1007/s12124-021-09622-y

Sakalys, J. A. (2003). Restoring the patient's voice. The therapeutics of illness narratives. *Journal of Holistic Nursing, 21*(3), 228–241. https://doi.org/10.1177/0898010103256204

Sandhu, H., Foote, D. C., Evans, J., Santosa, K. B., Kemp, M. T., Donkersloot, J. N., White, E. M., Mazer, L. M., & Sandhu, G. (2023). "The story I will never forget": Critical incident narratives in surgical residency. *Annals of Surgery, 277*(3), e496–e502. https://doi.org/10.1097/SLA.0000000000005219

Ulrich B. (2018). Listening. *Nephrology Nursing Journal: Journal of the American Nephrology Nurses' Association, 45*(4), 323.

Wilson, E. O. (2013). *The social conquest of earth*. W. W. Norton & Co.

Yeh, V. J-H, Sherwood, G., Schwartz, T., Kardong-Edgren, S., Durham, C., & Beeber, L. (July 2020). Online simulation-based mastery learning with deliberate practice: Developing interprofessional communication skill. *Clinical Simulation in Nursing, 32*(27–38).

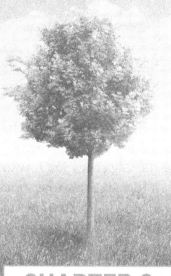

CHAPTER 8

REIMAGINING PRACTICING TOGETHER: REFLECTION IN SIMULATION-BASED LEARNING

–Jennifer Alderman, PhD, RN, CNL, CNE, CHSE
Ashley A. Kellish, DNP, RN, CCNS, NEA-BC

LEARNING OBJECTIVES/SUBJECTIVES

- Describe application of simulation-based learning in nursing education and practice across the professional learning continuum.

- Distinguish types of reflective-practice theoretical models related to simulation learning.

- Determine best practices for simulation-based learning in interprofessional education.

- Delineate goals for a preferred future of simulation in nursing education and practice.

OVERVIEW

In a post-pandemic world, there is a call to action for educators in nursing education and practice. The pandemic was a disrupter in unexpected ways, providing a rare opportunity for educators to innovate and move nursing education forward despite the simultaneous challenges created. The pandemic reinforced that learners must be prepared to face a variety of challenges in the workplace including short staffing, increasingly complex care environments, a lack of resources, and competing priorities.

More than 4 million licensed nurses practice in the United States, with a median age of 52 years (Smiley et al., 2021). In five years, approximately 20% of nurses plan to retire (Smiley et al., 2021). The shortage of registered nurses is projected to spread across the US through 2030. The most significant shortage will be in the West (Juraschek et al., 2019). From 2020 to 2021, the total supply of registered nurses in the US decreased by over 100,000. This was the most significant decrease over the last 40 years. Most nurses leaving the profession were under age 35, and most of these nurses were working in hospitals (Auerbach et al., 2022). The latest *Future of Nursing* report from the National Academies of Sciences, Engineering, and Medicine (2021) reinforces that nursing as a profession is facing a critical juncture. The next few years will require a more robust and diverse workforce to meet the complex needs of the society that nurses serve. Nurses stand in the gap, ready to address the inequities created by systems that have resulted in unparalleled health disparities. Given these expectations and demands, nurses need to be equipped with reflective practice skills to combat the emotional exhaustion and turnover currently plaguing irreplaceable members of the healthcare team. These skills are not developed only in the lecture hall; simulation and reflective practices are effective resources to educate the nurses needed in a post-pandemic era.

Nurses provide care individually and increasingly in teams. Nurses must be educated in a manner that allows them to confront the challenges of the healthcare system. Successful navigation of complex healthcare environments requires strong skills in interprofessional collaboration. Strong evidence supports simulation-based learning as impacting interprofessional education in building team behaviors and outcomes in bold ways (Walsh & Sethares, 2022). Simulation-based learning allows educators to teach critical reflective thinking skills. Simulation-based experiential learning allows learners to apply knowledge and practice skills in a realistic but simulated, safe environment. Critical aspects of simulation-based learning include reflection, reflective practice, and guided reflection (Walsh & Sethares, 2022).

SIMULATION-BASED LEARNING

Simulation-based learning is a type of experiential learning in which learners are charged with solving complicated problems in directed environments through carefully curated clinical scenarios (Lateef, 2010).

The American Association of Colleges of Nursing (AACN) has reimagined the Essentials for nursing education with the goal of bridging the gap between education and practice, and providing domains, concepts, and spheres of care through which competency-based nursing education can be achieved (AACN, 2021). The AACN endorses simulation-based learning as a method by which competency-based education can be attained. Of note, competency-based evaluation methods used in simulation-based learning need to include theoretical scaffolding approaches to evaluation, objective faculty assessments and learner self-assessments, and outcome evaluation based on knowledge and performance instead of learner satisfaction and self-confidence (Cole, 2023). Still, many validated tools used for evaluating simulation do not include components of all 10 domains of the AACN's competency-based Essentials (Cole, 2023), an area demanding improvements.

Nurse educators are emboldened to provide a transformative education for learners from pre-licensure nursing education to continuing professional development in nursing practice. To this end, it is no longer an option to include simulation in any aspect of nursing curricula—it is a requirement for a successful transition into any level of practice. This chapter will describe best practices in simulation-based learning in nursing education and practice and interprofessional education, examine reflective practices used in simulation-based learning, and offer future simulation education goals for advancing nursing education and practice.

SUPPORTING THEORETICAL FRAMEWORKS AND EVIDENCE

Theoretical frameworks that underpin the use of reflection in simulation-based learning include classic theories such as Knowles' Adult Learning Theory and Kolb's Experiential Learning Theory. Recent theories that apply more directly to reflection in simulation-based learning include Tanner's Model of Clinical Judgment, Ignatian Pedagogy, and situated cognition theory.

KNOWLES' ADULT LEARNING THEORY AND EXPERIMENTAL LEARNING THEORY

Knowles' Adult Learning Theory includes the understanding that adult learners are self-motivated and use past experiences to build new knowledge (Knowles et al., 2015). Kolb's Experiential Learning Theory holds the basic premise that through exploration and reflection, learners learn from their experiences (Kolb, 1984). Considering those two ideals alone makes it easy to understand how a simulated activity provides the foundation of an experience. The learner holds this experience and anything that comes from a reflection in their memory bank as something they went through. Future experiences then pull from this muscle memory to guide the learner in practice application; this coincides with the idea of gaining tacit knowledge, consciously or unconsciously, using simulated experiences (Gasaway, 2023).

TANNER'S MODEL OF CLINICAL JUDGMENT

According to Tanner's Model of Clinical Judgment, reflection is the key component for nurses to develop clinical judgment because reflection allows time to consider all possibilities after engaging in a scenario (Tanner, 2006). In fact, some educators hold that the reflective part of a simulation is more important than the scenario itself (Palaganas & Rock, 2014). *Clinical judgment* can be defined as "an interpretation or conclusion about a patient's needs, concerns, or health problems, and/or the decision to take action (or not), use or modify standard approaches, or improvise new ones as deemed appropriate by the patient's response" (Tanner, 2006, p. 204). Clinical judgment can be built upon with each simulation experience by reflecting post-event. Tanner proposes that the development of clinical judgment begins with noticing, proceeds to interpreting and responding, and concludes with reflecting. Learners bring personal frames to simulation that affect what they notice, how they respond, and their reflection on what they learn (Lesa et al., 2021). Tanner refers to reflection-in-action that occurs during the patient interaction or other activity and reflection-on-action that occurs after the interaction.

IGNATIAN PEDAGOGY

Ignatian Pedagogy is based on a centuries-old Jesuit philosophy steeped in spirituality with an emphasis on ethics, social justice, and integrity (Mountin & Nowacek, 2012). Its aim is to help learners move beyond focusing on self to focus on the larger picture and the needs of others. It aligns well with the holistic model of care that nursing provides (Pennington et al., 2013). The Ignatian pedagogical paradigm contains five principal elements—context, experience, reflection, action, and evaluation (Mountin & Nowacek, 2012), as shown in Figure 8.1.

- **Context:** Context has two dimensions: 1) The context that comes with the learner in the educational setting, including the learner's sense of self as well as the life circumstances the learner is facing, and 2) The learner's immediate surroundings such as classroom, organization, local, national, and worldwide concerns (Mountin & Nowacek, 2012). The key in this model is that reflection is a core component of every interaction between learner and educator, whether in the classroom or in a simulation setting. This theory ensures that reflective practices engage the learner throughout all experiences.

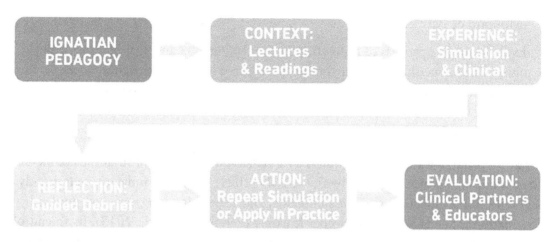

FIGURE 8.1 The five elements of the Ignatian Pedagogy.

Figure 8.1 provides a map for planning simulation activities to promote reflection. Learners become engaged in a context, helping them understand clinical diagnoses, nursing care, pathophysiology, and other content. Once placed in the simulation realm, scenarios are tailored to meet the objectives in their current learning context. Simulation provides a safe space for practicing the application of what they have learned. The overall learning effects are solidified in the guided reflection or debrief between facilitators and learners. Learners demonstrate the effects of the simulation learning in real-world practice visible to preceptors or educator evaluations, or even through another simulation.

- **Experience:** Experience is emphasized in the Ignatian pedagogical method. Experience is the heart of the learning that occurs in the educational setting. Examples of experiential learning in this paradigm include service learning, clinical, lab, or research (Mountin & Nowacek, 2012).

- **Reflection:** Reflection is meant to be a time in which learners examine their experiences to understand them more clearly. The role of the educator in the reflection process is to ask guiding questions during post-experiential learning activities (Jablonski et al., 2020). Asking questions related to the five senses (see, hear, taste, touch, smell) aligns with the Ignatian philosophy. Encouraging a more corporal reflection leads learners to have a more lived experience rather than a more disengaged experience (Mountin & Nowacek, 2012).

- **Action:** Action refers to when learners reflect on their experiences and use their new knowledge to spark action or actions. Attaining a more comprehensive understanding of others is one example of how the Ignatian philosophy is intended to play out (Mountin & Nowacek, 2012).

- **Evaluation:** The process of evaluation is a critical final element of Ignatian philosophy. The learner has had an experience, reflected on that experience, acted on the learning that resulted from the reflection, and then is expected to evaluate the entire process. The intent is to move past concept mastery and more to internal growth (Mountin & Nowacek, 2012).

Ignation pedagogy aligns with emphasis on reflection threaded through the competency-based education guidance provided by the AACN (2021). Evidence indicates that weekly clinical reflections, didactic writing assignments, and service-learning activities guided by Ignatian reflection pedagogy elicits deeper learning (Pennington et al., 2013). In an end-of-life simulation, Ignatian reflection pedagogy was used in a later stage of the simulation debrief to elicit further reflection about the lived experience of the simulation (Jablonski et al., 2020).

SITUATED COGNITION THEORY

Situated cognition theory, also known as *situated learning,* is foundational to simulation-based learning (Lave & Wenger, 1991). According to the theory, learning is influenced by the situation in which it occurs and is most effective in authentic environments. Learning requires learner engagement in authentic activities resembling the real world. This theoretical framework has been used to support augmented reality simulations (Anderson et al., 2021). Reflection is critical to situated cognition theory; as learners participate in authentic activities, time must be held for them to pause and reflect on the experience to identify and reinforce what they have learned from the experience (Lave & Wegner, 1991; Yu & Mann, 2021).

RETHINKING NURSING EDUCATION ACROSS THE PROFESSIONAL CONTINUUM: SIMULATION-BASED LEARNING

Simulation-based learning is utilized across the spectrum of nursing education programs and in practice settings. In nursing education, simulation is used in onboarding clinical instructors and across all nursing programs. In practice, simulation is used to train newly licensed healthcare professionals and to improve team communication. Simulation-based learning is associated with improvements in clinical judgment and critical thinking, self-confidence, and clinical skills (Nagle & Foli, 2022). Reflection guided by educators during simulation debriefs contributes to these outcomes (Nagle & Foli, 2022).

CLINICAL INSTRUCTOR TRAINING

In nursing education programs, simulated clinical experiences can be used to facilitate the transition into the role of clinical instructor. In one multisite study, clinical instructors received the traditional orientation plus a simulation in which they encountered six scenarios based on Quality and Safety Education for Nurses competencies. Each scenario presented a unique student challenge that instructors may encounter during their clinical teaching. Challenges included unprofessional behavior, incorrect application of evidence, student unpreparedness, and supervision of student skill performance. After debriefing and reflection, clinical instructors noted that the simulation allowed them to think about different ways to resolve any conflicts that could arise based on the scenarios. They appreciated learning from their peers and receiving feedback from experienced educators. Instruments measured increases in self-perceived confidence and decreases in anxiety for all participants (Ross et al., 2022).

PRELICENSURE NURSING EDUCATION

Prelicensure nursing students can utilize reflection post-simulation to gain muscle memory for future experiences. Through simulated activities that not only help build technical skills but also support experiential learning through action, students are exposed to events, ideas, mindsets of other professionals, and so forth. Post-simulation reflection can allow students to uncover their own biases, erroneous assumptions, and ways they are connecting concepts to practice. Simulation should be utilized in as many ways as it can be during pre-licensure programming.

A positive outcome of the pandemic is that it catapulted virtual simulation into nursing education. With the shortage of clinical sites and nursing faculty, an advantage to virtual simulation is that it can be used as clinical time, and learners can complete the simulation independently. A systematic review showed that virtual simulation improves learners' knowledge, skills, and affective outcomes (Tolarba,

VIRTUAL SIMULATION

Virtual simulation is a computer-created three-dimensional image or environment in which learners interact by using specialized equipment such as a helmet, goggles, or gloves with sensors (Tolarba, 2021).

2021). Using this model assures all pre-licensure students are exposed to experiential learning and reflection despite the challenges in the clinical setting.

In the current healthcare environment, chronic disease management makes up a large component of healthcare delivery. Almost two-thirds of adults over age 65 have multiple chronic health conditions. The AACN (2021) has stated that nursing graduates are coordinators of care and must be competent in all spheres of care, including chronic disease care. Simulation-based learning is a method by which prelicensure nursing students have an opportunity to provide care to patients in a home visit setting (Perry et al., 2022). The focus of this simulation was for nursing students to practice conducting a thorough medication history, called best possible medication history. They practiced communication skills with standardized patients as part of a simulated home visit. Students were able to identify omitted and transposed medications, as well as incorrect usage of medications. Using reflective debriefing, students identified how they could improve their communication by asking more open-ended questions to gain a better understanding of patients' health literacy and medication adherence. Knowing how to obtain a proper medication history from a population who typically experiences polypharmacy because of multiple chronic conditions is a required competency for prelicensure nursing students (Perry et al., 2022).

End-of-life care is also challenging to grasp without direct experience working with dying patients. A simulation designed to expose a pre-licensure learner to caring for the patient at the end of life—but more importantly, caring for the patient's family—provides a powerful lesson. The use of standardized actors to play supporting roles and engage with learners both during the simulation and during the debriefing reflection can open the learner's eyes to what patients and families are going through at the end of life. Through this experience, learners develop a paradigm to guide them when faced with this situation in clinical practice. The myriad of experiences required for nurses' continuing growth and development toward professional maturity can be addressed through post-simulation reflective practices.

GRADUATE NURSING EDUCATION

Prior to the pandemic, securing clinical sites for nurse practitioner clinical practica had reached a critical mass of intense need. While many nursing schools began paying preceptors in some areas, scarcity of resources prevented other schools from doing the same, thus limiting equal opportunities and diversity. The geographical area in which nurse practitioner students attend clinical practica has been expanded, although this increases financial and transportation burdens on students. Practicing across state lines can be problematic from a regulatory perspective. The pandemic exacerbated the problem as sites limited the number of students they work with to control the spread of infection. Thus, a perfect storm essentially created a favorable environment for increasing the amount of simulation-based learning in nurse practitioner programs.

In a graduate program that launched its online courses right at the start of the pandemic out of necessity, the use of online case studies provided an opportunity for learners to practice simulation debriefing after a sentinel event. Using online tools like Zoom and a structured reflection model based on debriefing with good judgment, learners were able to engage in role-play as interprofessional team members who had experienced the sentinel event themselves. They then debriefed one another in teams using an advocacy/inquiry approach to gain experiential learning in not only the event but in how to lead a difficult conversation and learn from errors to improve a healthcare system. This all occurred successfully in the virtual environment (Rudolph et al, 2007).

Some sample strategies use advocacy/inquiry (Rudolph et al., 2007):

- Engage the group by asking how they feel after the event. This allows the debriefer to have a needs assessment of the group after the event.

- Use the Plus/Delta model to engage in what went well and what might be done differently next time.

- Use advocacy/inquiry methodology by engaging in direct observations of what you say and asking curious questions like:

  - Tell me more about what happened when...

  - I observed X. I am curious about what your frame of mind was during that time?

  - I hear you discussing X. I wonder how you could do that differently next time?

- Conclude the debrief by summarizing major takeaways and/or engaging the team in sharing one key learning point they have gained.

Hussein and Favell (2022) conducted a scoping review to examine simulation-based learning in nurse practitioner programs. Results showed that through simulation-based learning, nurse practitioner students were able to increase confidence, improve clinical skills, and enhance knowledge. Simulation-based learning for nurse practitioner students is a viable option to help offset the lack of clinical practica sites and act as a bridge between theory and practice. Much more research is needed in this area to discern the outcomes of simulation-based learning for nurse practitioner students (Hussein & Favell, 2022).

Simulation can enhance leadership development. Engaging in role-play and reflecting on how one interacted during difficult situations can be very powerful to the developing nurse leader. Simulation provides opportunities to engage in best practices for interviewing. These reflective experiences enable leaders to conduct interviews with more confidence and skill; through reflection they could engage in cognitive rehearsal in responding to questions, engaging with candidates, and seeking the requirements of the new hire.

INTERPROFESSIONAL EDUCATION AND PRACTICE

Interprofessional education (IPE) is a required component of program accreditation in health professions education. *Interprofessional education* is defined by the World Health Organization (WHO) as occurring when "students from two or more professions learn about, from, and with each other to enable effective collaboration and improve health outcomes" (WHO, 2010, p. 7). For IPE to be effective, educators must be well prepared to deliver IPE course content, manage interprofessional groups of learners, develop appropriate learning objectives, and adapt instructional strategies to address the diversity among the learners (INACSL Standards Committee, 2021). Simulation-enhanced IPE provides a way in which competencies can be developed and assessed for health professions learners. Best practices in the implementation of simulation-enhanced IPE include the incorporation of a conceptual theoretical framework, use of a systematic approach to the design of the simulation, acknowledgment of and addressing any possible barriers to the simulation, and creation of an appropriate evaluation plan for the simulation (INACSL Standards Committee, 2021). It is essential that learners in health professions interact with and learn from individuals in other professions. Interprofessional simulations should integrate the Interprofessional Collaborative Practice Competencies as outlined in the Core Competencies for Interprofessional Collaborative Practice report (Interprofessional Education Collaborative, 2016):

- Interprofessional Teamwork and Team-based Practice

- Interprofessional Communication Practices

- Roles and Responsibilities for Collaborative Practice

- Values/Ethics for Interprofessional Practice

Interprofessional simulation in healthcare may include a variety of learners representing practice disciplines such as nursing, medicine, pharmacy, social work, allied health, and dentistry. Learners may be enrolled in educational programs or be licensed professionals in the workforce, or a combination of both. In one example, pre-health professions students participated in a simulation that taught donning and doffing of personal protective equipment (Fifolt et al., 2021). This simulation included pre-health professions from underrepresented minorities with the aim of preparing them for successful matriculation into their respective health professions schools. Learners reflected on their experience and identified two things they learned and two things they could improve upon in the future (Fifolt et al., 2021).

IPE in-situ simulations occur in practice settings and include participants who work together on a healthcare team. A common type of in-situ simulation is one related to resuscitation programs. In one example, a neonatal resuscitation simulation training program was implemented in a children's hospital. Scenarios in the simulation are based on common emergencies in neonatal care. Nurses and physicians participated together in the simulation. Results indicated that nurses and physicians felt the simulation training improved teamwork, communication, and professional development. Simulation training was also associated with improved neonatal outcomes in this setting (Bhatia et al., 2021).

IPE is ideally accomplished through multiple opportunities for learners to engage in simulated clinical experiences. Repeated interactions allow participants from varied professions to learn from and about each other and to learn how to interact, communicate, and collaborate. There are multiple methods to accomplish this work, but it is important to have an interprofessional team of educators to plan, implement, evaluate, and refine the IPE activities based on the Healthcare Simulation Standards of Best Practice (INACSL Standards Committee, 2021).

COGNITIVE BIAS SIMULATION TRAINING

Within the context of the current social justice movement, many educators have made great strides in creating interprofessional simulations aimed at increasing awareness of personal biases. These biases threaten effective communication and collaboration and thus patient outcomes through delays in care or poor management of care (Smith et al., 2022). In one example, three phases of a cognitive bias simulation were conducted with physical therapy, nursing, and radiation therapy learners. The first phase consisted of online learning related to increasing understanding of cognitive biases. This phase included video and reading assignments. In the second phase, learners were divided into two groups, with one group visiting a room set up as a "House of Horrors" in which various stations were set with patient safety violations. The second group viewed team perception videos with varying instructions related to the videos. In the third phase, learners shared their experiences in the simulation during a debriefing session. In follow-up, they responded to three key reflection questions in a required reflective writing assignment (Smith et al., 2022, p. 31):

- "How do cognitive bias and situational awareness apply to your work in healthcare?"

- "How would you describe an example of cognitive bias that you have experienced or witnessed in clinical?"

- "What is one example of a solution to help resolve or increase your awareness of cognitive biases?"

The most common biases identified across the learner groups were overconfidence and confirmation bias. The goal of the simulation was to use a situational awareness sim-IPE pedagogical approach to demonstrate how cognitive biases affect patient safety and quality. Learners realized that seeing things through their own perspective alone allows important safety concerns to be overlooked. Learners saw the value of interprofessional collaboration to gain multiple perspectives and uncover assumptions. Understanding debiasing strategies helps improve judgment and decision-making, thus leading to improved patient outcomes (Smith et al., 2022).

TELEHEALTH

An impactful sequelae of the pandemic was the explosion of telehealth education that became widely used as a vehicle for simulation in education and practice (Cook et al., 2022). Telehealth became a critical way to deliver healthcare in the throes of the pandemic and has continued to be a method of care delivery more so than it was before the pandemic. The pandemic identified a large gap in healthcare provider education—telehealth was not typically a robust component. Educators at one university created an interprofessional telehealth simulation that included nurse practitioners, physician assistants, and medical students—a didactic component accompanied by an objective structured clinical examination simulation. Standardized patients were utilized, and students were observed by a faculty member. Faculty from all three professional schools participated in the observations. After a reflective debriefing, students reported that they benefited from completing the simulation in interprofessional teams, as they noted a better understanding of roles and how team-based care can improve the patient experience (Cook et al., 2022)

APPLICATION IN PERSONAL AND PROFESSIONAL PRACTICE

Reflection and simulation-based learning form an ideal partnership, working synergistically to maximize the effectiveness of the simulated practice environment. Simulation-based learning is founded on the principles of adult learning, Experiential Learning Theory, and narrative pedagogy, thus providing a rich learning opportunity in safe spaces to prepare nurses for real-world practice. Reflection is important for planning and debriefing simulation learning experiences. Alden and Durham (2017) describe four reflective strategies for developing personal and professional learning goals to maximize learning opportunities and for translating to real-world practice:

- Pre-simulation planning is described as **reflection-before-action** (Alden & Durham, 2017). Providing time to orient to the environment, explain the process, discuss the objectives of the activity, assign roles, and present the simulation case are important planning activities for reflection-before-action.

- **Reflection-in-action** occurs in team huddles during the activity, pausing for clarification and making sure everyone is on the same page.

- **Reflection-on-action** is the guided debriefing led by the educator following the simulation. Questions guide learners in reflecting on individual and group performance, communication among participants, decision-making, emotional responses, the overall care of the simulated patient, and teamwork.

- **Reflection-beyond-action** is to help learners sustain what they learned for integration into their professional practice. One strategy is to have learners write a two-page debriefing paper on the experience, describing challenges, ways to apply what they learned into practice, and what questions remain.

Learning for the real world of a practice-based discipline is complex. Multiple learning approaches are necessary to prepare novice nurses for the dynamics of working in any healthcare delivery setting. Learning is not only an academic responsibility; learning occurs across the professional lifespan. Simulation-based learning grounded in adult learning and experiential learning theories is effective pedagogy for any stage of the nurse's career. To be effective in developing individual and team skills, however, applying Alden and Durham's four stages of reflective practice provides learners a way to rethink, reimagine, recreate, and continuously improve their professional practice.

REFLECTIVE SUMMARY

The global pandemic led to reimagining the way nursing education is delivered in academic and practice settings. Answering the call created by the pandemic, educators pivoted to provide robust learning opportunities virtually and in-person. Taking a toll on the nursing workforce, the pandemic also created opportunities for innovation and forward-thinking on the part of educators and administrators alike. For an exhausted and, in some cases, decimated workforce, educators and administrators must create meaningful learning experiences to prepare learners for practice, orient new nurses to practice, and provide continuing education for those who have been practicing. Simulation-based learning is a method that provides a safe environment for optimal learning to occur. Robust, reflection-laden debriefs give learners the space needed to process their experiences and take concepts learned directly to patient care settings.

1. How has the current healthcare environment impacted nursing education and why?

2. How does reflection improve nursing practice?

3. How does interprofessional simulation impact the practice of healthcare professionals?

4. What impact has the pandemic had on simulation-based learning?

5. What new directions could simulation-based learning in nursing education and practice go in due to the innovative spirit brought on by the pandemic?

LEARNING NARRATIVE

The AACN has determined that the 21st-century nurse must practice as a skilled care coordinator across four spheres of care: disease prevention/promotion, chronic disease care, regenerative and restorative care, and hospice/palliative care while simultaneously maintaining safety and quality of care (AACN, 2021). Given these expectations, nurses are met with many competing priorities while providing patient-centered care. Pre-licensure nurses frequently enter the workforce underprepared to face these pressures. Nurse educators are required to provide opportunities for pre-licensure nurses to practice leadership skills such as effective communication, managing conflict, and increasing self-awareness. The purpose of the following leadership simulation was to improve the communication, conflict management, and self-awareness knowledge, skills, and attitudes of pre-licensure nursing students (Alderman & Durham, 2022).

In collaboration with the university's Business School, the School of Nursing developed the *Peak Performance* leadership simulation to help pre-licensure nursing students improve their leadership skills. During the simulation, the learner responds to a variety of patient care, team-based, and personal situations utilizing various means of communication such as emails, voice messages, and texts, in the context of six patient care rounds. The learner must address as many scenarios per round as possible, being as efficient with time as possible. Small group debriefings were held in virtual breakout rooms. Students described their rationales for prioritizing and how they would handle conflicts they encountered. Students completed a reflection workbook after the debriefing and were offered the opportunity for one-on-one coaching sessions with the executive coaches from the Business School. Students completed pre/post assessments in which they evaluated their personal skills in self-awareness, communication, collaboration, openness, managing conflict, and managing others. The reflection workbook provided qualitative data related to self-evaluation of the following core values: empathy, integrity, and respect, along with a three-step action plan for improvement. Students noted improvement in knowledge and skills around communication and managing conflict, but they expressed frustration in the inability to complete all rounds of the simulation. Students were surprised by the complexity of care coordination awaiting them as they entered nursing practice.

Pre-licensure students increased their communication skills and obtained a better understanding of how to manage conflict in real-world circumstances fraught with competing priorities. Effective communication, conflict management, and self-awareness are critical to patient safety and providing quality care. Exposing students to the complex care coordination role of the nurse aligns well with the new AACN Essential Domains 2.9a–e and 5.2a–f (AACN, 2021).

The success of the nursing-focused Peak Performance simulation led educators to spread the model to an interprofessional version. Prelicensure nursing students, graduate nursing students, and medical students participated in a newly designed Peak Performance simulation focused on a discharge-planning case. The format was the same in that students received some introductory didactic information and then completed the simulation individually, answering reflection and prioritization questions. Business coaches led the debrief, and the simulation closed with a panel of interprofessional faculty discussing and reflecting on the challenges they faced when they transitioned to practice. All student participants completed pre/post surveys. Results showed significant gains in six leadership skills: self-awareness, communication, collaboration, openness, managing conflict, and managing others (Alderman & Durham, 2022).

The major points to take away are:

- Nursing shifts are fraught with competing priorities amid complex care environments every day.
- Nurse educators are obligated to prepare nurses for complex care environments.
- Teamwork, communication, and conflict management are cornerstones of patient quality and safety.
- Providing high-quality leadership simulations with debriefing methods grounded in reflection led by skilled educators can improve the competencies of learners in the areas of teamwork, communication, conflict management, and self-reflection.

REFLECTIVE QUESTIONS

1. How have you handled competing priorities encountered in your nursing practice?

2. After reflecting on your practice, what behaviors that you deem effective would you continue performing in your daily workflow and why?

3. After reflecting on your practice, what behaviors would you stop doing?

4. How has your thinking changed because of any insights you have obtained from this simulation?

REFERENCES

Alden, K., & Durham, C. (2017). Reflective practice in simulation-based learning. In S. Horton-Deutsch & G. Sherwood (Eds.), *Reflective practice: Transforming education and improving outcomes* (2nd ed., pp. 181–214). Sigma Theta Tau International.

Alderman, J. T., & Durham, C. F. (2022). *Enhancing patient safety through a simulation focused on improving communication and self-awareness*. Oral presentation. Quality and Safety Education for Nurses International Conference, Denver, Colorado.

American Association of Colleges of Nursing. (2021). *The essentials: Core competencies for professional nursing education*. https://www.aacnnursing.org/Portals/42/AcademicNursing/pdf/Essentials-2021.pdf

Anderson, M., Guido-Sanz, F., Diaz, D., Lok, B., Stuart, J., Akinnola, I., & Welch, G. (2021). Augmented reality in nurse practitioner education: Using a triage scenario to pilot technology usability and effectiveness. *Clinical Simulation in Nursing, 54*, 105–112. https://doi.org/10.1016/j.ecns.2021.01.006

Auerbach, D. I., Buerhaus, P. I., Donelan, K., & Staiger, D. O. (2022). A worrisome drop in the number of young nurses. *Health Affairs Forefront*. https://doi.org/10.1377/forefront.20220412.311784

Bhatia, M., Stewart, A. E., Wallace, A., Kumar, A., & Malhotra, A. (2021). Evaluation of an in-situ neonatal resuscitation simulation program using the new world Kirkpatrick Model. *Clinical Simulation in Nursing, 50*(C), 27–37. https://doi.org/10.1016/j.ecns.2020.09.006

Cole, H. S. (2023). Competency-based evaluations in undergraduate nursing simulation: A state of the literature. *Clinical Simulation in Nursing, 76*, 1–16. https://doi.org/10.1016/j.ecns.2022.12.004

Cook, C., Becklenberg, A., Kendall, A., Leppke, A., & Vohra-Khulla, P. (2022). An interprofessional telehealth educational and simulation program for primary care student providers: A research pilot study. *Nursing Economics, 40*(5), 230–236.

Fifolt, M., White, M. L., & McCormick, L. (2021). Using simulation to teach biosafety and interprofessional principles to students underrepresented in the healthcare professions. *Journal of Best Practices in Health Professions Diversity, 12*(1), 46–57.

Gasaway, R. (2023). *Tacit knowledge and situational awareness*. https://www.samatters.com/tacit-knowledge-and-situational-awareness/

Hussein, M. T. E., & Favell, D. (2022). Simulation-based learning in nurse practitioner program: A scoping review. *The Journal for Nurse Practitioners, 18*(8), 876–885. https://doi.org/10.1016/j.nurpra.2022.04.005

INACSL Standards Committee, Rossler, K., Molloy, M., Pastva, A, Brown, M., & Xavier, N. (2021, September). Healthcare simulation standards of best practice™ simulation-enhanced interprofessional education. *Clinical Simulation in Nursing, 58*, 49–53. https://doi.org/10.1016/j.ecns.2021.08.015

Interprofessional Education Collaborative. (2016). *Core competencies for interprofessional collaborative practice: 2016 update.*

Jablonski, A., McGuigan, J., & Miller, C. W. (2020). Innovative end-of-life simulation: Educating nursing students to care for patients during transition. *Clinical Simulation in Nursing, 48*(C), 68–74. https://doi.org/10.1016/j.ecns.2020.08.009

Juraschek, S. P., Zhang, X., Ranganathan, V., & Lin, V. W. (2019). United States registered nurse workforce report card and shortage forecast. *American Journal of Medical Quality, 34*(5), 473–481. https://doi.org/10.1177/1062860619873217

Knowles, M. S., Holton, E. F., & Swanson, R. A. (2015). *The adult learner: The definitive classic in adult education and human resource development* (8th ed.). Routledge, Taylor, & Frances Group.

Kolb, D. (1984). *Experiential learning: Experience as a source of learning and development.* Prentice-Hall.

Lateef, F. (2010). Simulation-based learning: Just like the real thing. *Journal of Emergency, Trauma, and Shock, 3*(4), 348–352. https://doi.org/10.4103/0974-2700.70743

Lave, J., & Wenger, E. (1991). *Situated learning: Legitimate peripheral participation.* Cambridge University Press.

Lesa, R., Daniel, B., & Harland, T. (2021). Learning with simulation: The experience of nursing students. *Clinical Simulation in Nursing, 56,* 57–65. https://doi.org/ 10.1016/j.ecns.2021.02.009

Mountin, S., & Nowacek, R. (2012). Reflection in action: A signature Ignatian Pedagogy for the 21st century. In N. Chick, A. Haynie, & R. Gurung (Eds.), *Exploring more signature pedagogies: Approaches to teaching disciplinary habits of mind* (pp. 129–142). Stylus Publishing.

Nagle, A., & Foli, K. J. (2022). Student-centered reflection during debriefing. *Nurse Educator, 47*(4), 230–235. https://doi.org/10.1097/NNE.0000000000001140

National Academies of Sciences, Engineering, and Medicine. (2021). *The future of nursing 2020-2030: Charting a path to achieve health equity.* The National Academies Press.

Palaganas, J. C., & Rock, L. K. (2014). Simulation-enhanced interprofessional education: A framework for development. In J. C. Palaganas, J. C. Maxworthy, C. A. Epps, & M. E. Mancini (Eds.), *Defining excellence in simulation programs* (pp. 108–119). Wolters Kluwer.

Pennington, K., Crewell, J., Snedden, T., Mulhall, M., & Ellison, N. (2013). Ignatian pedagogy: Transforming nursing education. *Jesuit Higher Education: A Journal, 2*(1), 34–40.

Perry, J., Powers, S. C., Haskell, B., & Plummer, C. (2022). Simulated home visits to promote chronic disease management competencies in prelicensure nursing students. *Nurse Educator, 47*(6), E132–E135. https://doi.org/10.1097/NNE.0000000000001229

Ross, J. G., Dunker, K. S., Duprey, M. D., Parson, T., & Humphries, L. (2022). The use of simulation for clinical nursing faculty orientation: A multisite study. *Clinical Simulation in Nursing, 63,* 23–30. https://doi.org/10.1016/j.ecns.2021.11.001

Rudolph, J. W., Simon, R., Rivard, P., Dufresne, R. L., & Raemer, D. B, (2007). Debriefing with good judgment: Combining rigorous feedback with genuine inquiry. *Anesthesiology Clinics, 25*(2), 361–376. https://doi.org/10.1016/j.anclin.2007.03.007

Smiley, R. A., Ruttinger, C., Oliveira, C. M., Hudson, L. R., Allgeyer, R., Reneau, K. A., Silvestre, J. H., & Alexander, M. (2021). The 2020 National Nursing Workforce Survey. *Journal of Nursing Regulation, 12*(1), S1–S96. https://doi.org/10.1016/S2155-8256(21)00027-2

Smith, L., Turkelson, C., & Hollenbeck, J. (2022). Exploring cognitive bias in health care using a simulation-enhanced interprofessional education activity. *Radiation Therapist, 31*(1), 27–39.

Tanner, C. A. (2006). Thinking like a nurse: A research-based model of clinical judgment in nursing. *Journal of Nursing Education, 45*(6), 204–211. https://doi.org/10.3928/01484834-20060601-04

Tolarba, J. E. L. (2021). Virtual simulation in nursing education: A systematic review. *International Journal of Nursing Education, 13*(3), 48–54. https://doi.org/10.37506/ijone.v13i3.16310

Walsh, J. A., & Sethares, K. A. (2022). The use of guided reflection in simulation-based education with prelicensure nursing students: An integrative review. *Journal of Nursing Education, 61*(2), 73–79. https://doi.org/10.3928/01484834-20211213-01

World Health Organization. (2010). *Framework for action on interprofessional education & collaborative practice.*

Yu, M., & Mann, J. S. (2021). Development of a virtual reality simulation program for high-risk neonatal infection control education. *Clinical Simulation in Nursing, 50*(1), 19–26. https://doi.org/10.1016.j.ecns.2020.10.006

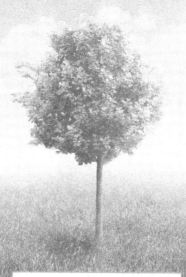

CHAPTER 9

REFLECTIVE LEARNING: RECALIBRATING COLLABORATION AND EVALUATION FOR SAFETY AND QUALITY COMPETENCIES

–*Gail Armstrong, PhD, DNP, RN, ACNS-BC, CNE, FAAN*
Gwen Sherwood, PhD, RN, FAAN, ANEF

LEARNING OBJECTIVES/SUBJECTIVES

- Apply various learning theories to nurses' professional development from academic learning across the professional lifespan.

- Describe reflective approaches reimagining ways to expand emotional intelligence and appreciative inquiry.

- Demonstrate reflective practices as a change model based on experiential learning, inquiry, and self-assessment for developing professional maturity.

- Examine reflective processes to make sense of contradictions in practice.

"We do not learn from experience; we learn from reflecting on experience."

–John Dewey

OVERVIEW

The centrality of reflective practice as a pivotal tenet of effective nursing education holds true for clinical nurses as well: Regardless of where one is on the professional journey, a practice of reflection strengthens a nurse's capacity for self-awareness, mindfulness, and situational awareness. Best developed in one's educational program, reflective practice is valuable to all nurses in a variety of clinical settings. Pedagogical approaches used with nurse learners are often highly relevant and effective in supporting the reflective practice of nurse clinicians. Pairing reflective practice with standards of quality and safety facilitates an awareness of the disconnect that often accompanies a compromise to quality and safety. In this disconnect lies the opportunity for understanding and improvement. Similar to nurse learners, nurse clinicians need time, space, and facilitation to debrief a safety event (Salik & Paige, 2022). Building intellectual muscle memory in reflective practice for nurse learners positions nurse clinicians to optimize the benefits of this essential skill set. Furthermore, evaluation modalities employed with nurse learners in educational programs are well-suited for the evaluation of vital aspects of the practice of nurse clinicians.

Among the healthcare professions, nursing has the most sustained application of reflective practices to support clinicians and prepare learners (Scheel et al., 2021). Reflective practice is entrenched in all healthcare professions for its value in establishing a reflective learning framework for clinicians. Medical educators have identified that reflective learning pedagogies foster moral development and enhance professional identity formation (Branch & George, 2017). Dental educators coalesce around an appreciation that deep reflection is a key requirement of dental education at all stages (Campbell & Rogers, 2022). Pharmacy educators have put out the call for increased reflective practice in their educational models (Mantzourani et al., 2019). Educators in physical therapy have identified the valuable contribution of reflective practice as a core component of PT education and identified the need for explicit linkages between reflective practice and the epistemologies of the PT discipline (Ziebart & MacDermid, 2019). With the flourishing of the appreciation of reflective practice across healthcare professions, there is abundant opportunity to integrate reflective practice pedagogy into interprofessional education for healthcare professionals.

This chapter applies various learning theories for co-creating reflective learning in interactive experiences to appreciate and develop ways to better understand nurses' work, explore and make sense of contradictions, and apply self-assessment to propel professional growth and development. Reflective practices that illustrate emotional intelligence and appreciative inquiry guide deep reflections to analyze work experiences for developing tacit and other forms of knowledge. Examples showcase strategies and prompts that educators and mentors can use to help learners and nurses develop reflective practice skills and explore how to integrate reflective approaches into learners' formative and summative clinical assessments and evaluative feedback.

SUPPORTING THEORETICAL FRAMEWORKS AND EVIDENCE

Van Schalkwyk et al. (2019) defined transformative learning theory as a complex metatheory. Transformative learning challenges prevailing thoughts, assumptions, and ways of doing things, leading to new knowledge and ways of doing and being. Transformative learning is characterized by change, blending the goals of reflective practice as a change agent particularly relevant in clinical learning experiences across the learning spectrum (Johns, 2022). Other chapters in this book have integrated the work of Mezirow with transformative learning and its demonstration of reflective practice; Van Schalkwyk et al. stated that 70% of studies reporting transformative learning referenced Mezirow and even more cited reflection as a key learning process (2019). Transformative learning highlights learning from mistakes, which fits the exemplary learning narratives for developing quality and safety competencies in this chapter.

Transformative learning theory melds well with situated learning theory (O'Brien & Battista, 2020) by considering the social and cultural considerations of an experience; thus, reflection examines the situated context of what happened. Situated learner theory departs from cognitive or behavioral educational methods and situates within everyday activities and culture to concentrate on relationships and identity formation that fits educating for practice-based disciplines such as nursing (Day & Sherwood, 2022). Nurse educators in both academic and practice settings apply transformative learning and situated learning theories using narrative pedagogies (Armstrong et al., 2022) implemented through reflective practices, bringing the learner into inquiry, asking questions for deeper learning through case studies representing the real world, or in simulation-based learning scenarios (see Chapter 8).

Johns (2022), a pioneer in developing reflective practice in nursing, explored reflective practice as the process of exposing contradictions in practice followed by reflection to confront the conditions in practice that limit the achievement of "good" work in which one "does the right thing." In exposing contradictions, nurses use a reflective process first to understand their definition of ideal practice, then examine the multiplicity of factors within the clinical interaction that either hindered or enhanced their ability to reach that ideal and determine alternative actions for the future (Johns, 2022). This process of exposing contradictions is especially heightened for nurse learners early in forming their professional identities. The potential of "creative tension" in the uncomfortable experience of contradiction lies in the search for improvement toward the ideal goal.

Freshwater (2008) describes three models that build into deeper reflective practices:

- **Descriptive practice** helps one develop consciousness of one's actions with a focus on reflection-on-action through journaling or critical incident reporting.

- **Dialogic reflection** is deliberate, and it includes talking with peers or clinical supervision.

- **Critical reflection,** perhaps the most difficult, brings changes in practice; practitioners can provide reasoning for actions by engaging in critical conversations about practice with self and others.

QUALITY AND SAFETY: PRAXIS AND REFLECTION

Nurses' value systems inherently recognize that safe practice and quality improvement represent "right action" within the mechanics of quality and safety at the systems level. New clinicians often experience cognitive dissonance when facing an incongruity between the standards they have learned and what they observe in practice. Compromises and lapses in quality and safety initiate inner conflict when nurses recognize potential adverse consequences for specific patients. For example, witnessing a medication error potentially harming Mr. Smith in Room 204 is transformed from an impersonal statistic to an important facet of an individual clinician's bedside practice and into how the system problem is addressed both at the individual and system levels. The tension between risk for harm and system redesign for error prevention is an ongoing aspect of nursing and relies on reflective practices to lead to redesign.

CONTRADICTION AND REFLECTIVE PRACTICE

Quality and safety and reflective practice overlap in the concept of *contradiction*. Reflective practice provides an ongoing process for nurses to consider their responses to practice contradictions they see in practice. Learners are educated about evidence-based standards, which they envision within well-organized patient care delivery systems operating in ideal circumstances. Nurses are disillusioned when they are exposed to the profound divide between the ideal values they have been taught about healthcare systems and the flawed care delivery systems they encounter in practice (Goulet et al., 2016).

Learners and experienced clinicians struggle with the limits of their own abilities yet feel a unique gravity as they observe contradictions in quality and safety standards that transcend other realities presented in educational scenarios. The contradictions they see in how patients are safeguarded amid lapses in quality demand attention because of the potential for patient harm. Nurses practice with continuing concern that they might harm a patient. Reflective practice is a tool for analyzing imperfect systems and their response within their own imperfect practice. Contradictory circumstances in how healthcare systems protect patient safety force nurses to examine their practice by pausing, reflecting on actions, and rethinking their contributions.

Learning reflective practices for managing these uncomfortable realities guides nurses in sustaining their professionalism, sense of renewal, and finding hope in working towards what they intend to achieve within any situation and improving the way they practice. Contradiction creates a sense of internal conflict, an uneasy sense deep within the practitioner, which erodes trust in the system, disillusions meaning and purpose, and lends itself to emotional fatigue. In teaching a reflective approach to practice, we help nurses recognize that contradictions exist because, for whatever reason, practitioners and systems are unable to always act congruently according to their beliefs (Johns, 2022). By helping nurses develop reflective practice skills in the early stages of becoming a nurse, these habits are ingrained in how they become aware of the realities of practice, act on discomfort by alleviating incongruities, and practice in alignment with their values (Johns, 2022; Patel & Metersky, 2021).

REFLECTIVE PRACTICES: RETHINKING QUALITY AND SAFETY COMPETENCIES

Competency-based curricula are replacing content-based curricula (American Association of Colleges of Nursing [AACN], 2021). Competencies are assessed by defining the knowledge, skills, and attitude objectives for each competency. Learners and nurses demonstrate achievement of competency through their plan to integrate the knowledge into their work, revealing changes in attitudes for adjusting future clinical situations and the specific actions involved in the patient's care. Domain 5 of AACN's Essentials, Quality and Safety, demonstrates the goals and mission of the Quality and Safety Education for Nurses (QSEN) competency framework by applying improvement principles in care delivery, defining nurses' contributions to patient safety, and helping create a safety of culture within the work environment (AACN, 2021). The AACN's Essentials is leveled for both pre-licensure and graduate education, as is the national initiative QSEN, which guided extensive curricula transformation incorporating quality and safety competencies (Cronenwett et al., 2007;

Cronenwett, Sherwood, Pohl et al., 2009). These competencies encompass patient-centered care, safety, teamwork, quality improvement, evidence-based practice, and informatics (accessible at www.qsen.org). QSEN's groundbreaking work surfaced the need for faculty, learner, and clinician development to integrate reflective practices in academic and clinical settings as a means to quality and safety improvement (Cronenwett, Sherwood, & Gelmon, 2009).

RECALIBRATING COLLABORATION: STRUCTURING REFLECTION IN CLINICAL LEARNING

Clinical learning experiences take place within complex healthcare environments. Clinical experiences examined through reflection on narratives and case studies require alternative types of assessment of performance (Sherwood & Day, 2022). Didactic and workplace learning are intrinsically linked; it is a new nurse's capacity for applying competencies in the clinical context that determines the quality and safety of their practice. Nursing as a practice-based discipline has a long history of apprentice training (see Chapter 12). A historical review of nursing apprenticeship models describes how rigorous academic practice partnerships are necessary for redesigning apprenticeships in nursing (Tesseyman et al., 2022). The complexity of nursing education is the integration of the intellectual level (knowledge), psychomotor skills, and values. Reflective practice expands a nurse's awareness of this shift to applying knowledge, not just acquiring knowledge, in learning efficacy (Bono-Neri, 2019).

In the 2010 Carnegie Foundation study, *Educating Nurses,* Benner and colleagues describe the three-apprenticeship model for nursing education. It explains nurses' need for ongoing support in knowledge development, clinical reasoning and skilled know-how, and ethical formation. In earlier apprenticeship models, learners in diploma programs were primarily educated through training that focused on the tasks of a nurse's "job." The report clarified that "higher apprenticeships" emphasize competence in learning over time, using a variety of pedagogies, with built-in processes for reflective practice. The inclusion of reflective practice is crucial, laying the foundation for enduring nursing praxis. This updated definition of apprenticeship learning emphasizes a multifaceted approach to phased learning in nursing, where apprenticeship captures the "experiential learning that requires interaction with a community of practice, situated coaching by teachers, and demonstration of aspects of complex practice that are not easily translated" (Benner et al., 2010, p. 24). This mirrors the theories introduced earlier in this chapter.

The three apprenticeships for nursing education (Benner et al., 2010) are:

- Acquiring and Using Knowledge and Science

  Knowledge (Domain 1 of AACN Essentials) of science is core to all aspects of competent nursing practice, in all clinical settings. Nursing practice requires scientific subject matter expertise (e.g., anatomy, physiology, pathophysiology, microbiology, chemistry, genetics, pharmacology); this scientific foundation is needed for patient care, interpretation of diagnostics, and staying current with practice.

- Using Clinical Reasoning and Skilled Know-How

  Making decisions in the context of the complexities of practice requires the synthesis of knowledge and intellectual agility in prioritizing key concerns. Managing a patient's dynamic condition over time while utilizing various resources requires complex clinical reasoning skills and effective communication skills with patients, families, and the healthcare team. Effective clinical decisions require rapid interpretation of clinical indicators and synthesizing information from multiple sources.

- Ethical Comportment and Formation

  Nurses need the skills of ethical decision-making, ethical reflection, and the ability to use moral reasoning in navigating complex care situations.

THE TIME AND SPACE TO REFLECT

Nurses are bombarded by stimuli. Reflective practice provides temporal distance from an experience. Within this time and space, learners and nurses can intentionally review an experience in the context of their professional values (Patel & Metersky, 2021). Without encouragement to consciously reflect on discrete experiences, overwhelmed nurses often bypass this rich learning opportunity. Inviting nurses to engage in reflection and mindful practice gives them vital avenues to make sense of their complex practice. By making space for reflection, nurses can deconstruct an incident observed in practice to harvest insights. Midwifery education and practice has embraced the value of reflective practice, encouraging scaffolding throughout midwifery education and practice (Bass et al., 2020). Reflective practice means rethinking practice, one's relationships with others, and feelings about performing certain tasks. Reflective practice is becoming more self-aware of one's own practice. Reflective practice in the clinical setting with pediatric clinicians highlights the vital importance of discrete time and a specific place for clinicians to engage in reflective practice (Plant et al., 2017).

REIMAGINING REFLECTIVE PRACTICE TO PROMOTE CLINICAL LEARNING

Effective tools that facilitate reflective practice are relevant for nurse learners and nurse clinicians. Quality and safety are value-laden concepts forming the foundation of nurses' professional values. Doing good work, doing the right thing, and being a good team member are core values in nursing. To improve outcomes requires both a mindset (i.e., the will) and the skills to use a set of tools (i.e., the ideas and execution). Emotional intelligence and appreciative inquiry are two reflective frameworks influential in nurses' personal and professional development across the learning continuum.

REFLECTIVE PRACTICE AND EMOTIONAL INTELLIGENCE

Learners and nurses need content and background to develop reflective practice skills. Reflective practice content gives learners schemata and language in developing a foundation to guide their reflective work. Reflective practice skills provide an effective approach to developing emotional intelligence (EI; Kaiafas, 2021). *Emotional intelligence* involves recognizing your own feelings as well as those of others and employing this insight in managing yourself and your relationships. Four realms describe EI: self-awareness, self-management, social awareness, and relationship management. Higher levels of increasing EI increase awareness of self, others, and the environment, which can inform effective practice.

EMOTIONAL INTELLIGENCE

EI is the ability to monitor feelings and emotions, to discriminate among them, and then use that information to guide your thinking and actions (Goleman et al., 2002).

EI fosters professional maturity and is the trademark of effective leaders. Reflection helps people make sense of experience, self-monitor feelings and emotions, and discriminate this information to guide their thinking, action, and way of responding. Reflective self-assessment encourages learners and nurses to reflect on their actions in practice and in relation to others (Horton-Deutsch & Sherwood, 2008). EI raises consciousness of self, others, and the situational context or environment, and, in turn, effective practice. Learners and nurses can use the reflective process, informed by elements of EI, to begin a sense-making process to understand their practice and the people and environment where they work.

REFLECTIVE PRACTICE: A FOUNDATION FOR APPRECIATIVE INQUIRY

Appreciative inquiry (AI) creates an open and affirming educational process by including learners in determining successful strategies for the learning environment (Stulz et al., 2021).

An appreciative approach focuses on what learners desire versus what learners do incorrectly (e.g., focusing on desired practice versus a gap analysis). Rather than clinical educators setting rules for behavior in the clinical situation, educators and learners apply AI principles to establish agreed upon elements of engagement (Chauke et al., 2015). The goal of AI is to reflect on strengths or what is working well for the individual, team, course, or system to expedite improvement work; strength-based approaches are inclusive, lessening fears and criticisms (Merriel et al., 2022).

MICROPRACTICES: CONNECTING QUALITY AND SAFETY AND REFLECTIVE PRACTICE

"Rather than learning to write, reflection is writing to learn."
–Freshwater, 2008

Learners and nurses find an easy pairing between reflective practice and quality and safety in ways that are often surprising. The following exemplar outlines a learning strategy to create space for learners and nurses to engage in reflection and develop mindful practice. Because of the integration of the quality and safety competencies defined in the QSEN project (www.qsen.org; Cronenwett et al., 2007; Cronenwett, Sherwood, Pohl et al., 2009) into nursing education essentials, all nurses should be exposed to learning opportunities in their educational program to understand quality and safety science (Sherwood & Day, 2022). The reflective practice strategy described here is an example of *reflection-on-action*, a retrospective reflection that helps make sense of an experience, thus influencing future understanding and practice (Schön, 1987).

Reflection papers guide learners and nurses in applying the process of reflective practice useful in academic settings, with new graduates in a transition-to-practice program or as part of a professional development portfolio. One- or two-page reflections completed weekly or as needed reinforce that all experiences can be part of the learning process. The practice of regular writing taps all ways of knowing that learners and nurses employ in building a knowledge base on which to base future actions. The papers can become requisite parts of the learners' course of study, nurses' professional development portfolio, or the basis of an annual performance assessment. Educators or nurse managers can see the focus of the learner or nurse in providing care. Educators, mentors, or others who review the papers return written responses offering support, ongoing dialogue, or coaching to continue to explore questions and encourage learners to listen to their emerging inner voices. By opening the door for increased awareness and consciousness (Johns, 2009) of their experiences, learners and nurses gradually come to trust the space provided and settle into a habit of reflecting. Reflective practice provides a framework through which nurses can articulate and understand the uneasiness and distress that compromise quality safe care, which, if left unexpressed, can lead to a sense of helplessness about their practice.

Providing prompts helps learners and nurses establish a purpose or goal of their reflection paper. For example, learners or nurses may be invited to write a reflection paper that outlines the three top values shaping their practice, which provides a forum for exploring the contradictions encountered in their experiences. Safety is a core value for practice, so this prompt facilitates developing mindfulness about risks to patient safety. Table 9.1 outlines the subsequent open-ended prompts as serial reflection papers that create a consistent, safe space for learners or nurses to examine emerging practice questions. Every nurse has questions about experiences; repeated writing invites them into a habit of inquiry and thereby facilitates self-awareness, practice awareness, and ultimately a foundation in mindfulness.

TABLE 9.1 WRITING PROMPTS FOR WEEKLY REFLECTION PAPERS

- Tell me about your top three priorities for your nursing practice. What barriers are you encountering in achieving these priorities?
- How do your current observations of caregiving challenge quality and safety?
- Describe a clinical experience that affirmed your decision to enter nursing.
- What was a notable experience from your time at the bedside today? Why do you think it was important for you?
- What are similarities among those individuals you consider to be positive role models?
- When today were you unsure of what to do? How did you feel? What steps did you take to be able to make an informed decision?

Reflective practice involves a distinct process for revisiting one's experiences. A variety of models describe, deconstruct, and employ reflective practice in nursing education (Patel & Metersky, 2021). Guiding learners or nurses in the process of reflective practice ensures more consistency and less circling, unable to get to the point. Educators or mentors can pose a pointed question to help the learner or nurse to phrase and reanalyze to land a conclusion. Feedback, encouragement, and support from a clinician, mentor, or educator reinforce a progressive process, encouraging learners and nurses to stay with a practice question until its natural conclusion.

CRITICAL REFLECTION: RECONSIDERING PRACTICE DEVELOPMENT AMONG LEARNERS AND NURSES

Through the process of reflection, learners often arrive at a deeper understanding of their practice. Patient- (or person-) centered care is a core domain in the AACN Essentials (2021) and a QSEN competency that is both broad and complex. One learner who had written about her love of the "technicality of the machines" in nursing captured her reflections in caring for a patient hospitalized with burns to his hands:

> *I was assisting the burn nurse with changing the bandages and dressings and the removal of the staples that had been placed to adhere the artificial surface to his own flesh. It looked as though it was healing fairly well. At first, I was intrigued by the process that I was watching, and then I looked at the face of the patient. It was plain that this was the first time he had seen the extent of his injuries since he was admitted. He was horrified.*
>
> *This experience was rich in caring moments for me as a nurse…It was an awakening for me to put the human context to the clinical conditions that I have only read about in books or simulated in the lab. This was not a limb with second- and third-degree burns to be debrided and bandaged. This was a person with a family to support and a crew of men who looked to him for their livelihood. This was a man used to being in charge of his environment and able to create things with the work of his hands. Now his life will be changed forever.*

The striking part of this reflection paper was the learner's dramatic shift away from objectifying her patient as a diagnosis or a physiologic process to humanizing her patient as an individual person with a rich human context and life beyond the hospital. Freshwater (2008) describes such deep reflection as a *critical reflection*. You can hear the learner's own surprise in this shift. Even her use of the phrase "caring moments" was indicative of a transformation for this developing clinician in moving beyond her previous reflection that focused on the technical aspects of care.

When a learner observes an explicit compromise or contradiction in patient safety, the experience can be confusing and upsetting. The example that follows outlines a learner's observation of an extreme compromise in patient safety around the insertion of a Foley catheter and her multilayered response to the experience.

> *I had quite a striking experience at the bedside this week, one that I believe I won't ever forget. In my EBP class this week, we were discussing the*

*implementation of EBP, and these discussions have informed some of
my questions. As much as we wish it wasn't still happening, many of our
preceptors on the floor show us learners "the right way" to do a task and
then "the way they do it." When a nurse is showing me something "her way"
and I know from class or lab that it is not the right way, it can tend to make
me very emotional for the patient. For example, this week I inserted a Foley
catheter and of course took my time to do it the correct way that we were
shown in our lab, all the while talking to the patient. Then later I went into
a room with my preceptor who was inserting a Foley. She put the same Foley
completely in and out (all the way to the Y bifurcation) three times. She did
this regardless of the fact that it had the woman's menses on it, never once
talking to the patient to let her know what was happening (in fact she was on
the phone the whole time).*

*I was in shock by these actions. I had never felt so far from our fundamentals
lab. I kept thinking about the extreme risk of infection my nurse had created.
I have been wondering why nurses do things the wrong way when they
obviously know the right way. Is it a time constraint thing? Or did my nurse
not want to have to charge the patient for three separate Foley catheter trays?
Or did she not want to take the time to get off the phone and go down the
hall to get another sterile catheter? Would she even feel guilty if she knew
her actions had put her patient at risk for infection? As confused as I was by
this "role-modeling," it has made me think about my own responses to time
constraints, inconveniences, and putting patients at risk.*

One can hear and feel this learner's sense of contradiction, sensitivity, and questioning. This reflection is another example of critical reflection as this learner described how she would improve her practice now and in the future. In previous reflection papers, this learner had written about the "burden" of her sensitivity and how poignantly she felt compassion and empathy. She followed up with an insightful response to this very upsetting event, articulating her powerlessness in the learner role as she watched her preceptor compromise patient safety, vowing she would not be powerless in her own practice. She continued to express her commitment to safe practice, evidence-based practice, and doing things "the right way."

REFLECTIVE PRACTICE: DEVELOPING COLLABORATIVE RELATIONSHIPS

Many learners choose to write about the reality-based difficulties of effective teamwork and collaboration in the clinical setting—Domain 6, Interprofessional Education and Practice in the AACN Essentials (2021) and a QSEN competency. Not being educated alongside other health professionals, nurse learners are often surprised at the variety of models other healthcare disciplines employ in providing patient care. The following reflection illustrates learning about the varied roles and responsibilities for nurses and physicians and how it informs the learner's approach.

> *Doctors and nurses see the same patient through different lenses. Nurses can spend considerably more time with each patient than a doctor does and are able to witness the patient's abilities and hindrances in achieving recovery. It is not a matter of whether the doctor or nurse is right or wrong; it is about working together as a medical team to provide the care that is appropriate for each patient. In optimal patient care, the interventions necessary are seen through each lens and provide the patient with holistic care toward healing. But sometimes the picture of the patient is seen through different lenses and [we] do not agree.*
>
> *This was the case when I took care of a patient whose diagnosis was status-post-modified radical neck dissection and left tonsillectomy with parapharyngeal tumor removal. The patient's physician visited him in the hospital, saw how his incision was healing, and wrote orders for him to be discharged. From a nursing perspective, this patient was NOT ready to be discharged from the hospital. The patient continued to have difficulty swallowing (he was on a liquid diet) and used oral suction every couple of minutes to help clear his secretions. He had mild nausea that was not well relieved. His pain was not managed well despite receiving morphine slow IVP every two hours. And despite teaching, the patient had a knowledge deficit of how to manage the care of his two JP drains. The patient lived alone and stated that he did not have any family members or friends that would be able to assist him at home. As a nurse, part of my role is to be my patient's advocate. In observing his struggles, I did not feel comfortable with the order to discharge him. I spoke with the RN I was working with, and she called the physician to try to paint a picture of what our experience had been in caring for this patient all day.*

While the learner remained nonjudgmental about the physician's different assessment of the patient, he attributed the varying assessment of the patient as different "lenses," both as a logical thinker and a critical thinker. He provided clinical evidence supporting his judgment that the patient was not ready for discharge and was explicit in the professional value of being the patient's advocate and thinking carefully about how to live that value in this clinical situation. Nurses have prolonged exposure to patients, expanding their insights and awareness with a responsibility to communicate that information to the healthcare team as part of what nurses do.

In early clinical rotations, learners can begin to appreciate what they do not understand or know in their practice; however, reflection provides the opportunity for learners to see their own development. As learners and nurses develop, they cultivate an increased sensibility of their own growth. The following reflection from a learner just prior to graduation demonstrates this evolution:

> *I have learned, through the process of my nursing education, how to listen. All my life I have been a great talker. Sitting with my patient last week while the pain medication took effect, I was quiet. My patient was quiet. It was a great moment. I might choose to be quiet more often. Also connected to my increased sense of myself is my increasing comfort with not knowing. Patient safety has been emphasized in all my QSEN work. I ask better questions now. I know my limits. I understand that when I am given the responsibility of caring for people, part of that caring is saying when I don't know something.*

An example of critical reflection, this learner has increased their sense of self, their strengths, and areas still developing. Reflective practitioners value the process and outcomes of critically examining practice through engagement and critical reasoning to reconsider practice; thus, through critical reflection, they continuously improve their practice.

EXAMINING RESPONSES TO REFLECTION PAPERS

Few learners or nurses appreciate the expectation of regular reflection whether oral or written. Resistance wanes after learners and nurses receive the educator/mentor comments on their reflection, quickly recognizing the value of the individualized, substantive written dialogue with their educator or mentor. Though these examples are from an academic perspective, the same coaching approach can help new graduates in transition to practice or nurses progressing along the novice-to-expert continuum. Experienced nurses can use the same process because they are continually "making sense of practice" and incorporating new knowledge. As a practice-based discipline, nursing is a lifelong learning process, and reflection is a way to continually update awareness, actions, and responses.

Practicing nurses may use reflection papers as part of their development portfolio much like learners use course evaluations. In this excerpt from a learner evaluation of a course, appreciation for the opportunity for reflective learning emerges as an important part of the course:

> *I appreciate the time the professor took to respond to every assignment I submitted. It was refreshing to see that our papers were read and to receive individualized feedback. I started looking forward to the comments on my reflection papers. They were supportive yet encouraged me to stretch in my thinking and in my practice. I developed a familiarity with my inner clinical voice through these papers.*

> *I wish more professors would use reflection papers. I learned so much about my own thinking through this assignment. It felt like valuable work. I feel more aware of my own values as a nurse and how I want to enact those values in my emerging practice.*

> *I was a pretty big critic of the reflection paper assignment when I first learned about it. Weekly writing, really?? I could not imagine any value to such an overwhelming assignment. But I quickly came to love this weekly outlet. I started hearing "Stephanie the nurse." I didn't know she existed before this. I think the writing helped me see more clearly which values will guide my practice. There was a lot that I saw in my clinical rotation that upset me, but the weekly writing provided a place to figure out some of that confusion.*

Whether a learner or practicing nurse, the constant dialogue with educators or mentors becomes a simultaneous learning experience of feeling seen, known, and connected. The back and forth educators and mentors experience with learners/nurses expands their own capacity as "educators."

REFLECTIVE PRACTICES: REDESIGNING ASSESSMENT AND FEEDBACK

The dominant mode of instruction in nursing education (especially clinical education) has an expert-educator and novice-learner relationship. Changing the clinical learning paradigm to an open learning partnership aligned with transformative, interactive, experiential learning fits the goals and aims of reflection (Horsburgh & Ippolito, 2018). Engaging learners or nurses in reflective practice requires mutual openness to examine new ideas and the ability to listen and act appropriately; both learners and educators must adopt an open attitude. Innovative assessment strategies include narratives, unfolding cases, simulation, focus groups, rubrics, reflection-on-action, and appreciative inquiry.

Nurses do not learn from experience alone; deep learning comes from critically reflecting on experience.

Conditioning the reflective practice muscle early in the educational journey creates muscle memory, which can sustain them throughout their practice. Educators can role-model openness to learning from clinical experiences by applying reflective practices to assessment and feedback and promoting lifelong skills for continuously improving one's work.

Perspectives vary on assessing reflective assignments, especially assigning a grade. Rubrics are a helpful way to offer feedback to learners so that they can write deeper, more direct reflections and apply evidence to how they are thinking about their practice. Feedback may include additional questions for helping think more clearly or for future application. In this back-and-forth written dialogue, educators and learners mutually learn and grow.

The same rubrics can be adapted to assessing online assignments and fostering the relationship between educator and learner. Bauer (2002) shared questions for evaluating learner participation in an online leadership course. Learners were given the following knowledge work questions for reflecting on their readings each week:

- What concepts, theories, models, tools, techniques, and resources in the week's assigned readings did you find most valuable?

- How might you use this information in your practice?

- Why is the information important to your practice?

- How will the knowledge improve your effectiveness as a clinician?

- How does the knowledge and information help you understand the interdependence of system dynamics in terms of context, relationships, and trends?

- Why care about the knowledge? How does it help you clarify values and manage professional purpose?

- How does the knowledge gained advance your achievement of the nursing program outcomes and support your mastery of the essentials for preparation as a registered nurse?

- What other thoughts, reflections, or significant learning have influenced your personal and/or professional development these past few weeks?

- Create and pose a question of your own design to the members of your learning circle. Answer at least one question posed by a colleague in your learning circle.

New paradigms for learner-centered approaches in contemporary higher education create new challenges for assessment and evaluation. Shifting from traditional objective evaluation (judgment) and assessment (level of competence) to reflective approaches more closely matches competency-based learning. An appreciative philosophy applied to assessment and evaluation of learners is consistent with views of higher education that balance the learner and educator relationship for mutual learning. Similarly, when a mentor applies an appreciative inquiry model for nurses' reflection, there is explicit corroboration helping a nurse's growth in practice.

Reflective learning is predicated on openness and credibility between learner and educator; as such, educators need to pay greater attention to fairness and the exercise of academic power by being open to discussion, knowing when to be flexible on timelines, and adjudicating disputes among groups (Soffer et al., 2019). Reflective learning reduces hierarchy by opening the dialogue for continuously analyzing and reframing learning goals. The focus shifts from achieving objectives to assessing how well learners and nurses can internalize what is learned and translate changes into practice behavior.

REVIEWING REFLECTIVE WORK

Clear criteria for reflective writing enable learners and nurses to understand expectations for a more meaningful reflective experience. Criteria should represent the complex nature of practice and be fluid to accommodate evolving needs of the learner or nurse. The act of co-creating helps nurses continue to think about the topic in new ways. Educators or mentors can ask, "In this assignment, how would I know if you understood all that you needed to know?" Educators can follow with probing questions to stimulate deeper thinking and develop alternative possibilities. Both learners and nurses feel empowered when they are asked to co-create and engage in dialogue about learning expectations.

Burns and Bulman (2000) identified four potential outcomes of reflection that can be reframed to assess. How has the learner/nurse demonstrated: 1) a new perspective on experience, 2) change in behavior, 3) readiness for application, and 4) commitment to action? These four outcomes, which can be cognitive and affective in nature, can also be the foundation for developing assessment expectations for learners and nurses.

Clark (2011) proposes a set of reflective questions for educators to ask in setting expectations for evaluation of reflective activities that can be used in didactic or clinical learning experiences:

- Does the learner or nurse seek alternatives?

- Does the learner or nurse view the experience from various perspectives?

- Does the learner or nurse seek a framework, theoretical basis, or underlying rationale (of behaviors, methods, techniques, programs)?

- Does the learner or nurse compare and contrast?

- Does the learner or nurse put the experience into different or varied contexts?

- Does the learner or nurse ask, "What if . . .?"

- Does the learner or nurse consider consequences?

RECREATING EDUCATOR EVALUATIONS OR ANNUAL NURSE EVALUATIONS

In conventional pedagogy, evaluation questionnaires are the principal means by which the quality of teaching/learning is gathered from learners, typically at the end of the semester. The same is true in clinical settings where nurses have annual evaluations to assess clinical competence, effectiveness as a team member, and overall practice quality. While best practices recommend a multi-perspective approach, an appreciative evaluation focuses on what went well. These questions are useful in formative evaluation:

- What went well for you in class (clinical) today? What is going well in your practice?

- What do you want more of?

- What, if anything, is frustrating you?

- What are you still worried about?

Appreciative questions provide valuable feedback yet engage learners and nurses in reflective practice to think about how they are learning and growing rather than identifying gaps. It encourages both learners and nurses to invest effort in improvement while encouraging collaboration in which all remain open to feedback and new ideas.

At the end of an activity, course, or clinical rotation, an appreciative evaluation may ask these questions:

- What gave life to this learning activity, course, or clinical rotation? What made it come alive for you?

- What were the most successful experiences you had in this course, rotation, or activity?

- How was this different from other learning experiences?

- What will you take from this course to apply elsewhere?

APPLICATION FOR PERSONAL AND PROFESSIONAL PRACTICE: REIMAGINING REFLECTION AND SELF-ASSESSMENT

Self-assessment raises awareness about how to make better choices in the future. Open-ended questions guide self-assessments and provide an opportunity to safely experience the range of emotions experienced in practice. Nurses who establish the practice of self-assessment during their clinical education are encouraged to incorporate it as part of lifelong professional development. Working through challenging or complex clinical situations, nurses develop the capacity to step back and look at their practice from a broader perspective, to see a situation from each participant's point of view.

SELF-ASSESSMENTS

Self-assessments encourage self-awareness and provide an opportunity for learners and nurses to explore and attend to feelings and attitudes, promoting their accountability.

The first step in change is asking questions about how they fit into the context of the situation and how well they are doing and being, which in turn leads to improved practice. Reflection is a transformational tool for individuals and their professional practice (Armstrong & Sherwood, 2022). During the COVID-19 pandemic, reflective practices facilitated self-care and resilience among healthcare providers; pairing reflective practice with mindfulness enhanced self-care outcomes for nurses to survive this challenging time (Graham, 2022; Wharton et al., 2021).

Reflection-before-action, -in-action, and -on-action can guide self-assessment. For example, self-assessment can be used at the beginning and end of an in-person or online class or learning activity to help participants mindfully engage by considering the purpose and goals for learning:

- Why am I here?

- What is my goal for learning?

- What commitment do I make for achieving my goals?

At the end of the session or clinical rotation, self-assessment questions deepen the capacity to continually assess professional development for lifelong learning. The habit of reflection encourages one's accountability for reflecting-on-action through three open-ended reflective questions:

- In what ways did the class/activity or clinical experience address my expectations?

- What did I learn?

- How will I use what I learned in my practice?

REFLECTIVE SUMMARY

Nurses are important members of the healthcare team in helping healthcare systems integrate ongoing improvement in quality and safety. Patient outcomes, quality, and safety are learned both at the systems level and at the personal level to advance professional development. When nurses understand those system improvements in the context of their individual patients, a transformation in mindset takes place, and quality and safety become an integral part of their daily work. Reflective practice pedagogy, whether in academic or clinical settings, provides important opportunities for nurses to explore their professional and individual commitment to quality and safety in their emerging practice. Written reflective dialogue with teachers, mentors, or other nurses provides systematic learning; this reflection-on-action is a process of sense-making of experience, thus building tacit knowledge to move toward professional maturity. Insights into improved systems begin in a nurse's own practice; improved systems are often the result of collaboration among professionals who are first committed to improving their own practice.

LEARNING NARRATIVE

Table 9.2 provides examples for learners and nurses in developing competencies defined both by QSEN skills and attitude elements, which are also exemplified in several domains from the 2021 AACN Essentials (adapted from Armstrong, Horton-Deutsch, & Sherwood, 2017). Review the competency element in column two describing the competency in column one. Use the prompts in column three to reflect on your own practice.

TABLE 9.2	QUALITY AND SAFETY EDUCATION FOR NURSES' (QSEN) COMPETENCY ELEMENT AND AACN DOMAIN FOR CLINICAL REFLECTION PROMPTS	
QSEN AND AACN COMPETENCY	COMPETENCY ELEMENT	PROMPT FOR CLINICAL REFLECTION
Patient-Centered Care (AACN Domain 2: Person-Centered Care)	Value the patient's expertise with own health and symptoms (Attitude)	• What observable behaviors in your practice demonstrate this attitude? • How do you balance the need for efficiency in your practice and the time/space for this attitude and corresponding behaviors? • Are there clinical situations where this attitude is in conflict with another practice value?
	Value continuous improvement of own communication and conflict-resolution skills (Attitude)	• Consider nurses you have observed who role-model this attitude in their practice and describe what it looks like. • What are the difficult or uncomfortable aspects of this attitude? How does your own self-awareness help with the improvement process included in this attitude?
Teamwork and Collaboration (Domain 6: Interprofessional Education and Practice)	Demonstrate awareness of own strengths and limitations as a team member (Skills)	• How do clinicians demonstrate this skill? How would this look to their colleagues? • How does this skill facilitate healthy teamwork?

continues

TABLE 9.2 QUALITY AND SAFETY EDUCATION FOR NURSES' (QSEN) COMPETENCY ELEMENT AND AACN DOMAIN FOR CLINICAL REFLECTION PROMPTS (CONT.)

QSEN AND AACN COMPETENCY	COMPETENCY ELEMENT	PROMPT FOR CLINICAL REFLECTION
	Respect the unique attributes that members bring to a team, including variations in professional orientations and accountabilities (Attitude)	• How might you gain awareness of the varied professional approaches and accountabilities of colleagues on your healthcare team? Why is this important? • What examples have you observed of "respect" acted out on the healthcare team? How has this attitude enhanced team functioning (from a colleague perspective)? From a patient perspective?
Evidence-Based Practice (Domain 4: Scholarship for Nursing Practice)	Question rationale for routine approaches to care that result in less than desired outcomes or adverse events (Skills)	• This skill requires individuals or teams to speak up. What are your observations of an individual's or a team's comfort with speaking up to question rationale for routine approaches that are ineffective? • As a nursing leader, how can you impact the culture of a microsystem so that individuals and teams feel free to speak up about ineffective care?
Quality Improvement (Domain 5: Quality and Safety)	Appreciate that continuous quality improvement is an essential part of the daily work of all health professions (Attitude)	• How is this attitude promoted among nurse leaders? • What is your experience of the adoption of this attitude among all team members? • What are supporting and disabling factors for this attitude in the work processes or habits you have observed? How do you integrate this attitude as a core part of your nursing practice?

REFLECTIVE QUESTIONS

1. What do you value most about nurses' work? What do you value most about the contributions you make to nursing?

2. What are the core values and best practices evident/absent in the reflections shared in this chapter?

3. Examine the reflections shared in this chapter from the perspectives of the people involved. For example, the reflection paper describing the learner's experience in caring for a patient with burns can be examined from the learner perspective or the educator, nurse, or patient perspective to further explore the nuances of the experience.

4. Describe three things that you commit to for improving patient safety What are the challenges and opportunities for achievement?

5. What are ways to integrate reflective practices more effectively into your teaching in both didactic and workplace learning?

REFERENCES

American Association of Colleges of Nursing. (2021). *The essentials: Core competencies for professional nursing education.* https://www.aacnnursing.org/Portals/42/AcademicNursing/pdf/Essentials-2021.pdf

Armstrong, G., Horton-Deutsch, S. & Sherwood, G. (2017). Reflection and mindful practice: A means to quality and safety. In S. Horton-Deutsch & G. Sherwood (Eds.), *Reflective practice: Transforming education and improving outcomes* (2nd ed., pp. 29–49). Sigma Theta Tau International.

Armstrong, G., Sherwood, G., Ironside, P., Cerbie Brown, E., & Wonder, A. (2022). Reflective practice: Using narrative pedagogy to foster quality and safety. In G. Sherwood & J. Barnsteiner (Eds.), *Quality and safety in nursing: A competency approach to improving outcomes* (3rd ed., pp. 301–320). Wiley-Blackwell.

Bass, J., Sidebotham, M., Creedy, D., & Sweet, L. (2020). Midwifery students' experiences and expectations of using a model of holistic reflection. *Women and Birth: Journal of the Australian College of Midwives, 33*(4), 383–392. https://doi.org/10.1016/j.wombi.2019.06.020

Bauer, J. F. (2002). Assessing student work from chatrooms and bulletin boards. *New Directions for Teaching and Learning, 2002*(91), 31–36.

Benner, P., Sutphen, M., Leonard, V., & Day, L. (2010). *Educating nurses: A call for radical transformation.* Jossey-Bass.

Bono-Neri, F. (2019). Pedagogical nursing practice: Redefining nursing practice for the academic nurse educator. *Nurse Education in Practice, 37*, 105–108. https://doi.org/10.1016/j.nepr.2019.04.002

Branch, W. T., Jr., & George, M. (2017). Reflection-based learning for professional ethical formation. *AMA Journal of Ethics, 19*(4), 349–356. https://doi.org/10.1001/journalofethics.2017.19.4.medu1-1704

Burns, S., & Bulman, C. (2000). *Reflective practice in nursing: The growth of the professional practitioner* (2nd ed.) Blackwell Science.

Campbell, F., & Rogers, H. (2022). Through the looking glass: A review of the literature surrounding reflective practice in dentistry. *British Dental Journal, 232*(10), 729–734. https://doi.org/10.1038/s41415-022-3993-4

Chauke, M. E., Van Der Wal, D., & Botha, A. (2015). Using appreciative inquiry to transform student nurses' image of nursing. *Curationis, 38*(1), 1–8. https://doi.org/10.4102/curationis.v38i1.1460

Clark, D. R. (2011). *Learning through reflection.* http://www.nwlink.com/~donclark/hrd/development/reflection.html

Cronenwett, L., Sherwood, G., Barnsteiner, J., Disch, J., Johnson, J., Mitchell, P., Sullivan, D. T., & Warren, J. (2007). Quality and safety education for nurses. *Nursing Outlook, 55*(3), 122–131. https://doi.org/10.1016/j.outlook.2007.02.006

Cronenwett, L., Sherwood, G., & Gelmon, S. B. (2009). Improving quality and safety education: The QSEN learning collaborative. *Nursing Outlook, 57*(6), 304–312. https://doi.org/10.1016/j.outlook.2009.09.004

Cronenwett, L., Sherwood, G., Pohl, J., Barnsteiner, J., Moore, S., Sullivan, D. T., Ward, D., & Warren, J. (2009). Quality and safety education for advanced nursing practice. *Nursing Outlook, 57*(6), 338–348. https://doi.org/10.1016/j.outlook.2009.07.009

Day, L., & Sherwood, G. (2022). Transforming education to transform practice: Using unfolding case studies to integrate quality and safety in subject-centered classrooms. In G. Sherwood & J. Barnsteiner (Eds.), *Quality and safety in nursing: A competency approach to improving outcomes* (3rd ed., pp. 268–300). Wiley-Blackwell.

Freshwater, D. (2008). Reflective practice: The state of the art. In D. Freshwater, B. Taylor, & G. Sherwood (Eds.), *International textbook of reflective practice in nursing* (pp. 1–18). Blackwell Publishing.

Goleman, D., Boyatzis, R., & McKee, A. (2002). *Primal leadership: Realizing the power of emotional intelligence.* Harvard Business School Publishing.

Goulet, M. H., Larue, C., & Alderson, M. (2016). Reflective practice: A comparative dimensional analysis of the concept in nursing and education studies. *Nursing Forum, 51*(2), 139–150. https://doi.org/10.1111/nuf.12129

Graham, M. M. (2022). Navigating professional and personal knowing through reflective storytelling amidst Covid-19. *Journal of Holistic Nursing, 40*(4), 372–382. https://doi.org/10.1177/08980101211072289

Horsburgh, J., & Ippolito, K. (2018). A skill to be worked at: Using social learning theory to explore the process of learning from role models in clinical settings. *BMC Medical Education, 18*(1), 156. https://doi.org/10.1186/s12909-018-1251-x

Horton-Deutsch, S., & Sherwood, G. (2008). Reflection: An educational strategy to develop emotionally competent nurse leaders. *Journal of Nursing Management, 16*(8), 946–954. https://doi.org/10.1111/j.1365-2834.2008.00957.x

Johns, C. (2022). *Becoming a reflective practitioner* (6th ed.). Wiley-Blackwell.

Kaiafas, K. N. (2021). Emotional intelligence and role-modeling nursing's soft skills. *Journal of Christian Nursing: A Quarterly Publication of Nurses Christian Fellowship, 38*(4), 240–243. https://doi.org/10.1097/CNJ.0000000000000881

Mantzourani, E., Desselle, S., Le, J., Lonie, J. M., & Lucas, C. (2019). The role of reflective practice in healthcare professions: Next steps for pharmacy education and practice. *Research in Social & Administrative Pharmacy: RSAP, 15*(12), 1476–1479. https://doi.org/10.1016/j.sapharm.2019.03.011

Merriel, A., Wilson, A., Decker, E., Hussein, J., Larkin, M., Barnard, K., O'Dair, M., Costello, A., Malata, A., & Coomarasamy, A. (2022). Systematic review and narrative synthesis of the impact of Appreciative Inquiry in healthcare. *BMJ Open Quality, 11*(2), e001911. https://doi.org/10.1136/bmjoq-2022-001911

O'Brien, B. C., & Battista, A. (2020). Situated learning theory in health professions education research: A scoping review. *Advances in Health Sciences Education, 25*, 483–509. https://doi.org/10.1007/s10459-019-09900-w

Patel, K. M., & Metersky, K. (2021). Reflective practice in nursing: A concept analysis. *International Journal of Nursing Knowledge, 33*(3), 180–187. https://doi.org/10.1111/2047-3095.12350

Plant, J., Li, S. T., Blankenburg, R., Bogetz, A. L., Long, M., & Butani, L. (2017). Reflective practice in the clinical setting: A multi-institutional qualitative study of pediatric faculty and residents. *Academic Medicine: Journal of the Association of American Medical Colleges*, 92(11S), S75–S83. https://doi.org/10.1097/ACM.0000000000001910

Salik, I., & Paige, J. T. (2022). *Debriefing the interprofessional team in medical simulation.* StatPearls Publishing.

Scheel, L. S., Bydam, J., & Peters, M. D. J. (2021). Reflection as a learning strategy for the training of nurses in clinical practice setting: A scoping review. *JBI Evidence Synthesis*, 19(12), 3268–3300. https://doi.org/10.11124/JBIES-21-00005

Schön, D. A. (1987). *Educating the reflective practitioner.* Jossey-Bass.

Sherwood, G., & Day, L. (2022). Quality and safety in clinical learning environments. In G. Sherwood & J. Barnsteiner (Eds.), *Quality and safety in nursing: A competency approach to improving outcomes* (3rd ed., pp. 321–348). Wiley.

Soffer, T., Kahan, T., & Nachmias, R. (2019). Patterns of students' utilization of flexibility in online academic courses and their relation to course achievement. *International Review of Research in Open and Distributed Learning, 20*(3). https://doi.org/10.19173/irrodl.v20i4.3949

Stulz, V., Francis, L., Pathrose, S., Sheehan, A., & Drayton, N. (2021). Appreciative inquiry as an intervention to improve nursing and midwifery students transitioning into becoming new graduates: An integrative review. *Nurse Education Today*, 98, 104727. https://doi.org/10.1016/j.nedt.2020.104727

Tesseyman, S., Peterson, K., & Beaumont, E. (2022). The nurse apprentice and fundamental bedside care: An historical perspective. *Nursing Inquiry*, e12540 [Advance online publication]. https://doi.org/10.1111/nin.12540

Van Schalkwyk, S. C., Hafler, J., Brewer, T. F., Maley, M. A., Margolis, C., McNamee, L., Meyer, I., Peluso, M. J., Schmutz, A. M., Spak, J. M., Davies, D., & Bellagio Global Health Education Initiative. (2019). Transformative learning as pedagogy for the health professions: A scoping review. *Medical Education*, 53(6), 547–558. https://doi.org/10.1111/medu.13804

Wharton, C., Kotera, Y., & Brennan, S. (2021). A well-being champion and the role of self-reflective practice for ICU nurses during COVID-19 and beyond. *Nursing in Critical Care*, 26(2), 70–72. https://doi.org/10.1111/nicc.12563

Ziebart, C., & MacDermid, J. C. (2019). Reflective practice in physical therapy: A scoping review. *Physical Therapy*, 99(8), 1056–1068. https://doi.org/10.1093/ptj/pzz049

PART IV

REFLECTIVE PRACTICE IN ORGANIZATIONS AND COMMUNITIES

10 Rethinking How We Work Together: Reflective Practices
    Using Emergent Strategy, Liberating Structures, and
    Clearness Committees.................................... 207

11 Pluralistic Possibility: Reflective Practices
    to Reframe Our World.................................. 227

12 Redesigning Academic and Practice Partnerships:
    Reflective Communities That Learn and Practice
    Together 249

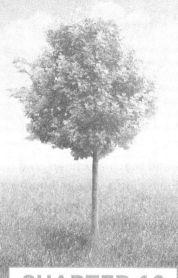

CHAPTER 10

RETHINKING HOW WE WORK TOGETHER: REFLECTIVE PRACTICES USING EMERGENT STRATEGY, LIBERATING STRUCTURES, AND CLEARNESS COMMITTEES

–*Sara Horton-Deutsch, PhD, RN, FAAN, ANEF, SGAHN*

Gwen Sherwood, PhD, RN, FAAN, ANEF

LEARNING OBJECTIVES/SUBJECTIVES

- Identify the characteristics of effective and inclusive ways of working together in groups to help all belong.

- Describe theoretical frameworks that support reflective ways of working together.

- Discuss the value of reflection for creative problem-solving.

- Explore how emergent strategy, liberating structures, and clearness committees expand our capacity for creating more inclusive, engaging, adaptive, and resourceful learning and practice environments.

OVERVIEW

Healthcare is often referred to as a team sport. No one profession or discipline can manage the myriad conditions of those seeking care. Working in groups or teams is complex, built on relationships, can be confusing, and may be counterproductive. Mastering innovative processes for improving organizational culture through more effective teamwork is both more satisfying for caregivers and can improve patient outcomes through clearer communication, shared purpose, and better relationships. Organizations are defined by their culture. Culture is defined by the way people in the culture relate, communicate, and act towards one another (Mallette & Rykert, 2018). These deep-seated behaviors, attitudes, and values are entrenched and difficult to reshape. Reflective practices using innovative strategies can interrupt interactions to make space for change and create inclusive environments where everyone belongs.

This chapter proposes ways to rethink working together to change relationships, improve outcomes, and invite everyone to participate. We propose three processes for engaging groups in identifying what is most important to be able to chart a new path forward. We explore the dynamics and importance of working together in groups in ways that involve listening, creating authentic connections, providing support, and evolving to see possibility and wholeness. We challenge conventional approaches to group interaction by drawing on complexity theory and highlighting how emergent strategy, liberating structures, and clearness committees represent more meaningful and effective ways of working together.

SUPPORTING THEORETICAL FRAMEWORKS AND OTHER EVIDENCE

Reflective ways of working together in groups are supported by several theoretical frameworks that emphasize the importance of self-reflection, critical thinking, and collaborative learning. We describe Experiential Learning Theory, transformative learning theory, and Complexity Science.

EXPERIENTIAL LEARNING THEORY

Experiential Learning Theory (Kolb, 2014) emphasizes the importance of learning through direct experience, reflection, and application. In group settings, this framework involves engaging in activities that challenge assumptions, promote critical thinking, and facilitate self-reflection. This theory proposes that people learn best when they are actively engaged in the learning process, rather than simply receiving information passively. By providing opportunities for learners to reflect on and make meaning of their experiences, experiential learning can promote deeper learning, increased retention of information, and the development of practical skills that can be applied in real-world settings.

TRANSFORMATIVE LEARNING THEORY

As explored in earlier chapters, transformative learning theory (Mezirow & Taylor, 2009) explains learning as a process of personal and social transformation that involves critically examining assumptions, beliefs, and values. From this perspective, group members engage in dialogue and activities that challenge assumptions and promote critical reflection on personal and societal values and beliefs. Similarly, communities of practice view learning as a social and collaborative process that involves participation in a shared practice or domain of knowledge. From this perspective, working together involves engaging in dialogue, sharing experiences and expertise, and reflecting on collective practice to support ongoing learning and development.

COMPLEXITY SCIENCE

Complexity science advocates emphasize the importance of self-organization, adaptation, and emergence in complex systems. From this perspective, groups are viewed as complex adaptive systems that exhibit emergent behaviors that cannot be predicted by studying the behavior of individual members in isolation. Complexity science suggests that effective group work involves creating conditions that support self-organization and emergence. This involves fostering diversity, encouraging experimentation, and promoting distributed leadership. Rather than relying on centralized control and top-down decision-making, complexity science suggests that groups should operate in a more decentralized and collaborative manner, with individuals taking on leadership roles based on their expertise and interests (Jensen, 2023).

Complexity science also emphasizes the importance of feedback loops in promoting learning and adaptation in groups. By continuously monitoring and reflecting on group processes and outcomes, individuals can adjust and adapt to improve group performance and support ongoing learning and development. Overall, complexity science suggests that working together in groups involves embracing complexity, uncertainty, and ambiguity and creating conditions that support self-organization and emergence. Much like experiential and transformative learning theories, this requires a willingness to experiment, take risks, and engage in ongoing learning and adaptation.

COMPLEXITY SCIENCE: RETHINKING ORGANIZATIONAL RELATIONSHIPS

The application of complexity science to the study of organizations is a recent addition to this array of perspectives and is most relevant to this discussion of new and more reflective ways of working with each other. According to Lindberg and colleagues (2008, p. 32), "Complexity science is not a single theory, but rather an interdisciplinary field that recognizes multiple theoretical frameworks. Complexity science examines [complex adaptive] systems comprised of multiple and diverse interacting agents." Lindberg et al. continue their discussion of complexity science:

> Complex situations display properties of uniqueness and thus must be approached and understood individually. A high degree of uncertainty is inherent in complex problems and situations, and outcomes are not predictable. Solutions cannot be assured through the application of known formulas. Likewise, expertise and experience are helpful, but do not always ensure a successful resolution. Complex problems call for unique solutions. (2008, p. 27)

When complexity is the interpretive lens for organizational life, the relationships in that organization become the most important focus. Complexity science teaches different ways of examining groups and organizations—simply put, the more complex the organization, the less effective linear and hierarchical leadership and communication will be. Westley et al. (2006) describe the elements of working from a complexity stance:

COMPLEXITY SCIENCE

Complexity science is based on a view of systems that includes highly interrelated and rapidly adaptable parts. Each element in these complex adaptable systems affects the behavior of all other elements, and small changes can lead to large effects.

> Questions are key. In complex situations there are no final answers. But certain key questions illuminate the issues of social innovation.
>
> Tensions and ambiguities are revealed through questioning. Social innovation both reveals and creates tensions. Once understood these tensions can then be engaged not simply managed in the interests of amplifying the desired change.
>
> Relationships are key to understanding and engaging with the complex dynamics of social innovation. For social innovations to succeed, everyone involved plays a role. As systems shift, everyone—funders, policymakers,

social innovators, volunteers, and evaluators—are affected. It is what happens between people, organizations, communities, and parts of systems that matter—"in the between" of relationships.

A certain mindset is crucial—framed by inquiry, not a certainty, one that embraces paradoxes and tolerates multiple perspectives. (Westley et al., 2006, pp. 21–22)

Beneath all the theoretical language lives a deceptively simple premise:

. . . If it is changing, we are after, and when we see the patterns and our role in their creation, we can make different choices in how we participate in a conversation . . . In complexity terms, this introduction of diversity into a pattern of interaction may represent the small change that triggers an entirely new pattern of relating or meaning. This emergence happens through a self-organizing process we can influence but not control. This self-organization is happening all around us and we are active players. (Lindberg et al., 2008, p. 42)

Historically, nursing scholars have examined groups and organizations from various perspectives, including systems theory, cultural theory, group process, political theory, and change theory, among others. While each approach has contributed valuable insights and brought distinctive strengths and weaknesses to the table, we propose using emergent strategy, liberating structures, and clearness committees as alternative approaches to articulate regenerative viable futures.

EMERGENT STRATEGY FOR SHAPING THE FUTURES WE WANT TO LIVE

Emergent strategy (Brown, 2017), which builds on complexity science, shares a focus on the importance of adaptation in complex systems. In the context of complexity science, emergent strategy is seen as a natural outcome of self-organization and adaptation in complex systems. As individuals interact and exchange information within a group or organization, new patterns, and behaviors emerge that cannot be predicted by studying the behavior of individual members in isolation. These emergent patterns may involve new ways of working together, new products or services, or new ways of understanding and responding to changing conditions.

Emergent strategy is viewed as more effective than traditional, top-down planning approaches in uncertain and rapidly changing environments. By encouraging experimentation, learning, and adaptation, the emergent strategy allows groups and organizations to respond more quickly and effectively to changing circumstances and opportunities. Complexity science provides a theoretical foundation

EMERGENT STRATEGY

An emergent strategy is one that emerges over time through ongoing experimentation, learning, and adaptation, rather than being predetermined or planned.

for understanding the dynamics of emergent strategy and the importance of self-organization, adaptation, and emergence in complex systems. By embracing these principles and fostering conditions that support ongoing learning and experimentation, groups and organizations can develop effective emergent strategies that respond to changing circumstances and support long-term success. According to Brown (2017), emergence notices and attends to how small actions and connections create complex systems and patterns that become ecosystems. Emergence is how we change and "emergent strategy is how we intentionally change in ways that grow our capacity to embody the just and liberated worlds we long for" (Brown; 2017, p. 3). Emergent strategy core principles guide change toward a vision of sustainability, regeneration, and inclusion. Through these principles, we begin to see our values and uncover the root cause of problems. They help us in asking important questions such as: "What are the root problems in nursing, in my community, and what do deep, foundational, rooted solutions look like?" This way of thinking, asking these questions, comes from and seeks healing, rather than dominating others with our beliefs (Brown, 2017).

The core principles of emergent strategy (Brown, 2017, pp. 41–42):

- Small is good; small is all.

- Change is constant.

- There is always enough time for the right work.

- There is a conversation in the room that only these people in this moment can have. Find it.

- Never a failure, always a lesson.

- Trust the people.

- Move at the speed of trust. Focus on critical connections over critical mass. Build resilience by building relationships.

- Less prep, more presence.

- What you pay attention to grows.

Emergent strategy as a practice and toolset requires a fundamentally different way of being with each other and in the community. Further reading and reflecting on these principles are the first steps in beginning to understand how emergent strategy principles can shift a conversation, challenge values, and shape a more positive future. Building on the core principles of emergent strategy are four universal tools to guide implementation (Brown, 2017):

- **Trust the people:** This involves goal and intention settings, inviting the right people, individual participant articulation of what they want to prioritize and discuss, developing an adaptable agenda so participants can shape the meeting, listening with love by seeking understanding and help participants to understand each other, knowing when to say yes and no (yes to what deepens the gathering and no to efforts to silence others), give the group time to be in its process (don't hover), and always ask, "What's the best, most elegant step?"

- **Principles:** Have a set of shared principles to work together, and as circumstances change, be open to revisiting common understandings of what matters most. Examples of shared principles include inclusivity, emphasizing bottom-up organizing, letting people speak for themselves, working in solidarity, building just relationships, and committing to self-transformation.

- **Protocols:** These are ways principles look in action including the boundaries, practices, and paths that can be articulated through group agreements. What are standing agreements for working together? To create emergent spaces, Brown recommends (2017, p. 229–230):

  - Listening from the inside out (a gut feeling matters)
  - Engage tension; don't indulge in drama
  - W.A.I.T.: Why am I talking?
  - Make space, take space–; balance speaking with listening
  - Confidentiality
  - Being open to learning
  - Being open to someone else speaking your truth
  - Building, not selling
  - Yes/and, both/and
  - Value the process as much as the outcome

- Assume the best intent

- Self-care and community care

- **Consensus:** This means ensuring the people who are doing the work agree on what is being done, why, and how. Doing so helps to ensure nothing is slowing or diverting the energy of the work.

LIBERATING STRUCTURES: RECREATING HOW WE INTERACT AND REFLECT

Like emergent strategy, *liberating structures* (LS) are non-hierarchical ways of working together based on complexity science that can "unleash" the power of everyone to think and act in new ways. Lipmanowicz and McCandless (2013) developed LS to provide access to the benefits of complexity science without the associated theoretical burden. Business and healthcare organizations around the world have used LS with a widespread positive effect (Holskey & Rivera, 2020; Mahoney et al., 2016; Mallette & Rykert, 2018). Because LS were created from field experience, they operate at the ground level of people's daily experience of their work.

LS are a collection of methods designed for easy use by anyone to shift the interaction patterns and "unleash the collective wisdom and creativity of nearly everyone in an organization" (Lipmanowicz & McCandless, 2010, p. 7). An important ground rule of LS is to provide everyone with the opportunity to share views and participate actively in the process; LS invite belonging. LS involve acting our way into new thinking, rather than thinking our way into action. LS lead us to "unlearn" old habits and biases for better engagement in our personal and professional experiences (Swenson et al., 2017).

The list of LS in Figure 10.1 is itself a reflection of adaptability and emergence—new ones are being invented all the time and old ones are modified as they are used. "The basic idea is that Liberating Structures are combinations of freedom and control—they provide minimal structures or rules to maximize engagement by all. They are easy to learn and use and need not be implemented perfectly to produce results and change the pattern of interactions. Many of them create conversational spaces for people to self-organize and discover latent innovations that remain hidden when too many decisions and controls are imposed from the top. They make it easy for people at all levels to speak up, participate, and contribute" (Lipmanowicz & McCandless, 2010, p. 10). They are intended to allow groups to create solutions through "informal social networks and decentralized communities-of-practice" (p. 6). LS work in large and small groups, require a few minutes, or can be designed to encompass whole days.

Liberating Structures Menu: Including and Unleashing Everyone v 2.2

Impromptu Networking
Rapidly share challenges and expectations, building new connections

9 Whys
Make the purpose of your work together clear

What, So What, Now What?
Together, look back on progress to-date and decide what adjustments are needed

TRIZ
Stop counterproductive activities & behaviors to make space for innovation

Appreciative Interviews
Discover & build on the root causes of success

1-2-4-All
Engage everyone simultaneously in generating questions/ideas/suggestions

User Experience Fishbowl
Share know-how gained from experience with a larger community

15% Solutions
Discover & focus on what each person has the freedom and resources to do now

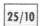
25-To-10 Crowd Sourcing
Rapidly generate & sift a group's most powerful actionable ideas

Troika Consulting
Get practical and imaginative help from colleagues immediately

Conversation Café
Engage everyone in making sense of profound challenges

Min Specs
Specify only the absolute "Must do's" & "Must not do's" for achieving a purpose

Wise Crowds
Tap the wisdom of the whole group in rapid cycles

Wicked Questions
Articulate the paradoxical challenges that a group must confront to succeed

Drawing Together
Reveal insights & paths forward through non-verbal expression

Improv Prototyping
Develop effective solutions to chronic challenges while having serious fun

Agreement-Certainty Matrix
Sort challenges into simple, complicated, complex and chaotic domains

Shift & Share
Spread good ideas and make informal connections with innovators

Heard, Seen, Respected
Practice deeper listening and empathy with colleagues

Social Network Webbing
Map informal connections & decide how to strengthen the network to achieve a purpose

Design StoryBoards
Define step-by-step elements for bringing projects to productive endpoints

Open Space
Liberate inherent action and leadership in large groups

Discovery & Action Dialogue
Discover, spark & unleash local solutions to chronic problems

Integrated~Autonomy
Move from either-or to robust both-and solutions

Generative Relationships
Reveal relationship patterns that create surprising value or dysfunctions

Critical Uncertainties
Develop strategies for operating in a range of plausible yet unpredictable futures

Purpose-To-Practice
Define the five elements that are essential for a resilient & enduring initiative

Ecocycle Planning
Analyze the full portfolio of activities & relationships to identify obstacles and opportunities for progress

Panarchy
Understand how embedded systems interact, evolve, spread innovation, and transform

What I Need From You
Surface essential needs across functions and accept or reject requests for support

Celebrity Interview
Reconnect the experience of leaders and experts with people closest to the challenges at hand

Helping Heuristics
Practice progressive methods for helping others, receiving help, and asking for help

Simple Ethnography
Observe & record actual behavior of users in the field

Keith McCandless & Henri Lipmanowicz www.liberatingstructures.com

FIGURE 10.1 Liberating structures menu.
Source: Lipmanowicz & McCandless, 2013, p. 68

Figure 10.2 illustrates two possibilities for organizational/group behavior: One pattern is centered on control; the other is focused on letting go. Control-centric cultures create a cycle of dependence, whereas cultures focused on letting go foster cycles of self-organization. Control tends toward a focus on tasks and alignment, whereas letting go tends toward a focus on engaging people. When control is ascendant, the culture fosters negative behaviors, such as aggression, forced "buy-in," secrecy, burnout, not taking responsibility, blame and mistrust, and caution. Dependency feeds back to the creation of ever more control. When letting go is predominant, the culture engages in interdependent work and shared accountability. Some commonly experienced behaviors in that kind of system include listening, asking for help, removing barriers to innovation, taking more responsibility, seeking full participation by all, information sharing, and risking action. LS can be the catalyst for moving from control to letting go.

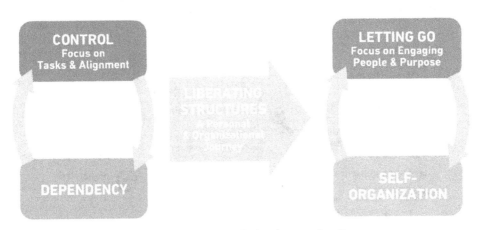

FIGURE 10.2   Shifting behaviors and culture.
Source: Lipmanowicz & McCandless, 2013

LS can be scaled up or down, depending on the size of the group and the nature of the work to be done. This approach works in teacher-learner dyads, in classrooms, in governance groups such as committees and task forces, or entire institutions.

LIBERATING STRUCTURES: REFLECTING-IN-ACTION AND REFLECTING-ON-ACTION

Reflection is integral to LS but emerges later in the process. The idea behind acting our way into thinking is that we can use LS to quickly make changes in our patterns of interaction, leading to reflection. Initial small changes may require time to realize what has happened; reflection takes time to develop. Changing the ways we communicate and interact with each other drives culture change and helps establish new habits and behaviors. Reflective practices help us notice how (and how much) our relationships have changed. A group conversation using What, So What, Now What cycles illustrates reflection-on-action:

- What? What stands out in the stories we have shared? What do you notice?

- So What? Is there a pattern underneath the stories? Does it make a difference?

- Now What? What action can help us move forward? Who else should be here?

The conversations guided by LS often involve telling, hearing, and thinking about stories, great and small. From a reflective perspective, engaging in conversations in this manner cues us to reflect on our thoughts and whether our responses within the experience were effective. Johns (2006) calls this dialogue between the retelling of the story (text) and other sources of knowing *theoretical framing,* helping us to uncover the relevance and validity to inform our practice. By conversing in a manner that involves sharing our own stories and incorporating relevant literature, we further inform and frame our ideas, and insights emerge (Swenson et al., 2017).

USING LIBERATING STRUCTURES: RESTARTING CONVERSATIONS

Considering the pandemic and socio-cultural-economic factors impacting our communities, healthcare organizations and academic settings are revisiting their vision, mission, and core values to find new ways forward. Three examples of LS are Conversation Cafés, 1-2-4-All, and TRIZ. *Conversation Cafés* (originating in Seattle soon after September 11, 2001) are open, hosted conversations where people gather to make sense of their world. Conversation Cafés have no agenda but are a simple process that helps shift participants from small talk to BIG talk, focusing on conversations that matter.

The Conversation Café website (www.conversationcafe.org) provides an introductory video and print resources. Starting a Conversation Café is based on three primary principles: 1) inclusivity and diversity (everyone can participate); 2) a designated host or hosts (but not a permanent host; anyone can host, and all are invited to try); and 3) open access to the conversation. The only rules or agreements are:

- What is said cannot be owned by anyone: Clarify that what is said in the Conversation Café must be in the public domain. No one at the table or outside the conversation can claim exclusive ownership of the ideas that emerge.

- Commercial-free (and agenda-free) zones: No one can attend primarily to promote or impose a particular agenda, point of view, outcome, or solution.

- No committees: No political networking, committee formation, or action groups allowed.

- Continuing to push our edges: Encourage people to become hosts in a wide variety of settings on their topics.

- Empowering hosts: Provide clear information to all hosts and participants about the mechanics of hosting Conversation Cafés and the open, inquisitive spirit of hosting.

Develop questions for conversation that will interest a broad range of participants. Provide a café atmosphere with refreshments and arrange chairs around a single table. Swenson and colleagues (2017) use a "talking stick" so that only one person talks at a time, enabling everyone to have time to talk and be heard. The host or facilitators encourage "deep listening" while the person talking is encouraged to say what they wish without comment or questions from others. All are provided a chance to respond once to the question, then respond again, in turn, after all had spoken (or "passed") once.

"Creative conversation happens in a generative space that lies between. Notions of leading or following dissolve. A keen attentiveness and responsiveness among participants take over. The process evokes a fine attunement to each other and what is happening in the moment."

–Keith McCandless (personal communication)

Swenson and colleagues (2017) provide an example of a Conversation Café stimulated by questions to discuss the school's newly developed core values: respect, responsibility, trust, and dialogue. Participants were invited to talk about a time when a core value was demonstrated by them or someone else. In the second round, each person could enlarge or clarify what they or another participant had said.

The discussion on each core value enabled participants to identify when the value had been demonstrated, what behaviors and language were used, and what feelings were evoked when the value was evident (or absent). Establishing a safe space for conversation, faculty and staff members were able to converse without hierarchy, without concern for repercussions or retaliation, and with the assurance of confidentiality of the discussions. Conversation Cafés can vary in time and typically last around 60 to 90 minutes. Scheduling some at the end of the day and others at midday enables different people with different schedules to participate.

1-2-4-ALL

The LS called *1-2-4-All* can be used to start a different kind of conversation. A 1-2-4-All conversation begins with self-reflection on a particular question. After this individual reflection, that person shares their thoughts with one other person. Each pair then shares with another group of two, and finally, each group of four shares their conversations with the whole group (All). The themes from the "All" conversation generate the next steps for the group. The initial conversation cycles (1-2-4) are designed to be short, perhaps five minutes for each cycle. The rapid cycles allow for "jointly shaping solutions and insights in the moment" (Lipmanowicz & McCandless, 2010). The whole-group conversation allows for the broadening and deepening of the themes from the rapid cycles. Mahoney et al. (2016) describe how the American Psychiatric Nurses Association used 1-2-4-All and other LS to identify priorities for their Research Council. Holskey and Rivera (2020) used 1-2-4-All and other LS to design a new professional practice model.

The facilitator begins by identifying an appreciative question. For example, within a school of nursing exploring program improvement, the question may be, "What opportunities do you see for making the relationship between graduate programs seamless?" Or, before a presentation at a conference, the presenter may ask, "What brought you to this presentation today?" The rapid cycle of conversations creates a friendly, collaborative, and inclusive environment. This LS encourages the sharing of ideas and perspectives, leading to a more diverse range of insights. By providing time for individual reflection, as well as small group and whole group discussion, the 1-2-4-All structure aims to promote active listening, collective learning, and shared ownership of outcomes. The structure also helps to break down hierarchies and power dynamics, ensuring that everyone has an opportunity to speak and be heard. Ultimately, the goal of the 1-2-4-All LS is to create a sense of community and engagement among participants, leading to more effective and sustainable outcomes.

TRIZ: TURNING IT UPSIDE DOWN

The *TRIZ* process is about creative destruction and making a space for something new to emerge. It allows participants to recognize and amplify the dysfunctional parts of a system, and then choose to eliminate them. Mallette and Rykert (2018) reported how they used TRIZ to promote a positive culture change in their nursing faculty.

For example, Swenson et al. (2017) started with a question: "What would a reliable system for making us all miserable at work look like? What is the most terrible result we could imagine?" Faculty and staff members worked in groups of four, using a rapid cycle process to answer these questions. This is often challenging at first because we are not used to thinking nonsensical thoughts about our organization or unit, but it encourages participants to let their minds go wild in this imagining and to have fun.

When the groups debriefed, several elements of a terrible workplace were generated. Ideas included everyone must always keep their doors shut. No one was allowed to talk to anyone else in person. If two people encountered each other in the halls, they were not allowed to greet one another or have any conversation. Everyone would be required to eat lunch in their own office, and always alone. The administrative assistants would make sure they never got work done on time, and they would make as many mistakes as possible. The best result would be that the faculty member would eventually stop giving administrative staff work—they would just do it themselves, behind closed doors. We would never acknowledge any elements of our lives away from school—no birthdays would be noted, no flowers or cards sent if someone was hospitalized, and no congratulations on significant life achievements. In short, the perfectly terrible system we designed would ensure that all of us would work in total isolation, with no humane or supportive interactions whatsoever.

The next step asks each person to reflect on whether any of the elements of the terrible system were like anything already happening. Participants were asked to identify what actions they could take to stop doing things that lead to isolation and dysfunction. Reflecting on this TRIZ process allowed participants to discover ways they were isolating themselves socially from one another and then described ways they could change behaviors. A collective decision was made to reserve a conference room every day for an hour to encourage eating lunch together. Reflecting on these behaviors to recognize opportunities for improving the organizational culture and ways of working together created space for something new to happen. Small differences such as these encourage us to change our habits of interaction, which in turn changes a culture of isolation into one of sustaining human connection.

LS are malleable and responsive to evolving circumstances. New structures are constantly emerging, changing, and revising. LS are context-specific representatives of the people, places, problems, and issues involved, providing innovative ways to recreate ways we work together.

CLEARNESS COMMITTEES FOR ENABLING DISCERNMENT AND COURAGEOUS, WISE ACTIONS

Another example of rethinking how we work together is through a clearness committee derived from a Quaker practice. Clearness committees originated in Quaker communities for decision-making and discernment but have extended to community groups and organizations as a form of peer support and guidance.

A *clearness committee* is a small group of individuals who come together to help someone find clarity or guidance on a particular issue or decision. The individual seeking clarity or guidance is the "focus person," and the committee members are "listeners." During a clearness committee session, the focus person presents their issue or decision to the listeners, who then ask open-ended questions to help the focus person explore their thoughts and feelings around the issue. The listeners do not offer advice or solutions but instead create a safe and supportive space for the focus person to find their clarity and discernment. The conversation is confidential.

The clearness committee aims to protect individual integrity in decision-making (discernment) while drawing on the resources of a supportive community. For example, a clearness committee can be used with someone early in their career to work through a decision on their career path, with doctoral students striving to determine their research focus, or with a nurse member considering retirement options. Discernment differs from telling someone what to do; discernment is reflecting on choices to differentiate between choices and directions consistent with one's values and beliefs. The goal is to enable an individual to listen to themselves, to their "inner compass" when faced with dilemmas or difficult choices. Listeners do not offer advice or suggestions but help remove pre-judgments and other interferences so that the individual can tune to their inner voices.

To use a clearness committee effectively, Palmer (2004) provides these guidelines:

1. The "focus person" chooses the members of the clearness committee, usually three to six trustworthy people who are diverse in gender and background.

2. Using the "What/So What/Now What" LS can provide an agenda for the clearness committee. The focus person describes the issue: what is the issue, what are the background issues, and what are our beginning speculations on approaches to the problem or dilemma? Members of the committee read this statement before the meeting.

3. Listeners and the focus person come together in a quiet, private place. Each listener keeps notes during the meeting and gives them to the focus person at the end of the session. Sessions are usually planned sessions for one to two hours. The session continues for the time agreed upon without any attempt to stop earlier.

4. The session begins in silence and a few contemplative moments. Listeners start by asking the focus person honest, open questions that only the focus person could answer. Only the focus person can answer, and only the focus person can have access to the "truth" of the situation. Questions might be, "What have you thought about this issue up until now?" or, "Have you ever faced a decision like this before?"

5. Questions might solicit ever deeper, more thoughtful, and reflective responses from the focus person. The person might choose not to answer.

6. Questions and deep listening must not be rushed; they must be gentle, quiet, calm, and humane. The group might have long periods of silence.

7. Listeners remain fully present and engaged with the focus person and the issues at hand without distractions.

8. In the last few minutes of the meeting, listeners might read back some of the notes about the issues and discussion. The focus person might respond and reflect, or not. Each listener has a few minutes to comment on the focus person's strengths that emerged, celebrating the ability of the clearness committee to open themselves up to the discernment process. All notes from the meeting are a gift to the focus person.

9. The goal is not to decide, solve any problems, or fix the focus person. The focus person can choose if they wish to discuss the "Now What" of the discernment process.

APPLICATION TO PERSONAL AND PROFESSIONAL PRACTICE

Academic and practice settings are increasingly complex. To be relevant, reimagining by using innovative approaches such as emergent strategies, LS, and clearness committees can engage and inspire their members to respond to change. Older linear models are no longer as effective or efficient as the world has evolved, changed, and redirected following the COVID-19 pandemic. A survey of institutions of higher learning (Harris et al., 2016) reported that 90% of the schools who explored these innovative approaches produced positive results by engaging groups, focusing on everyday solutions for big and small projects, suggesting design strategies, and transforming decision-making.

Harris (personal communication, August 26, 2016) reports that using LS can trigger a "healthy virus" effect. To stimulate personal and professional growth, try various structures in group or family meetings, classrooms, community settings, and informal conversations. Positive outcomes engage more people, and the move toward emergent and liberating ways of working together grows toward transformation. Through practice, the phenomenon can quickly spread throughout academic, practice, and community settings. Importantly, emergent strategies, LS, and clearness committees can be used for leadership and personal and professional development, clinical practice, adult education, and with students in a wide variety of fields (Harris et al., 2016).

The applications of emergent strategy, LS, and clearness committees to personal and professional practice are unlimited, as they provide frameworks for more collaborative, inclusive, and reflective ways of working. In education, they can guide interactive learning that unleashes the imagination needed to solve complex issues. In personal practice, these approaches can help individuals cultivate self-awareness, navigate uncertainty, and build resilience. In professional practice, they can be used to foster a more equitable and productive workplace culture, facilitate decision-making, and promote innovation. By embracing emergent strategy, LS, and clearness committees, individuals and organizations develop more agile and adaptable approaches to personal and professional challenges, leading to more sustainable and impactful outcomes.

REFLECTIVE SUMMARY

This chapter offered theory-based, practical, evidence-based ideas to reinvent group interactions regardless of size to enact reflective thinking. Guided by mindful ways of being, these ideas promote reflection-in-action and reflection-on-action. Principles from complexity science applied in emergent strategy, LS, and clearness committees create more reflective, inclusive, and effective working environments. Complexity science recognizes that organizations and systems are dynamic, interconnected, and constantly evolving, and it encourages a shift from traditional top-down approaches to more adaptive and emergent strategies. Emergent strategy focuses on experimentation, iteration, and learning from experience, rather than relying on preconceived plans and assumptions. Similarly, LS and clearness committees are participatory approaches fostering inclusivity, collaborative decision-making, and supporting individual and group reflection.

By applying these principles to workplace environments, individuals and organizations can become more responsive, resilient, and adaptable. These approaches encourage reflection and exploration of multiple perspectives, and allow for the emergence of creative solutions to complex problems. As a result, complexity science and emergent strategy enacted using LS and clearness committees can help create a more collaborative and inclusive workplace culture, where individuals are encouraged to share ideas and perspectives, and where the organization can become more effective in achieving its goals.

LEARNING NARRATIVE

The COVID-19 pandemic has left an indelible mark on our global society. As educators regrouped to return to in-person classes, and workers in all settings dealt with the impacts on how we work, emotions rose to the surface. Using What/So What/Now What, an LS, provided a discussion platform to share experiences and move towards new beginnings. The guided reflective process provided a semi-structured way for everyone to share their responses in an inclusive safe space free from judgment and allowed diverse views to surface. By using appreciative constructive questions, the group remained focused on discussing how they wanted to reimagine the work environment and sustain positive changes that emerged from the pandemic. Follow the questions for your benefit, or try the exercise with your family, a group of peers, or with learners.

1. **What: Understand the event.**

   The facilitator asked the group to reflect on the effects of the pandemic to identify the most striking impact on their personal and professional lives. Using 1-2-4-All, the group then shared first with another person, then in a duo, added another duo, and finally one person from each group of four shared a point with the entire group, going round robin until all points were reported.

2. **So what: Make sense of the facts and implications.**

   The facilitator now posed several reflective questions about what had been reported. For example:

   * Reflecting on the points reported, what were the things that surprised you the most?

   * What are the things you are most excited about that were unavailable during the pandemic?

   * What were the most important strategies for your personal sustainment?

   * What strengths did you discover in yourself? In those around you?

3. **Now what:** Set a course of action and new solutions.

   * What was the most important gift of the pandemic that you continue to treasure?

   * What change are you committed to maintaining?

   * What is your preferred future going forward that the pandemic helped you redefine?

REFLECTIVE QUESTIONS

1. What challenges and opportunities have you experienced working in nursing teams and interprofessional teams?

2. How would you design a staff or faculty meeting using one of the strategies in the chapter?

3. How do the theories presented help you to understand why the strategies are useful?

4. Identify a critical question in your organization and select one of the strategies from this chapter to organize for discussion. Whom would you include? Where would you hold the session? How would you frame the question? What outcome do you hope for?

5. Compare and contrast the strategies described in this chapter with the usual problem-solving strategies.

6. What are the strengths of the strategies described in this chapter?

REFERENCES

Brown, A. M. (2017). *Emergent strategy: Shaping change, changing worlds*. AK Press.

Harris, D., Lilly, C., Semura, J., & Johnston, R. (2016, Aug. 19). *LS: Scaling up across higher education*. Presentation at NCCI, Montreal, Quebec, Canada.

Holskey, M. P., & Rivera, R. R. (2020). Optimizing nurse engagement: Using liberating structures for nursing professional practice model development. *The Journal of Nursing Administration*, *50*(9), 468–473. https://doi.org/10.1097/NNA.0000000000000918

Jensen, H. J. (2023). *Complexity science: The study of emergence*. Cambridge University Press.

Johns, C. (2006). *Engaging reflection in practice: A narrative approach*. Blackwell.

Kolb, D. (2014). *Experiential learning: Experience as the source of learning and development*. Pearson FT Press.

Lindberg, C., Nash, S., & Lindberg, C. (2008). *On the edge: Nursing in the age of complexity*. PlexusPress.

Lipmanowicz, H., & McCandless, K. (2010). Liberating structures: Innovating by including and unleashing everyone. *E&Y Performance, 2*(3), 6–20.

Lipmanowicz, H., & McCandless, K. (2013). *The surprising power of liberating structures: Simple rules to unleash a culture of innovation*. Liberating Structures Press.

Mahoney, J. S., Lewin, L., Beeber, L., & Willis, D. G. (2016). Using liberating structures to increase engagement in identifying priorities for the APNA Research Council. *Journal of the American Psychiatric Nurses Association*, *22*(6), 504–507. https://doi.org/10.1177/1078390316663308

Mallette, C., & Rykert, L. (2018). Promoting positive culture change in nursing faculties: Getting to maybe through liberating structures. *Journal of Professional Nursing*, *34*(3), 161–166. https://doi.org/10.1016/j.profnurs.2017.08.001

Mezirow, J., & Taylor, E. (2009). *Transformative learning in practice: Insights from the community, workplace, and higher education*. Jossey-Bass.

Palmer, P. (2004). *A hidden wholeness: The journey toward an undivided life*. John Wiley & Sons.

Swenson, M., Sims, S., & McCandless, K. (2017). Reflective ways of working together: Using liberating structures. In S. Horton-Deutsch & G. Sherwood (Eds.), *Reflective practice: Transforming education and improving outcomes* (2nd ed., pp. 291–313). Sigma Theta Tau International.

Westley, F., Zimmerman, B., & Patton, M. Q. (2006). *Getting to maybe: How the world is changed*. Vintage Canada.

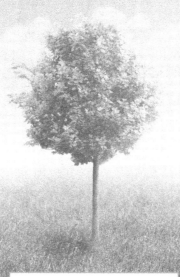

CHAPTER 11

PLURALISTIC POSSIBILITY: REFLECTIVE PRACTICES TO REFRAME OUR WORLD

–*Amber Young-Brice, PhD, RN, CNE*
Melissa Shew, PhD
Jennifer Maney, PhD

LEARNING OBJECTIVES/SUBJECTIVES

- Connect AACN Essentials, guidelines, and competencies for nursing education to liberatory education and caring sciences in the service of caring for others.

- Interrogate shortcomings in "diversity of thought" as it currently tends to be used in organizations.

- Justify thinking in terms of pluralistic possibility as a strength in higher education, nursing practices, and leadership.

- Promote cross- and interdisciplinary expertise and leadership possibilities through pluralistic possibilities.

"Education as the practice of freedom— as opposed to education as the practice of domination—denies that [a person] is abstract, isolated, independent and unattached to the world; it also denies that the world exists as a reality apart from people. Authentic reflection considers neither [an abstract person] nor the world without people, but people in their relations to the world."

–Freire, 1970, p. 81

OVERVIEW

The American Association of Colleges of Nursing (AACN) Essentials (guidelines and competencies for nursing education) provides a framework that reflects diversity in practice settings and the necessary collaboration across healthcare professions while reconfirming nursing as a unique discipline (AACN, 2021). To advance the discipline, the new AACN Essentials calls for an intentional approach in nursing education that "reflects a number of contemporary trends and values and addresses several issues to shape the future workforce, including diversity, equity, and inclusion" (AACN, 2021, p. 5).

This chapter develops a theoretical and practical model of pluralistic possibility to help nurses, educators, and leaders meet future needs in their fields that go beyond traditional conceptions of "diversity of thought." We identify pitfalls that can exist in current popular ways of conceptualizing "diversity of thought" that can preclude educators, practitioners, and leaders from confronting real issues head-on. We then provide a brief overview of the history of different concepts that have been discarded, revised, or borrowed from unexpected places to name experiences in empowering ways, especially for those who have been marginalized or excluded in our world. The dynamism of language mandates that we sometimes need to step back and reflect on which words and phrases are most appropriate and accurate to name our world and experiences.

For these reasons, we offer that "pluralistic possibility" may respond to shortcomings inherent in current ways of conceiving diversity of thought. This model draws on theories of liberatory education and consciousness-raising to show how a plurality of perspectives can help name, identify, and transform specific problems to meet futuristic needs. We conclude by anticipating what cross-disciplinary and interprofessional opportunities might look like in light of pluralistic possibility, with a specific focus on nursing, education, and leadership.

SUPPORTING THEORETICAL FRAMEWORKS AND OTHER EVIDENCE

We are always learning, even if we aren't fully aware of it (Hammond, 2021). We make meaning of our world based on beliefs, norms, cultural mental models, and experiences in addition to what is learned by student-teacher relationships and the educational process we find ourselves in as learners and educators (Beckett, 2013). We bring together two frameworks, *pluralist possibilities* and *liberatory education,* to challenge how we view language, the world, and our work as nurses. Reflective practices weave into the questions explored to transform our worldview, creating possibilities we never knew were available to us.

PLURALISTIC POSSIBILITIES AND CARING SCIENCE

It is difficult to maintain a current vocabulary as language gets revised, new words enter our shared lexicon, or phrases from one realm of our world transfer to another. In offering "pluralism" in response to "diversity of thought" to address nursing as a Caring Science and artistic practice, *pluralistic possibility* speaks to the ways that interprofessional and cross-disciplinary expertise is required to transform current realities and anticipate future ones. The triangulation of educators, healthcare professionals, and organizational leaders can adopt pluralistic possibility, which aligns with critical consciousness and reflective practices.

PLURALISTIC POSSIBILITY

Pluralistic possibility affirms the ideas that multiple perspectives and outcomes can exist simultaneously within a given situation or context, and that there can be more than one way of understanding or approaching a particular issue or problem.

Pluralistic possibility stems from the word *pluralism,* which means respecting the otherness of others including different races, ethnicities, cultures, and politics (Ghouse, 2022).

This way of thinking is not new and aligns with relational emancipatory education within Caring Science (Hills et al., 2021). It offers a fresh way of thinking about how to approach the triangulation of practitioner-educator-student. In this model of pluralistic possibility, each person enters relations with the other with their own standpoints, perspectives, experiences, and knowledge.

LIBERATORY EDUCATION AND CRITICAL CARITAS CONSCIOUSNESS

In alignment with Caring Science, liberatory education is an approach to teaching and learning that seeks to create a more just and equitable society by recognizing and addressing how traditional education disempowers students (Hills et al., 2021). Liberatory education requires that we acknowledge the plurality of perspectives that forge together in any educational setting, but especially in the caring sciences. Indeed, we may think of care ethics, an ethical theory developed late in the 20th century mainly by women who rejected the purely abstract nature of preceding ethical theories like utilitarianism and deontology. Care ethics considers the centrality of relationships in how we make ethical decisions. According to care ethics, there is no "absolute good" to which we ought to aspire as people look to an objective truth in abstract lived experiences. It recognizes that we are always in relation and exist only in a network of people, systems, and values to which we are obligated and from which we express our desires. In this way, there can be better or worse choices that a person can make, of course, but given that we exist in networks and folds of caring relations—even to ourselves—these perspectives, values, and realities ought to be considered valid and important. More specifically, these perspectives, values, and current realities invite healthcare professionals to work together toward an "evolved Critical Caritas Literacy as the ethical and scientific way of learning, growing and evolving as caring—loving humans in healing service to the world, sustaining humanity and our survival on planet earth" (Watson, 2017, pp. 3–4).

> *"Critical Caritas Literacy is an ontology of being/becoming that comes from the subjective inner world of each person, morally aroused for reflective and contemplative self-growth, self-care experiences that contribute to the whole of humanity."*
>
> –Watson, 2017, p. 7

A challenging aspect of what we are called to do across different realms of our lives—as practitioners, educators, and leaders—concerns the ways that we must maintain professional and personal coherence as an ethical duty not just as good in itself or abstractly, but importantly good for others with whom we are in relation. bell hooks (1994) says, "It was clear to audiences that I practiced what I preached. That union of theory and praxis was a dynamic example for teachers seeking practical wisdom" (p. 4). This idea echoes that of Paulo Freire (1970), who says, "The basis of our encounter ought to be a respect for the differences between us and an acknowledgment of the coherence between what I say and what I do" (p. 120). Caring—that is, embracing caring as a moral imperative to act ethically and justly by making just and ethical decisions (Hills et al., 2021)—must thus be kept squarely in view.

In liberatory education, reflective practices can help students to identify and reflect on their own experiences of marginalization and to connect these experiences to broader social justice issues, and use education as a political act (Hills et al., 2021). By reflecting on their own experiences, all involved can gain a deeper understanding of how power operates in society to develop the critical consciousness necessary to challenge systems of oppression.

Critical Caritas consciousness developed through reflective practices is a key component of liberatory education. Within a liberatory framework, *critical Caritas consciousness* is the ability to recognize and analyze how power operates in society and to take action to challenge systems of oppression. Metacognition is an important aspect of developing a critical consciousness, with the ability to think about one's thinking in a critically reflective way (Cara et al., 2020). Reflective practices can help individuals to recognize their own biases and assumptions and to question how these biases may contribute to systems of oppression and authoritarian behaviors (Hills et al., 2021). By engaging in reflective practices, individuals can become more aware of how their own thoughts and actions may perpetuate inequality and can work to challenge these patterns and hegemonic practices (Hills et al., 2021).

Reflective practices are an important tool for promoting self-awareness and critical thinking, which are key components of both liberatory education and critical consciousness (Cara et al., 2020; Hills et al., 2021). Those who have developed a critical consciousness have self-awareness of their own positionality and capacity to challenge contradictory ideas and guide others to also develop these capacities given the complex and intertwined social structures and expectations (Hills et al., 2021).

COMPLEXITIES OF "DIVERSITY OF THOUGHT"

We live in an increasingly diverse world, with people carrying all types of identity markers with them—race, ethnicity, language, religion, political affiliation, socioeconomic status, sexuality, gender orientation, and on and on. People do not leave those markers with them—when they go to college, when they enter the workforce, and certainly not when they seek medical attention. University instructors and healthcare workers interact with individuals and families from all walks of life, not always reflecting their own lived experiences. In addition, educators are teaching a more diverse group of students as institutions of higher education are being more intentional about the recruitment of diverse students and the rise in numbers of identity groups (e.g., Latino/a-identified Americans, African Americans, etc.).

To provide authentic and just care to students and patients, these realities require attention for reflecting on efforts around diversity, equity, and inclusion (DEI). The National Institutes of Health (NIH, 2017) defines *DEI* as "the range of human differences, including but not limited to race, ethnicity, gender, sexual orientation, age, social class, physical ability or attributes, religious or ethical value system, national original and political beliefs." The NIH continues to define *inclusion* to involve empowerment and appreciate the inherent worth and dignity of all people. *Equity,* according to the Annie E. Casey Foundation (2020), is defined as "the state, quality or ideal of being just, impartial and fair"(para. 3).

These terms are not useless. However, there are varying degrees of understanding of what DEI efforts should be, so it becomes important to recognize the objectivity of what DEI means. To one hospital administrator or college of nursing dean, DEI efforts include the training of white people to act without implicit bias. To another, it means intentional recruiting efforts to diversify the workplace or college classroom. Yet to another, it may involve a deep dive into a person's own identity and how they may hold privilege. Others feel that diversity of thought, meaning the different ways in which people express or exhibit their preferred way of thinking, holds the key to the appropriate way to proceed with diversity and inclusion efforts.

In contemporary workplace culture, it has become common to hear about various DEI efforts. One of those efforts includes the idea of diversity of thought. Pragmatically, this means that people in any group do not need to look or think or identify differently in order to bring diversity of inclusion into action. Sometimes that approach replaces traditional diversification efforts such as hiring for better representation in literal ways (identity). Others find that problematic and instead focus on hiring people who commit to this idea of thought diversity (Bastian, 2019). This new focus puts a priority on differences in perspective based on one's own identity markers and experience. One cannot argue that creating an environment—be it the classroom or an intake room in a healthcare system—that challenges people to respect others and attempt to understand their experience, is itself wrong.

It is worth noting, however, that according to the report on achieving health equity through nursing workforce diversity (National Advisory Council on Nurse Education and Practice, 2013), a more diverse nursing workforce will be better prepared to diverse an increasingly diverse patient population. This effort has been proven to help close the health equity gap in the United States by training and preparing healthcare professionals who more closely mirror their patients in terms of identity markers. A 2022 study found that racially minoritized patients to shared a similar racial identity as their healthcare provider improved communication, perceptions of care, trust, and ultimately better health outcomes (Moore et al., 2022).

Therefore, this approach of presuming diversity of thought being enough (versus a representation approach) becomes murky if the focus on thought comes at the expense of also looking at things like representation where people bring their authentic life experiences and lenses. What happens when people adhere to this rather simplistic view of DEI efforts at the expense of what we know to be true about equitable and just patient care across all identities, that being better health outcomes and addressing a health equity disparity between people of different racial identities? It may be a positive aspiration, to work on one's thought processes, but at what point does it become not only controversial to pursue this but risky to those most vulnerable to inequity and injustice whether that be in the college classroom, the workplace, or the patient room?

It is fair to assume that "diversity," meaning "representation," is a value add and has positive learning and performance outcomes for students. According to a Princeton University Trustee Report, experiences with diversity improve students' cognitive skills and performance along with their own self-confidence, attitudes about their college experience, and future performance in a variety of workplaces (Son Holoien, 2013). Students in the classroom or patients in a healthcare setting need to see people who look like them, so the narrative goes, and not without merit (one caveat to note is a warning to not seek representation only to fall back to the "equality as sameness") (Holck & Muhr, 2017). Hiring for representation and varying the skills, knowledge, and experiences of a diverse group of individuals to provide empathetic care to a growing population of people who look different from each other is the best way to provide person-centered care whether in academia or practice settings.

EMPATHY

Empathy is a critical tool in harnessing the relationship between patient and caregiver. Empathy allows healthcare workers to recognize and appreciate the patient's experiences, worries, and perspectives and contributes to better health outcomes (Moudatsou et al., 2020). Empathy is influenced by current beliefs and value systems, education and training, group influences, work experiences and culture, supervisory influences, and professional identity (Yu et al., 2022). We bring our values into whatever setting we are in, whether that is a clinical practice or a classroom setting which influences how we appreciate others' situations and experiences (Yu et al., 2022). It leaves the question of what happens when the individuals involved do not share common lived experiences or identity markers leading to very different life experiences, for example, the experience of racism or stereotypes of bias.

Pursuing diversity efforts in and of themselves can be dangerous if not done correctly and with great care. By valuing interactions and encounters with students, instructors, patients, supervisors, etc. who are from a different group than oneself (by race, ethnicity, gender identity, sexual orientation, language, or religion), encounters together greatly benefit those being served (and those providing those services). It is inherent in our professional responsibilities to respect, engage, and value those with different attitudes and life experiences to better prepare learners and nurses to provide fair, equitable, and just service/care (Son Holoien, 2013). The importance of being culturally sensitive with patients or students/learners is the core foundation of person-centered approaches to care and education (Kamrul et al., 2014). Reflecting on the ways we understand cultures that may be different from ours helps us have empathy for ways in which those differences and cultural identity markers impact their life, their health, and their perspective.

RETHINKING NURSING EDUCATION AND PRACTICE

Trends in nursing education are addressing the needs of the future (AACN, 2021), and DEI is at the forefront. With demographics shifting in many workplaces—classrooms, clinics, or the corporate world—the growing disparity in how different individuals with different markers experience the world and the ways in which they receive healthcare or schooling, DEI efforts must remain a priority (National Academies of Sciences, Engineering, and Medicine [NASEM], 2021). The global pandemic of 2020 continued to shine a spotlight on these inequities in an alarming manner.

Inequity in healthcare distribution is both a US national problem and a global problem. Many people do not recognize or understand the systemic and ongoing issues that both cause and exacerbate inequities, yet *The Future of Nursing 2020–2030* report focuses on these inequities, proposing many ways nurses can be part of the solutions (NASEM, 2021). The focus on DEI efforts is a value in nursing education hoping to better prepare future nurses and maybe even more importantly arm them with authentic information at the root causes of this disparity. "Evidence-based, institution-wide approaches focused on equity in student learning and catalyzing culture shifts in the academy are fundamental to eliminating structural racism in higher education" (Barber et al., 2020, by AAC, 2020, p. 6).

Advancing a shift in culture mandates a priority to recruit and retain nursing students who can best understand what it is like to grow up without the same access to proper healthcare as others. A population of diverse students and future educators and clinicians does not guarantee the elimination of inequity. Making a commitment to inclusion, examining structural racism and inequity, and applying a lens on how implicit bias and stereotypes are barriers to adequate healthcare reinforces the imperative to recruit a more diverse student population who can play a role in the pursuit of justice and equity.

Nursing educators and practitioners need to be aware of the dangers of a single story reflecting a Eurocentric curriculum or worldview or research agenda. Educators, students, and clinicians increasingly serve as culture brokers between their individual worldviews and those of their more diverse student peers and people in their care. It is more than simply becoming aware of one's tendency to stereotype or generalize or compare one's own experience to those of the "other"; it is reflecting from an emotionally intelligent stance to have self-awareness of self in relation to others, including those different from us.

WHAT'S IN A WORD? LANGUAGE AND NAMING THE WORLD

Shortcomings in the phrase "diversity of thought" do not limit the desire to bring together multiple voices and perspectives to identify and solve various problems. Across institutions of higher education, multiple initiatives bring together disparate disciplines working on topics such as climate change, artificial technology, and globalism. No one person or disciplinary expertise can completely solve a truly pressing problem. To begin to identify, transform, and solve large-scale problems related to healthcare or higher education is to consider the role that language plays in shaping and identifying how we understand these problems. Broadly speaking, language is what enables us to name specific experiences, keeping phrases if they are worth keeping, discarding them when they are not, and inventing new ones as new needs emerge. In this way, language sustains a powerful relationship with reality. When terms and phrases are invented and recognized, they allow people to say, "Yes! *That's* what happened!" or, "No, I don't think that's quite right. It was more like this."

Language also allows people to come together and name a variety of shared experiences in their lives, which is acutely important when it comes to naming injustices. Especially on system-wide levels, these injustices are often uncovered and discovered by talking about them with others. Issues in the workplace like racial discrimination, unequal pay, and gender inequalities are more able to be identified, explained, and addressed when they are named and pulled out from the background of our general experiences of the world. Indeed, training in developing the skill of identifying problems amid a complex web of situations and variables is becoming recognized as essential in fields like narrative medicine, which seeks to train healthcare professionals to use the arts and humanities to read the contexts (of a painting, say) to identify specific problems to be diagnosed. (See Chapter 5 for more on Visual Thinking Strategies.) Language training could help lessen the prominent issue of misdiagnosis by learning more accurate terms for communicating with patients. These points underscore the pronounced value that nursing places on liberal education, for "liberal education creates the foundation for intellectual and practical abilities within the context of nursing practice as well as for engagement with the larger community, locally and globally" (Zimmer, 2020). It is primary learning across the demands of a practice-based discipline.

Labeling or "diagnosing" happens in all aspects of our world. Language changes as the needs of a society change. As we come to understand the multilayered nature of reality, we grow by identifying opportunities to conceptualize experiences, knowledge, and expertise in new ways. As suggested in this chapter, reviewing the phrase "diversity of thought"—which, once identified, includes a multitude of identities beyond apparent or implied identity markers—considers whether we should conceive of a new phrase that does not imply virtue signaling or an empty phrase.

Consider two significant terms that have both historical and contemporary resonance: racism and homophobia. Since its first definition in 1938 and its revision in 1961, the definition of "racism" was again revisited in 2020. The reality of racism as experienced around the world is undeniable, with definitions emphasizing its harm in individual ways committed by individual people in the 1960s. Newer ideas about racism as systemic and institutional today are informing how people generally experience racism in our world now in ways that maintain individual harm but introduce an important kind of harm hitherto unemphasized—structural and institutional harm. Linguist and lexicographer Ben Zimmer (2020) put it this way: "The legacy of past editions meant that the entry was so broadly construed that it did not seem particularly applicable to systemic racism as experienced by Black Americans." Language needs to evolve and change in the ways that allow it to name more accurately people's lived experiences and our reality and how that reality impacts healthcare delivery at the individual and system levels.

"Homophobia" is a term developed in the 1960s, but as our shared understanding of antigay prejudice continues to grow, many think that the term is outdated and fails to capture what's happening when we say that someone is homophobic. Though "the widespread acceptance of the idea that hostility against gay people is a phenomenon that warrants attention...represented a significant advance for the cause of gay and lesbian human rights," preferred terms now include heterosexism and antigay prejudice (Herek, 2004, p. 9). By retaining the -*phobia* suffix of the word, those who hold antigay prejudices may appear to be released or relieved from their prejudices because it could seem to be a condition that they suffer, like any other phobic condition. In that way, the person is simply at the mercy of their phobia. While the word had meaning in identifying biases specifically directed toward certain populations, it also functions to let the biased person off the hook for their bias.

The history of these terms shows they are open to revision and reconceptualization. In a similar way, the five core competencies in nursing—human wholeness, health, healing and well-being, environment-health relationship, and caring—denote current perspectives of nursing as a discipline. Nursing takes its inspiration from Florence Nightingale but has historical twists and turns that lead us to highlight these principles in this way now. Future iterations of nursing may require different core competencies, for there may be different problems facing our world that nursing will need to address in other ways.

REDEFINING LANGUAGE: MOVING TO A CARING WAY OF BEING AND DOING

Language evolves, and its meanings can be transferred from one realm of experience to another. This transference of language creates opportunities for interprofessional dialogue that can identify and transform challenges now to anticipate solutions and realities that are more future-directed and life-giving (Watson, 2017).

New terms mostly from the social world of dating are seeping into mainstream thought. *Gaslighting* in philosophical psychology (Stark, 2019) names a particular experience people have in being manipulated, having their interpretations of reality questioned, and being told that what they know or think they know is not accurate. Through the lens of gaslighting, for instance, the phrase *work-life balance* might function to cover employer shortcomings to provide this kind of balance, effectively gaslighting employees into thinking that it is only their responsibility to work toward this balance—and that it is employees' fault if this balance is out of whack (Storm & Muhr, 2022). *Ghosting* is another psychological term (Freedman et al., 2022) applied to the phenomenon of abruptly ending communication at work and in the workplace (DePaul, 2021). *Breadcrumbing* refers to being strung along by a current or future employer (Neilson, 2021). These socially prevalent words name distinctive ways that people experience pain and harm in relationships and are used to indicate ways that people are unfairly denied access to opportunities and experiences that they might want and that might be good for them. The crossover of language from the dating world today to the workplace helps people make sense of negative experiences that happen to them.

By first naming specific kinds of negative experiences we create the possibility to change them. We might say that without naming—racism, homophobia, gaslighting, ghosting, etc.—people are left less credible as knowers. This undermining of credibility might result in what philosopher Miranda Fricker (2007) calls "cognitive disablement," which "prevents [a person] from understanding a significant patch of her own experience: that is, a patch of experience which it is strongly in her interests to understand, for without that understanding she is left deeply troubled, confused, and isolated" (p. 151).

We could imagine that this kind of experience is dispiriting on many levels—professionally, personally, affectively, mentally, and spiritually. Indeed, this person may be "gaslit" regarding their own understanding, denying their own curiosity and right to know in the first place. To help heal this "cognitive disablement" in which a person feels alienated from their own understanding and experience, we might think of the second domain in nursing education: person-centered care. This care holds the dignity of the patient as foremost and is a domain in *The Essentials of Nursing Practice* (AACN, 2021), included in the QSEN (www.QSEN.org) competencies and by the Institute of Medicine (2003) as an essential competency for all health professions. "Person-centered care focuses on the individual within multiple complicated contexts, including family and/or important others. Person-centered care is holistic, individualized, just, respectful, compassionate, coordinated, evidence-based, and developmentally appropriate" (AACN, 2021, pg. 10). Person-centeredness provides apt justification for moving toward the model proposed here of pluralistic possibility and embraces the whole of caring sciences in our world right now.

APPLICATION IN PERSONAL AND PROFESSIONAL DEVELOPMENT

We must center our work and nursing practice both at the university location or within healthcare settings on antiracist pedagogy and culturally responsive leadership practices (Gay, 2010; Khalifa, 2018).

RETHINKING EDUCATION AND PRACTICE THROUGH PLURALISTIC POSSIBILITIES

We, the authors of this chapter representing a plurality of different disciplines and expertise (nursing, philosophy, and education), sometimes struggle with an instinct in universities or institutions of higher learning to theorize these issues abstractly without thinking about what they might look like in our classrooms and with our students. Taking cues from the K-12 world of education can guide conversations about asset versus deficit approaches to the classroom—a conversation that is now gaining traction in colleges of education but far from implementation in various learning environments. In their germinal article, "Equity Traps" (2004), McKenzie and Scheurich implore educators to examine their own deeply held assumptions about race, socioeconomic class, and all the identity markers that students bring into a classroom (or that a patient brings into a room). Educators at all levels, they argue, need to be prepared to unearth their stereotypes and biases about the perceived deficits that students bring with them to the learning space—whether that is race, culture, class, language, behavior, etc. It is important to recognize that creating welcoming learning spaces maximizes student success, just as welcoming environments in healthcare promote patient healing. An asset-based approach to learning sees students as filled with possibilities and strengths. Likewise, it is hoped that education and practice focused on person-centered care can improve patient outcomes.

Commensurate with this idea, the term "culturally responsive teaching," coined by Geneva Gay (2010), proposes that students find learning to be more meaningful and interesting when it involves their lived experiences. Though much of the research around culturally responsive leadership emanated from teacher preparation programs, it is also key to health educators in the college environment. Teaching and mentoring future nurses or nurse educators using this approach increases the hope that healthcare providers will, in turn, provide equitable and just care to all patients across all identities. In essence, if we are intentional about recognizing all students' strengths, acknowledging our biases and keeping them in check, then we can capitalize on marginalized students' life experiences and see those as a positive.

REFLECTIVE PRACTICES TO REFRAME DEI

In the classroom, Freire (1970) says, "It is a posture of unconditional respect for the students, for the knowledge they have that comes directly from life and that, together with the students, I will work to go beyond. My coherence in the classroom is as important as my teaching of contents. A coherence of what I say, write, and do" (p. 94). Part of this coherence involves being fastidious about maintaining competence in one's subject matter, and the other part connotes the ongoing responsibility that educators have toward maintaining curiosity and study in their subject matter. That is, educators, like practitioners, must be devoted to growing their content knowledge and professional development. As Freire says, "I am a teacher proud of the beauty of my teaching practice, a fragile beauty that may disappear if I do not care for the struggle and knowledge that I ought to teach" (1970, p. 95). Without this competence, it is difficult to be coherent. But we can think about coherence in other ways, too, concerning an alignment between our personal and professional practices more generally.

HOW DO STUDENTS WANT TO LEARN?

Operationalization of equity and anti-oppression in nursing education are outlined in the AACN Essentials, which threads justice, equity, diversity, and inclusion throughout the 10 domains (AACN, 2021; Roy et al., 2022). A school of nursing conducted a quality improvement project that integrated the concepts of justice, equity, diversity, and inclusion (JEDI) into their prelicensure nursing program. After conducting a needs assessment of what concepts students and faculty felt were missing in the curriculum related to JEDI, a curriculum revision was completed. Students responded positively about the incorporation of JEDI concepts, yielding the following themes (Roy et al., 2022):

1. *Students had a greater awareness of the influence of social determinants of health.*
2. *Students appreciated the incorporation of different sexual orientations, genders, and ethnicities in case studies.*
3. *Students indicated the importance of correct pronoun use.*
4. *Students developed a better understanding of race, which is neither biological nor genetic.*
5. *Students were able to relate health disparities to social inequities rather than race.*

Students suggested that faculty consider adding more JEDI concepts across the curriculum, including more examples of the assessment and care of BIPOC individuals, and different disease manifestations be included (Roy et al., 2022).

A recent student survey (Student Voice Pulse Survey, N = 1,250 undergraduate students; Flaherty, 2023) revealed that students learn best through use of case studies (learning narratives) and discussions. How can you infuse JEDI concepts through a pluralistic lens in a manner consistent with what students are indicating they learn best?

In any model of education, we must be vigilant about how people in relative positions of power—educators, practitioners, and leaders of any kind—should aim to cultivate personal self-awareness. A lack of self-awareness can translate to superficial empathy in line with expectations of professionalism instead of being authentically empathetic. Authentic empathy is nurtured through awareness of the complex lives of our students, patients, and colleagues (Wong et al., 2021). Further, the current focus on evidence-based practice (versus a more caring approach of evidence-informed practice), outcomes, and standards de-emphasize human relationships, empathy, and compassion (Eckroth-Bucher, 2010). We must build a capacity for empathy through critical self-reflection and introspection toward exploring our positionality and breaking away from our biases toward fellow humans (Eckroth-Bucher, 2010; Ghouse, 2022).

PLURALISTIC POSSIBILITIES: REFLECTIONS FOR DEVELOPING SELF-AWARENESS, EMPATHY, AND IPE

"The significant problems we face cannot be solved at the same level of thinking we were at when we created them."

–Albert Einstein, in Mohr & Magruder Watkins, 2002

Pluralistic possibility is necessary to broaden our collective understanding of what constitutes health, illness, and healing (Wong et al., 2021). Pluralistic possibility in nursing and interprofessional practice is a process where we learn to value diversity in perspectives, opinions, and experiences of individuals within a healthcare organization and stop perpetuating systematic marginalization (Wong et al., 2021). The evidence informing the AACN Essentials (2021) considers the importance of a new social order of scientists, theorists, and practitioners coming together to inform nursing theory. The value of liberal education and integration of different disciplinary knowledge is key to understanding oneself and others as the basis of what nurses do in caring for others and making clinical judgments. The AACN Essentials (2021) aligns with what we are proposing in considering pluralistic possibility. It involves creating an inclusive and collaborative environment where every individual's voice is heard and respected and decision-making is a shared responsibility. To reach this pluralistic potential, higher levels of consciousness are necessary, and that begins with self-awareness.

To be open-minded to the otherness of others and experience another person's humanity, a person must be engaged in the task of self-knowledge (Eckroth-Bucher, 2010). In psychology, self-awareness is an interpersonal phenomenon. Social work literature states we add understanding of our own biases, values, and interests which stems from culture for integrating into our personal experiences and how we impact other people (Eckroth-Bucher, 2010). Developing one's own self-awareness is a lifelong journey. Educators can help learners and nurses develop the habit of this reflective process during nursing education programs and continue to evolve leading towards a higher level of awareness and critical consciousness.

While self-awareness is the ability to recognize and understand one's own emotions, thoughts, and behaviors, empathy is the ability to recognize and comprehend the mental and emotional state of another. When someone is empathetic, they can put themselves in another person's shoes and understand their perspective (McKinnon, 2018). To be truly empathetic, it is important to be self-aware. Self-awareness helps us understand our own biases and limitations, which can help us approach situations with an open mind and avoid projecting our own emotions onto others. This is important in practice and even more so in leadership roles when managing others. As we've discussed, pluralistic possibility appreciates multiple perspectives and the coming together of diverse minds. Empathy is a tool we can use for appreciating these multiple perspectives and identities in the teaching of students, care of patients, or leading within organizations. Pluralistic possibility can also enhance empathy as we understand different perspectives and how those perspectives manifest in different behaviors (McKinnon, 2018).

HOW IS EMPATHIC AWARENESS DEVELOPED?

Empathy in education and clinical practice stems from the development of a holistic, empathic practice (McKinnon, 2018). Fostering a holistic empathic practice means embodying the process of empathy and not merely using it in isolation (McKinnon, 2018).

McKinnon (2018) outlined the antecedents of empathy:

1. *Engagement*
2. *Listening and "echoing"*
3. *An informed awareness of another's circumstances (cognitive empathy)*
4. *A good imagination*
5. *Relating the product of that imagination to the self (affective empathy)*
   - *How can you foster these elements in your classroom or practice setting?*
   - *How can you develop imagination, which McKinnon indicates is at the heart of empathy as a way of being?*
   - *How can you incorporate reflective exploration that aids in building empathy skills?*

Pluralistic possibility leads us towards appreciating the insights and perspectives of those around us, feeling safe to challenge assumptions, and seeking out multiple solutions for problems. Within organizational development, a positive approach to organizational change is through the process of appreciative inquiry (Mohr & Magruder Watkins, 2002). Appreciative inquiry is a reflective practice approach with a similarly positive tone as a pluralistic possibility in encouraging a holistic approach to problem-solving and is discussed in more detail in Chapter 15. And like a pluralistic possibility, appreciative inquiry does not focus on changing people, but on inviting people to engage in collaborative discovery to problem-solving. Learning from the moments of excellence serves as the foundation for appreciative inquiry processes, where questions are focused on what is working versus the constant attention to what isn't. If we consider appreciative inquiry in an education context, it aligns with the asset-based pedagogy mentioned earlier in the chapter, in the "Rethinking Education and Practice" section.

In practice settings, either at the bedside or in leadership capacities, appreciative inquiry serves to inspire transformational change by focusing on "human ideals and achievements, peak experiences, and best practices, the things—not the conflicts—tend to flourish" (Mohr & Magruder Watkins, 2002, p. 2). Focusing on strengths rather than weaknesses, remaining positive in a tone of questions being asked, and seeking out success stories is a radical departure from current practice in education and nursing practice. When we constantly focus our attention on what isn't working, we cannot find the capacity for focusing on what does work. With appreciative inquiry, there is an increased motivation for pluralistic possibility, collaboration, and creativity to solve our most pressing problems in educating students, caring for others, or in leadership capacities.

Domain 6 of the new AACN Essentials emphasizes the importance of interprofessional partnerships and intentional collaboration across professions and within care teams (AACN, 2021). Integration of self-awareness, empathy, and using an appreciative inquiry lens provides a foundation to build capacity for pluralistic possibility within and across disciplines for collaboration and coordination of multiple professions to address complex problems. No one profession has all the answers. It takes self-awareness to the level of having critical consciousness to allow for vulnerability in admitting we do not have all the answers, or even to challenge the assumptions of others.

> *"Most of us have heard things about others from our friends, news, social media, or our knowledge of others, and we instantly form opinions about others. As responsible individuals, we must strive to strip stereotyping and build pathways to ensure our society's smooth functioning, whether in the workplace or in our neighborhoods."*
>
> –Ghouse, 2022, p. 157

LEARNING NARRATIVE: CREATING SELF-AWARENESS THROUGH STEAM

In nursing practice, even while a nursing student, compassion and self-awareness are essential to well-being and the ability to interact with others and provide care for others. "Becoming self-aware requires continuous reflection and learning about self in different situations" (Younas & Rasheed, 2018, p. 222). Consider the following reflective framework by Becker-Phelps (2023) that encourages the development of self-awareness through STEAM and how this framework could fit personally or professionally in a classroom or practice setting:

- **S-Sensations**

  What do I sense in my body? Think about a scenario or situation you've faced or anticipate facing in school or practice. How does your body feel when you think about this situation? Take a mindful approach and scan your body from your head to your toes.

- **T-Thoughts**

  What am I thinking? When you think about the scenario or situation, what sort of thoughts are you having? Are they self-critical thoughts including "should"? If you are having trouble thinking about your thoughts, try journaling or sharing with a trusted friend or colleague.

- **E-Emotions**

  What am I feeling? This is where you lean into what you're feeling when thinking about the scenario or situation. Self-critical thoughts can cause negative consequences and subsequent emotions which lead to stress, exhaustion, and possibly powerlessness (Younas & Rasheed, 2018).

- **A-Actions**

  How have I been acting/reacting? Pay attention to the impact of your thoughts and feelings and what sort of behaviors this situation has elicited. Negative thoughts and emotions can lead to drastic actions, whereas compassionate self-awareness of the thoughts and emotions can help you discern how to rationally navigate the situation.

- **M-Mentalizing**

  "Do I really get what's going on for me and understand what is motivating my actions?" Or "Do I really get what's going on for the other person and understand what is motivating their actions?" This aspect of the STEAM framework helps us get towards pluralistic possibility by considering ourselves but also others in this self-awareness process.

REFLECTIVE QUESTIONS

If no one person or disciplinary expertise is likely to completely solve in a lasting way a truly pressing problem, the task becomes how we might honor the expertise around us to identify, transform, and solve problems not only on a large scale but also in daily experiences in our classrooms, institutions, and organizations.

1. What other types of societal issues or concerns could be tackled by this approach?

2. Which disciplines could begin to address these issues in your context?

3. What are some specific collaborative strategies (or pluralistic possibilities) that could move these issues forward in meaningful ways?

4. Is diversity of thought enough to get individuals to consider systemic inequities in their settings, or is something more needed to serve populations in a just way? Why or why not?

5. How might the language in nursing education or healthcare settings evolve to best reflect all peoples' lived experiences?

6. How does the evolution of language impact our perspectives on caring for others?

REFLECTIVE SUMMARY

This chapter developed a theoretical and practical model of pluralistic possibility to help nurses, educators, and leaders meet future needs in their fields that go beyond conceptions of "diversity of thought." We identified pitfalls that can exist in current popular ways of conceptualizing "diversity of thought" that can preclude educators, practitioners, and leaders from confronting real issues head-on. The dynamism of language mandates that we sometimes need to step back and reflect on which words and phrases are most appropriate and accurate to name our world and experiences. For these reasons, we offered a model of "pluralistic possibility" as a response to the shortcomings of conceiving diversity of thought. This model draws on theories of liberatory education and consciousness-raising to show how a plurality of perspectives can help name, identify, and transform specific problems to meet futuristic needs. We provided an application to personal and professional contexts with reflective prompts to guide your development of pluralistic possibility for your own context, be it education, practice, or leadership.

REFERENCES

American Association of Colleges of Nursing. (2021). *The essentials: Core competencies for professional nursing education.* https://www.aacnnursing.org/Portals/42/AcademicNursing/pdf/Essentials-2021.pdf

Annie E. Casey Foundation. (2020, Aug. 24). *Equity vs. equality and other racial justice definitions.* https://www.aecf.org/blog/racial-justice-definitions

Barber, P. H., Hayes, T. B., Johnson, T. L., & Marquez-Magana, L. (2020). Systemic racism in higher education. *Science, 369*(6510), 1440–1441. https://www.science.org/doi/10.1126/science.abd7140

Bastian, R. (2019, May 13). Why we need to stop talking about diversity of thought. *Forbes.* https://www.forbes.com/sites/rebekahbastian/2019/05/13/why-we-need-to-stop-talking-about-diversity-of-thought/?sh=faefb8f67c37

Becker-Phelps, L. (2023). *Gain self-awareness through STEAM. Compassionate Self-Awareness.* https://drbecker-phelps.com/wp-content/uploads/2023/08/STEAM.pdf

Beckett, L. (2013). *Teacher education through active engagement. Raising the professional voice* (1st ed.). Routledge. https://doi.org/10.4324/9780203407660

Cara, C., Hills, M., & Watson, J. (2020). *An educator's guide to humanizing nursing education.* Springer Publishing. https://doi.org/10.1891/9780826190093

DePaul, K. (2021, May 12). So you got ghosted—At work. *Harvard Business Review.* https://hbr.org/2021/05/so-you-got-ghosted-at-work

Eckroth-Bucher, M. (2010). Self-awareness. A review and analysis of a basic nursing concept. *Advances in Nursing Science, 33*(4), 297–309. https://doi.org/10.1097/ANS.0b013e3181fb2e4c

Flaherty, C. (2023) *Survey: students cite barriers to success, seek flexibility.* Inside Higher Ed. https://www.insidehighered.com/news/2023/02/14/survey-top-five-barriers-student-success

Freedman, G., Powell, D. N., Le, B., & Williams, K. D. (2022). Emotional experiences of ghosting. *The Journal of Social Psychology.* https://doi.org/10.1080 /00224545.2022.2081528

Freire, P. (1970). *Pedagogy of the oppressed.* Continuum.

Fricker, M. (2007). *Epistemic injustice: Power and the ethics of knowing.* Oxford University Press. https://doi.org/10.1093/acprof:oso/9780198237907.001.0001

Gay G. (2010). *Culturally responsive teaching: Theory, research, and practice.* Teachers College Press.

Ghouse, M. M. (2022). Shaping pluralistic cohesive societies. *Academicus International Scientific Journal, 13*(26), 154–160. https://doi.org/10.7336/academicus.2022.26.10

Hammond, Z. (2021). Liberatory education: Integrating the science of learning and culturally responsive practice. *American Educator, Summer,* 4–39.

Herek, G. M. (2004). Beyond "homophobia": Thinking about sexual prejudice and stigma in the twenty-first century. *Sexuality Research & Social Policy: A Journal of the NSRC, 1*(2), 6–24. https://doi.org/10.1525/srsp.2004.1.2.6

Hills, M., Watson, J., & Cara, C. (2021). *Creating a caring science curriculum* (2nd ed). Springer Publishing. https://doi.org/10.1891/9780826136039

Holck, L., & Muhr, S. (2017). Unequal solidarity? Towards a norm-critical approach to welfare logic. *Scandinavian Journal of Management, 33*(1), 1–11. https://doi.org/10.1016/j.scaman.2016.11.001

hooks, b. (1994). *Teaching to transgress: Education as the practice of freedom.* Routledge.

Institute of Medicine. (2003). *Health professions education: A bridge to quality.* National Academies Press.

Kamrul, R., Malin, G., & Ramsden, V. R. (2014). Beauty of patient-centered care within a cultural context. *Canadian Family Physician, 60*(4), 313–318.

Khalifa, M. (2018). *Culturally responsive school leadership.* Harvard Education Press.

McKenzie, K. B., & Scheurich, J. J. (2004). Equity traps: A useful construct for preparing principals to lead schools that are successful with racially diverse students. *Educational Administration Quarterly, 40*(5), 601–632. https://doi.org/10.1177/0013161X04268839

McKinnon, J. (2018). In their shoes: An ontological perspective on empathy in nursing practice. *Journal of Clinical Nursing, 27*(21-22), 3882–3893. https://doi.org/10.1111/jocn.14610

Mohr, B., & Magruder Watkins, J. (2002). *The essentials of appreciative inquiry: A roadmap for creating positive futures*. Pegasus Communications.

Moore, C., Coates, E., Watson, A., de Heer, R., McLeod, A., & Prudhomme, A. (2022). It's important to work with people that look like me. Black patients' preferences for patient-provider race concordance. *Journal of Racial and Ethnic Health Disparities*, 1–13. Advance online publication. https://doi.org/10.1007/s40615-022-01435-y

Moudatsou, M., Stavropoulou, A., Philalithis, A., & Koukouli, S. (2020). The role of empathy in health and social care professionals. *Healthcare, 8*(1), 26. https://doi.org/10.3390/healthcare8010026

National Academies of Sciences, Engineering, and Medicine. (2021). *The future of nursing 2020–2030: Charting a path to achieve health equity*. National Academies Press.

National Advisory Council on Nurse Education and Practice. (2013). *Achieving health equity through nursing workforce diversity: Eleventh report to the Secretary of the Department of Health and Human Services and Congress*. https://www.hrsa.gov/sites/default/files/hrsa/advisory-committees/nursing/reports/2013-eleventhreport.pdf

National Institutes of Health. (2017). *NIH glossary*.

Neilson, K. (2021). *Breadcrumbing, ghosting and conscious uncoupling at work*. HRM Online. https://www.hrmonline.com.au/section/featured/breadcrumbing-ghosting-workplace/

Roy, K., Hunt, K., Sakai, K., & Fletcher, K. (2022). Social justice in nursing education: A way forward. *Journal of Nursing Education, 61*(8), 447–454. https://doi.org/10.3928/01484834-20220602-05

Son Holoien, S. (2013). *Do differences make a difference? The effects of diversity on learning, intergroup outcomes, and civic engagement*. Princeton University. https://inclusive.princeton.edu/sites/g/files/toruqf1831/files/pu-report-diversity-outcomes.pdf

Stark, C. (2019). Gaslighting, misogyny, and psychological oppression. *The Monist, 102*(2), 221–235. https://doi.org/10.1093/monist/onz007

Storm, K. I. L., & Muhr, S. L. (2022). Work-life balance as gaslighting: Exploring repressive care in female accountants' careers. *Critical Perspectives on Accounting*. https://doi.org/10.1016/j.cpa.2022.102484

Watson, J. (2017). Global advances in human caring literacy. In S. Lee, P. Palmieri, & J. Watson (Eds.), *Global advances in human caring literacy* (pp. 3–12). Springer.

Wong, S. H. M., Gishen, F., & Lokugamage, A. U. (2021). Decolonizing the medical curriculum: Humanizing medicine through epistemic pluralism, cultural safety, and critical consciousness. *London Review of Education, 19*(1), 1–22. https://doi.org/10.14324/LRE.19.1.16

Younas, A., & Rasheed, S. P. (2018). Compassionate self-awareness: A hidden resource for nurses for developing a relationship with self and patients. *Creative Nursing, 24*(4), 220–224. https://doi.org/10.1891/1078-4535.24.4.220

Yu, C. C., Tan, L., Le, M. K., Tang, B., Liaw, S. Y., Tierney, T., Ho, Y. Y., Lim, B. E. E., Lim, D., Ng, R., Chia, S. C., & Low, J. A. (2022). The development of empathy in the healthcare setting: A qualitative approach. *BMC Medical Education, 22*(245), 1–13. https://doi.org/10.1186/s12909-022-03312-y

Zimmer, B. (2020, Sept. 4). The evolution of racism. *The Atlantic*. https://www.theatlantic.com/culture/archive/2020/09/how-racism-made-its-way-into-dictionary-merriam-webster/615334/

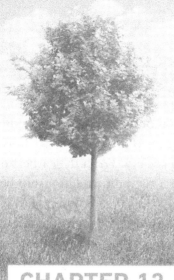

CHAPTER 12

REDESIGNING ACADEMIC AND PRACTICE PARTNERSHIPS: REFLECTIVE COMMUNITIES THAT LEARN AND PRACTICE TOGETHER

–Eileen Fry-Bowers, PhD, JD, RN, CPNP-PC, FAAN

LEARNING OBJECTIVES/SUBJECTIVES

- Examine theoretical frameworks and models defining "reflective learning community."

- Differentiate between an academic-practice partnership created for the purpose of developing a clinical placement agreement versus one created for the purpose of reflective learning.

- Discuss the attributes needed for a successful academic-practice partnership to function as a reflective learning community.

- Describe how reflective academic-practice partnerships support the implementation of guidelines and competencies for nursing education.

- Explore the role of design thinking in creating a well-functioning academic-practice reflective learning community benefiting learners, educators, and clinicians.

OVERVIEW

As a practice discipline, the education of nurses should be centered on the development of the knowledge, skills, and attitudes needed to provide care to individuals, families, communities, and populations in an ever-evolving society. From the earliest days of professional nursing education, this process has required a symbiotic relationship between those providing didactic content and those delivering clinical care. Initially, this existed as hospital-based apprenticeship programs where the superintendent of the nursing program and the chief nursing officer of the hospital were often one and the same (Whelan, 2011). By the mid-20th century, nursing education moved from these training programs to institutions of higher learning, and although this has been essential for the development of nursing as a scientific discipline, it has required nursing educational programs to align themselves with institutional healthcare providers to offer direct patient care experiences as an additional component of academic education.

This chapter explores the historical evolution of nursing education as a practice-based discipline and the necessity of integrating didactic and practice-based learning and proposes co-creating alternative solutions. Theoretical frameworks and models guide consideration of different purposes of academic-practice partnerships, characteristics of effective partnerships, and contributions of a reflective learning community. The chapter begins with deep reflections using hindsight, insight, and foresight perspectives on the evolution of academia's relationships with healthcare delivery systems and its reliance on workplace learning in preparing nursing's workforce.

HINDSIGHT, INSIGHT, AND FORESIGHT LEARNING PERSPECTIVES ON ACADEMIC-PRACTICE PARTNERSHIPS

A deep reflection on the history and evolution of the relationship between formal nursing education programs and healthcare delivery systems is long and complicated. The reflective process of *hindsight* (looking back for lessons learned), *insight* (lessons learned applied in current situations), and *foresight* (looking towards the future) can guide future directions in building reflective learning communities (Pesut, 2019). In looking back in *hindsight,* it is impossible to separate the function and impact of healthcare delivery institutions from the evolution of nursing education. Many say what happens in one is reflected in the other; this is certainly true in examining academic-practice partnerships. Figure 12.1 reflects this symbiotic relationship.

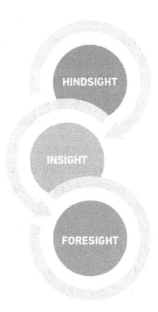

FIGURE 12.1 Hindsight, insight, and foresight reflective framework for perspective setting on history within the context of the present and forecasting the future.

The long-standing nursing faculty shortage and continuing changes in clinical agency processes for hosting non-employee learners has substantially impacted the ability of schools and programs of nursing across the country to offer high-quality clinical learning experiences that ensure the development of a competent registered and advanced practice nursing workforce. In response, the American Association of Colleges of Nursing (AACN, 2016) commissioned Manatt Health to complete a comprehensive national study on how academic nursing could more fully contribute to the larger healthcare system. The final report, *Advancing Healthcare Transformation: A New Era for Academic Nursing,* issued in 2016, called for greater integration of nursing education, practice, and research and called on leaders in higher education and clinical practice to intentionally work synergistically towards developing the nursing workforce, improving healthcare delivery, and innovating healthcare systems.

While important for shifting the paradigm regarding the interaction between academia and clinical practice, there were limitations. The report predominantly focused on aligning academic health science centers and affiliated schools and programs of nursing, which, at the time of the report, accounted for only 11.7% of academic nursing institutions (Enders et al., 2016; Sebastian et al., 2018). In addition, the report was primarily informed by nurse leaders from institutions located east of the Mississippi River, and the exemplars emphasized large health systems that have historically prioritized clinical placements in acute care services. Regional differences such as political or regulatory obstacles, institutional power dynamics, or cultural variation in the delivery of healthcare services were never fully acknowledged as substantive practical challenges to forming academic-practice partnerships, especially for nursing programs not affiliated with health systems. Establishing academic-practice partnerships emphasizing improvements in educational experiences and practice capacity acknowledges that these relationships can be difficult to develop and sustain due to time and resource constraints and cross-institutional knowledge deficits (Baptiste et al., 2022).

An *insight* perspective is useful to examine current academic practice partnerships. Notably, the need for a specific number of prelicensure direct care experiences in acute care settings frequently dominates nursing schools' efforts to align with institutional healthcare providers and often drives, and perhaps limits, the possibility and characteristics of any academic-practice relationship. Assumptions around the type and quantity of clinical experiences has constrained thinking about the types of real-world experiences learners need to gain competency necessary for nursing practice and, as such, have influenced the kind of academic-practice partnerships that nursing schools and programs pursue.

Although Kardong-Edgren et al. (2021) report a lack of evidence identifying a prescribed number of direct care hours to prepare learners to be registered nurses, most direct care learning hours are to be obtained in the acute care setting. In fact, significant variability in required hours exists among state boards of nursing in the US. Twenty-six states define clinical experiences, and only ten states require a specific number of hours, ranging from 400 to 750, with an average of 510 (Bowling et al., 2018). To address the need for direct care hours, numerous centralized academic-clinical practice consortiums across the country have the express goal of coordinating the clinical placement process to benefit both nursing service providers and nursing programs, primarily in acute care agencies. These systems distribute the limited supply of clinical placements, yet the question arises whether membership in these consortiums limits options for the development of innovative relationships between entities outside of this consortium.

The Essentials: Core Competencies for Professional Nursing Education (AACN, 2021) recently revised and adopted by AACN membership schools, acknowledges that healthcare delivery increasingly occurs within four spheres of care:

- **Disease prevention/promotion of health and well-being,** which includes the promotion of physical and mental health in all patients as well as management of minor acute and intermittent care needs of generally healthy patients

- **Chronic disease care,** which includes management of chronic diseases and prevention of negative sequelae

- **Regenerative or restorative care,** which includes critical/trauma care, complex acute care, acute exacerbations of chronic conditions, and treatment of physiologically unstable patients that generally requires care in a mega-acute care institution

- **Hospice/ palliative/supportive care,** which includes end-of-life care as well as palliative and supportive care for individuals requiring extended care, those with complex, chronic disease states, or those requiring rehabilitative care

Acknowledging the imperative of clinical learning in these four spheres of care has profound implications and introduces new possibilities for the variety of relationships that academic nursing needs to forge to ensure that learners can achieve competency according to the curricular guidelines accredited schools follow.

Foresight points to the growing need for practice-ready nurses and demands that nursing education and clinical practice engage in new and collaborative ways to ensure that learners are prepared for the practice environment. Most nursing education programs have focused on imparting knowledge to learners, especially the knowledge required to pass licensing and certification examinations, yet addressing the demands of complex 21st-century healthcare delivery systems requires learners to master the *competencies* (or knowledge, skills, and attitudes) nurses need for successful practice. Evidence indicates that new nurses at all levels face challenges moving from the learning environment of their educational experience to the practice environment of their professional role, a phenomenon amplified in recent years (Stegman & Woods, 2021). Although this mismatch may result from outdated educational approaches, another explanation may be attributed to the receptivity of the clinical environment to new graduate nurses and the readiness of the workplace to support them (Masso et al., 2022).

The COVID-19 pandemic exposed the profound dependence of nursing schools and programs on healthcare facilities and agencies to provide experiential learning opportunities, especially in the acute care environment. When facilities closed their doors to learners, classifying them as visitors, nursing schools and programs across the country scrambled to develop alternatives to direct care experiences. While some of these alternatives were innovative and of high quality, others were not. These changes raised the real possibility of new nurses entering the workforce without ever having touched a real patient. The pandemic confirmed the necessity of a fully functioning nursing educational pipeline, especially given the dire nursing workforce deficits (Spector et al., 2021). The pandemic also revealed academic nursing's growing awareness that learning experiences must promote an understanding of health equity, social determinants of health, and population health, amplifying the need to prepare learners to recognize their own implicit biases. The unfolding pandemic affirmed the imperative for schools to participate in interprofessional collaboration and multi-sector partnerships to provide learners with meaningful experience in delivering care in diverse community settings, including public health departments, schools, libraries, workplaces, and neighborhood clinics (National Academies of Sciences, Engineering, and Medicine [NASEM], 2021a).

Supervised direct care experiences in all settings have been and continue to be the cornerstone of pre-licensure and advanced practice nursing education, high-quality simulated experiences notwithstanding. Ensuring that learners in all program levels can participate in clinical experiences and develop the competencies necessary to enter the nursing workforce in all settings requires that schools and programs of nursing develop collaborative partnerships with entities that provide services across the four spheres of care. Such partnerships can also serve as a foundation for career advancement, promote lifelong learning, provide structure for pre-licensure and advanced practice nurse residency programs, and support the nursing workforce pipeline (Phillips et al., 2019). Educators and practitioners must routinely engage and share information to determine how to best educate and prepare clinicians needed to support evolving systems of care. Nursing schools and programs must "adapt to not just what the market is, but to what it will be" (NASEM, 2019, p. 30). Similarly, practice must recognize current forces in higher education, from budget deficits to demand for greater online learning options, with nursing education sitting squarely within a Venn diagram of higher education and healthcare (Figure 12.2). Thus, "there needs to be *continuous* [emphasis added] dialogue between the workplace and education in order to facilitate these changes" (NASEM, 2019, p. 30).

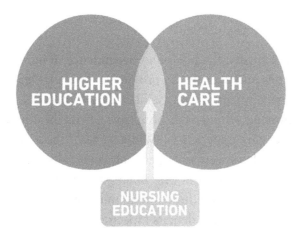

FIGURE 12.2 Nursing education at the intersection of higher education and healthcare.

The literature provides myriad evidence for guiding schools and programs of nursing in working with community partners condensed to the following seven principles (NASEM, 2021b):

- Recognize the need to partner.
- Value and respect each other.
- Accept each other.
- Set clear expectations.
- Provide feedback.
- Expect impact, product, or outcome.
- Trust each other.

Less commonly noted is an emphasis on *collaborative learning* among the partners. Often, especially in nursing education and practice, partners come together for each entity to achieve a particular predetermined goal, such as developing a faculty practice or procuring a clinical site for experiential learning. The process is designed to support achieving that particular outcome—and this outcome becomes the preferential measure of the success of the partnership. Is an opportunity missed when educators and practitioners each come to the table with this predetermined goal in mind rather than the goal of collaborative learning among all partners?

THEORETICAL FRAMEWORKS AND SUPPORTING EVIDENCE

Meeting the current needs of the nursing academic and healthcare delivery environments requires building a bridge between education and practice that transcends specific goals such as establishing a faculty practice, securing clinical placements, or developing clinical faculty. Preparing and supporting the current and future nursing workforce—learners, educators, and practitioners alike—requires acknowledging that few specific problems have explicit solutions. Rather, multiple tensions, competing priorities, and misaligned incentives create complex issues that must be managed by different sectors in society at large, including higher education and healthcare, and compel innovation in thinking and interaction, especially between practice and academia. If nursing academia and practice are to meet the future, they must come together regularly in the present.

Design thinking, a method for creative problem-solving, has gained traction in many sectors in recent years. The tenets of *design thinking,* a non-linear, iterative process used to understand users, challenge assumptions, redefine problems and create innovative solutions to prototype and test, have also begun to permeate nursing. For example, the University of Pennsylvania School of Nursing offers a course titled "Innovation in Health: Foundations of Design Thinking" (University of Pennsylvania School of Nursing, n.d.), and while nursing education and practice alike are adopting this approach for solving specific problems, especially relating to quality improvement, structures to support collaboration in this process are not common. In addition, design thinking itself has been criticized for its lack of attention to designer positionality. While empathy is the first stage of the process, the needs of users or communities are "refracted through the [designer's] personal experience and priorities" (Iskander, 2018). This is a particularly important consideration when bringing nursing education and practice together to solve a problem when there are inherent power dynamics, controlled access, and limited resources, as in the case of clinical placement distribution.

DESIGN THINKING

Design thinking is a non-linear, iterative process used to understand users, challenge assumptions, redefine problems, and create innovative solutions to prototype and test for application.

The design-thinking process can preserve the status quo and may limit problem-solving to those in the position to engage in the process. Iskander (2018) argues when the "designer acts as a gatekeeper for the meanings that are included in the design process, the potential for connections becomes limited not only to what the designer views as significant, but also to the relationships she can imagine" (para. 13). She also suggests that the design-thinking process is ill-suited to solving problems in rapidly changing areas or areas with a lot of uncertainty; that design thinking as implemented today risks underestimating the "complexity of the systems that are at play" (para. 14).

Health and the systems that support its development are exceedingly complex and subject to social, economic, and political pressures. The design thinking approach may be useful in nursing for addressing clearly defined problems that require a particular solution, yet adapting nursing education, practice, research, and regulation for the 21st century requires more than solution-oriented processes. Effective learning communities require a new way of *thinking and being* that integrates and aligns nursing education with the reality of nursing practice at all levels across all settings gained through a reflective process. It requires more than coming together to solve a problem—it requires coming together to build a reflective community that learns and practices together.

Merriam-Webster defines *partnership* as "a relationship resembling a legal partnership and usually involving close cooperation between parties having specified and joint rights and responsibilities" (Merriam-Webster, 2023). Under this definition, most schools and programs of nursing and most healthcare entities may have hundreds of partnerships potentially rendering further discussion of academic-practice partnership moot. Why, then, is this attention on academic-practice partnerships?

A search of PubMed using "nursing" and "academic-practice partnerships" reveal 248 results over 20 years, while a Google Scholar search yields over 10,000 results. Certainly, the nursing faculty shortage and increasingly limited supply of clinical sites available for learning experiences incentivize academic and practice entities to forge relationships that meet each institution's needs, often formalized through "clinical affiliation agreements" or "memoranda of understanding." Even so, many of these relationships do not create or facilitate conditions that foster the actualization of the AACN Academic Nursing report or implementation of the new Essentials. The promise of these documents, as well as other reports such as *The Future of Nursing 2020–2030* report (NASEM, 2021a), lies not in staid legal agreements but in the transformation of how academia and practice work with one another. What would happen if nursing education and nursing practice joined one another in community?

Consider the following definition of *community:* "a feeling of fellowship with others, as a result of sharing common attitudes, interests, and goals" (Google, n.d.). Sustaining relationships between schools and programs of nursing and clinical partners first require that interactions are based on satisfying mutual needs. Partnerships must also be intent on creating symbiotic learning communities that support learners from beginner through lifelong learning while also adapting to ever-evolving healthcare delivery systems and bridging processes that benefit both nursing education and nursing practice.

Learning itself has taken on great importance over the past several decades. Companies are interested in becoming learning organizations, higher education has embraced learning communities as a pedagogical tool, learning networks are common in research, and learning health systems are spreading throughout the industry. *Learning* is "a process that leads to change, which occurs as a result of experience and increases the potential for improved performance and future learning" (Ambrose et al., 2010, p. 3). Learning involves understanding, relating, and connecting ideas, critical thinking, and transferring knowledge to new and different contexts, resulting in a change in knowledge, attitude, or behavior. Dewey asserted that learning (education) is a social process rooted in community and espoused that "education is not preparation for life; education is life itself" (Dewey, 1916, p. 239). Dewey emphasized social interaction and active learning. Dewey (1933) also emphasized the importance of reflection, describing it as an "active, persistent, and careful consideration of any belief or supposed form of knowledge in the light of the grounds that support it and further conclusions to which it tends" (p. 9).

While references to Dewey are most often found in educational or philosophical spaces, his theories are equally applicable to nursing and healthcare. Building on Dewey, Schön (1983) asserted that when professionals possess practice-based knowledge, situational responses become spontaneous, constructed, and informed by previously experienced reflections. As a practice discipline, the delivery of nursing care is an inherently social process. A rapidly evolving healthcare landscape, as well as concomitant post-pandemic changes in society, requires all nurses (educators and practitioners) to regularly reflect and adjust their knowledge, skills, and attitudes in collaboration with colleagues across sectors and disciplines to meet the demands of healthcare delivery.

Professional learning communities provide a structured space for people to connect, collaborate, and align around shared aspirational and practical goals and work across boundaries while holding members accountable to a common agenda, values, metrics, processes, and outcomes. Participants share and reflect on experiences and learn from each other, deepening collective knowledge and thereby improving their ability to achieve goals, make change, and potentially transform their industries. Learning communities provide a mechanism for connecting organizations, agencies, and philanthropies to engage in collective inquiry and action and promote scaling of promising practices (Stoll et al., 2006).

Structured professional learning communities already exist in nursing. Quality improvement collaboratives have been widely used as an approach to sharing knowledge and resources to solve problems, improve practices, and achieve quality improvement goals (Wells et al., 2018). For example, the Quality and Safety Education in Nursing project employed collaborative learning communities to bridge academic and clinical partnerships (Cronenwett et al., 2009). In 2010, the American Nurses Credentialing Center Magnet Recognition Program® established a Magnet learning communities program, piloting it with 21 hospitals (Morgan, 2011). This exchange of ideas resulted in the adoption of new practices by increasing accessibility to innovations and new knowledge emerging regularly in Magnet institutions.

The nursing literature provides many examples of academic-practice partnerships; many of these papers describe a relationship between a nursing school or program and a healthcare facility designed to support clinical placements or clinical projects for learners. Few describe moving the partnership to a sustainable reflective learning community that *adapts* to learners' needs, faculty needs, and institutional needs across programs *over time*. In fact, current models of academic-practice partnerships, while effective, are not without substantial challenges (Paton et al., 2022) and as a result, may not be reaching their full potential.

ACADEMIC-PRACTICE PARTNERSHIPS AS REFLECTIVE RELATIONSHIPS

The AACN has developed substantial resources to support the development of academic-practice partnerships, including the *Guiding Principles for Academic-Practice Partnerships* developed in 2012 by the AACN-AONL Task Force on Academic-Practice Partnerships (AACN, n.d.). The Principles emphasize that these relationships should be intentionally created, formalized, and based on mutual goals, respect, shared knowledge, and clear communication. In a foundational study that informed the development of the Principles, Beal and colleagues (2011) determined that successful academic-practice partnerships were based on mutual investment and commitment to the relationship that promoted shared decision-making and problem-solving, rooted in trust and respect, and founded on personal relationships. Specifically, they stated, "To be effective and sustainable, there must be 'open and free communication' where there is a level of comfort and trust that allows for dialogue on any issue with the ultimate goal being a 'shared commitment to excellence and meaningful outcomes'" (p. e92). Barriers included time, resources, workload, communication, organizational culture conflict, and politics.

Investigators assessing the long-standing Veterans Affairs Nursing Academic Partnership highlighted the importance of inter-organizational collaboration, as well as addressing challenges arising from blending different cultures, altering clinical and faculty roles, ensuring the promotion of evidence-based practice, and "recognizing that stable relationships must be based on long-term commitments rather than short-term changes in the demand for nursing care" (Dobalian et al., 2014, p. 36). Certainly, many academic-practice partnerships may, in fact, already exist as learning communities. They may be intentional about coming together regularly to learn from one another in a supportive, integrative, and holistic manner—not simply for the purpose of solving a problem but for the purpose of an ongoing dialogue that is as much learning oriented as it is solution oriented. Structured engagement values the involvement of all stakeholders, with a focus on sustained learning over time. These learning communities are primed to transform into *reflective learning communities* where participants regularly engage in reflective practice within the community experience.

A *reflective academic-practice learning community* makes space for descriptive, dialogic, and critical reflection, which supports deep thinking, by individuals and the collective, about what is known and what is assumed. It promotes conscious and deliberate discussion of challenging issues, encourages sense-making of relationships and experiences, fosters insight, and stimulates innovation (Horton-Deutsch & Sherwood, 2017). As the profession of nursing moves through the 21st century, it is imperative that nursing academia and nursing practice engage in reflective practices in the community to ensure that learners are prepared for the increasingly complex workplace environment rife with professional and interpersonal challenges. While Dewey and Schön emphasized reflection at the time of an action (reflection-in-action) or reflection after an event has occurred (reflection-on-action), which are concepts essential for nursing practice, forward-looking academic-practice partnerships should also look to transcend a current state (sustainability) and instead strive to become regenerative organizations—organizations that embrace reflection-for-action. Reflection-for-action requires contemplation of future action with the intention of improving or changing practice. When academic-practice partnerships move toward thinking about how future actions will impact outcomes, there is an opportunity for deeper collaboration and innovation. Reflection-for-action fosters a regenerative process of seeking to create more equitable and sustainable systems that promote human well-being and resilience. This approach recognizes that knowledge and circumstances are constantly evolving, and this more expansive concept promotes not only collaboration, innovation, and sustainability but supports efforts to renew, restore, and incorporate equity, well-being, and lifelong learning.

REFLECTION-FOR-ACTION

Reflection-for-action fosters a regenerative process, creating more equitable and sustainable systems that promote human well-being and resilience.

APPLICATION FOR PERSONAL AND PROFESSIONAL PRACTICE

The AACN Principles and substantial evidence-based literature offer guidance for creating successful academic-practice partnerships. Even so, for a partnership to evolve as a reflective learning community, shared values and shared commitment are essential, as is ensuring involvement from all stakeholders within each organization. The rapid pace of change in society, and healthcare specifically, requires that learners be prepared to work in evolving systems that promote human well-being and resilience. Designing appropriately resourced, practical educational processes that benefit learners, the health system, and society requires frank discussions about deeply challenging issues. These conversations can only take place where there is an alignment about what is important, what is a priority, and what is valued within organizations. It requires a commitment of time and resources to process. It also requires empathy for the demands placed on each institution and the incentives driving decisions within organizations. Lastly, as a reflective learning community, the members of a nursing academic-practice partnership must be willing to critically interrogate their individual and collective work in a continuous, collaborative, inclusive, learning-oriented, growth-promoting manner.

REFLECTIVE LEARNING COMMUNITIES

Reflective learning communities have shared values and shared commitment, ensuring involvement from all stakeholders with each organization.

Adoption of the new Essentials (2021) by the AACN membership schools provides an excellent impetus for the formation of reflective academic-practice learning communities. "The Essentials serve to bridge the gap between education and practice" and support a "collective understanding [that] allows all nurses to have a shared vision [and] promotes open discourse and exchange about nursing practice" (AACN, 2021, p. 1). The move toward competency-based education necessitates partnership between nursing schools and programs and health-related entities in ways not often present today. The Essentials promotes shared ownership of nursing education and practice by encouraging co-design of these environments.

As nursing schools and programs evaluate their curricula and experiential learning opportunities, it is critical that they engage with practice partners beyond the clinical placement or faculty practice relationships. Practice partners can offer valuable insight into the evolving needs and opportunities in the healthcare delivery setting, ensuring that curricula remain relevant. Education partners can share pedagogical and andragogical approaches adopted to serve evolving learner populations and capitalize on advances in educational technology. Collaborative inquiry, discussion, and reflection on the Essential's four spheres of care can lead to creative approaches to providing direct care learning experiences and decompress demands in acute care settings for placements as well as faculty. (The four spheres of care are discussed in "Hindsight, Insight, and Foresight Learning Perspectives on Academic-Practice Partnerships" earlier in this chapter.) Moreover, sustained and deep analysis can assist participants in naming assumptions and acknowledging personal and professional biases of each other's environments, which can impede innovative thinking. Importantly, while a theoretical end date exists for a school or program for implementation of the Essentials (i.e., when the curricula shift to a full competency-based educational model), ongoing interaction between academia and practice will remain important to ensure that learners enter the workforce ready to practice.

REFLECTIVE SUMMARY

Nursing schools and programs and healthcare systems and related entities have long worked together and relied upon each other to meet specific institutional needs in preparing the nursing workforce. The rapidly evolving nature of higher education and healthcare delivery systems exerts significant pressure on nursing education and nursing practice environments. These pressures require these partners to adapt their relationships and move from what have often been time-limited or goal-focused transactional relationships to deeper, continuous, reflective, and evolutionary learning relationships. Although nursing has moved on from its early roots of an apprenticeship educational model, remnants of these structures remain. The very nature of nursing as a practice discipline requires that academia and practice co-design the learning process; each informing the experience through collaborative inquiry, reflective learning, and deliberative action.

LEARNING NARRATIVE

Designing a reflective learning community requires an intentional commitment to creating a shared space to promote connection, collaboration, and clear communication. Partners in the community must be willing to continuously examine their individual and collective efforts, which requires trust, respect, and sharing of common values and goals.

A large public safety-net metropolitan health system has served as a clinical practice site for a private school of nursing for more than 20 years. The director of the prelicensure nursing program regularly communicates with the health system's director of professional education to arrange clinical experiences for learners. While cordial and professional, their relationship exists only to support this clinical placement function. They have no other regular interaction. Several nurses in the health system serve as adjunct clinical instructors for the school's nursing programs, and many direct care nurses routinely precept learners during their clinical experiences. Each entity faces significant challenges brought on by the rapid pace of change in the healthcare industry and higher education. The chief nursing officer of the health system and the dean of the school of nursing believe that each organization has much to offer the other organization, and they wish to form a partnership that will enable both entities to thrive in the future. They hope to design a reflective learning community that learns and practices together.

- What should the leaders consider as they begin to form this academic-practice part-nership?

- What questions should they be asking? And of whom?

- What organizational characteristics require consideration?
- Who are the stakeholders and what role will they play in this partnership?
- What resources are available to them as they design this learning community?
- How will the leaders and stakeholders measure the success of this effort?

REFLECTIVE QUESTIONS

1. How can the theoretical frameworks and models explored in this chapter guide the development of a reflective learning community for enhancing collaboration and building evolutionary learning relationships?

2. What are some key differences between a partnership focused on developing a clinical placement agreement and one focused on creating a reflective learning environment? How can these differences impact the overall goals and outcomes of the partnership for all stakeholders involved?

3. What personal attributes do you think are essential for creating a successful reflective learning community? In what ways can you cultivate these attributes within yourself and collaborate with other stakeholders to foster a supportive and effective academic-practice partnership?

4. How can reflective academic-practice partnerships support the implementation of guidelines and competencies for nursing education?

5. What specific strategies promote collaboration, shared learning, and continuous improvement of nursing education within the context of academic-practice partnerships?

REFERENCES

Ambrose, S. A., Bridges, M. W., DiPietro, M., Lovett, M. C., & Norman, M. K. (2010). *How learning works: Seven research-based principles for smart teaching.* John Wiley & Sons.

American Association of Colleges of Nursing. (n.d.). *Academic-practice partnerships: Guiding principles for academic-practice partnerships.* https://www.aacnnursing.org/Academic-Practice-Partnerships/The-Guiding-Principles

American Association of Colleges of Nursing. (2016). *Advancing healthcare transformation: A new era for academic nursing.* https://www.aacnnursing.org/Portals/0/PDFs/Publications/AACN-New-Era-Report.pdf

American Association of Colleges of Nursing. (2021). *The essentials: Core competencies for professional nursing.* https://www.aacnnursing.org/Portals/42/AcademicNursing/pdf/Essentials-2021.pdf

Baptiste, D., Whalen, M., & Goodwin, M. (2022). Approaches for establishing and sustaining clinical academic partnerships: A discursive review. *Journal of Clinical Nursing, 31*(3-4), 329–334. https://doi.org/10.1111/jocn.15830

Beal, J. A., Breslin, E., Austin, T., Brower, L., Bullard, K., Light, K., Millican, S., Pelayo, L. W., & Ray, N. (2011). Hallmarks of best practices in academic-practice partnerships in nursing: Lessons learned from San Antonio. *Journal of Professional Nursing, 27*(6), e90–e95. https://doi.org/10.1016/j.profnurs.2011.07.006

Bowling, A. M., Cooper, R., Kellish, A., Kubin, L., & Smith, T. (2018). No evidence to support number of clinical hours necessary for nursing competency. *Journal of Pediatric Nursing, 39,* 27–36. https://doi.org/10.1016/j.pedn.2017.12.012

Cronenwett, L., Sherwood, G., & Gelmon, S. (2009). Improving quality and safety education: The QSEN Learning Collaborative. *Nursing Outlook, 57*(6), 304–312. https://doi.org/10.1016/j.outlook.2009.09.004

Dewey, J. (1916). *Democracy and education: An introduction to the philosophy of education.* MacMillan Company.

Dewey, J. (1933). *How we think: a restatement of the relation of reflective thinking to the educative process.* Heath and Company.

Dobalian, A., Bowman, C. C., Wyte-Lake, T., Pearson, M. L., Dougherty, M. B., & Needleman, J. (2014). The critical elements of effective academic-practice partnerships: A framework derived from the Department of Veterans Affairs Nursing Academy. *BMC Nursing, 13,* 36. http://www.biomedcentral.com/1472-6955/13/36

Enders, T., Pawlak, B., & Morin, A. (2016). *Advancing health care transformation: A new era for academic nursing.* American Association of Colleges of Nursing.

Google. (n.d.). Community. In *Google dictionary.* https://g.co/kgs/zrQEJb

Horton- Deutsch, S., & Sherwood, G. (2017). *Reflective practice: Transforming education and improving outcomes.* Sigma Theta Tau International.

Iskander, N. (2018, Sept. 5). Design thinking is fundamentally conservative and preserves the status quo. *Harvard Business Review.* https://hbr.org/2018/09/design-thinking-is-fundamentally-conservative-and-preserves-the-status-quo

Kardong-Edgren, S., Leighton, K., McNelis, A. M., Foisy-Doll, C., Sharpnack, P. A., & Kavanagh, J. M. (2021). Evidence vs. eminence: Clinical hours in nursing education. *Journal of Professional Education, 37*(5), A1–A2. https://doi.org/10.1016/j.profnurs.2021.07.008

Masso, M., Sim, J., Halcomb, E., & Thompson, C. (2022). Practice readiness of new graduate nurses and factors influencing practice readiness: A scoping review of reviews. *International Journal of Nursing Studies,* 104208. https://doi.org/10.1016/j.ijnurstu.2022.104208

Merriam-Webster. (2023). Partnership. In *Merriam-Webster online dictionary.* https://www.merriam-webster.com/dictionary/partnership?utm_campaign=sd&utm_medium=serp&utm_source=jsonld

Morgan, S. H. (2011). Magnet learning communities. *Journal of Nursing Care Quality, 26*(3), 197–198. https://doi.org/10.1097/NCQ.0b013e31821e08ee

National Academies of Sciences, Engineering and Medicine. (2019). *Strengthening the connection between health professions education and practice: Proceedings of a joint workshop.* The National Academies Press. https://doi.org/10.17226/25407

National Academies of Sciences, Engineering and Medicine. (2021a). *The future of nursing 2020–2030: Charting a path to achieve health equity.* The National Academies Press.

National Academies of Sciences, Engineering and Medicine. (2021b). *Health professions faculty for the future: Proceedings of a workshop.* The National Academies Press. https://nap.nationalacademies.org/read/26041/chapter/1

Paton, E. A., Wicks, M., Rhodes, L. N., Key, C. T., Day, S. W., Webb, S., & Likes, W. (2022). Journey to a new era: An innovative academic-practice partnership. *Journal of Professional Nursing, 40*, 84–88. https://doi.org/10.1016/j.profnurs.2022.03.006

Pesut, D. J. (2019). Anticipating disruptive innovations with foresight leadership. *Nursing Administration Quarterly, 43*(3), 196–204. https://doi.org/10.1097/NAQ.0000000000000349

Phillips, J. M., Phillips, C. R., Kauffman, K. R., Gainey, M., & Schnur, P. (2019). Academic–practice partnerships: A win-win. *The Journal of Continuing Nursing Education, 50*(6), 282–288. https://doi.org/10.3928/00220124-20190516-09

Schön, D. (1983). *The reflective practitioner.* Temple Smith.

Sebastian, J. G., Breslin, E. T., Trautman, D. E., Cary, A. H., Rosseter, R., & Vlahov, D. (2018). Leadership by collaboration: Nursing's bold new vision for academic-practice partnerships. *Journal of Professional Nursing, 34*(2), 110–116. https://doi.org/10.1016/j.profnurs.2017.11.006

Spector, N. M., Buck, M., & Phipps, S. (2021). A new framework for practice-academic partnerships during the pandemic and into the future. *American Journal of Nursing, 121*(12), 39–44. https://doi.org/10.1097/01.NAJ.0000803192.68710.8f

Stegman, J., & Woods, A.D. (2021, Jan. 20). *Closing the education gap: Building confidence and competence.* Wolters Kluwer. https://www.wolterskluwer.com/en/expert-insights/survey-nursing-readiness

Stoll, L., Bolam, R., McMahon, A., Wallace, M., & Thomas, S. (2006). Professional learning communities: A review of the literature. *Journal of Education Change, 7*(4), 221–258. https://doi.org/10.1007/s10833-006-0001-8

University of Pennsylvania School of Nursing. (n.d.). *Design thinking for nurses.* https://www.nursing.upenn.edu/details/news.php?id=1369

Wells, S., Tamir, O., Gray, J., Naidoo, D., Bekhit, M., & Goldman, D. (2018). Are quality improvement collaboratives effective? A systematic review. *BMC Quality & Safety, 27*(3), 226–240. https://doi.org/10.1136/bmjqs-2017-006926

Whelan, J. (2011). *American nursing: An introduction to the past.* PennNursing. https://www.nursing.upenn.edu/nhhc/american-nursing-an-introduction-to-the-past

PART V

REGENERATION AND RENEWAL

13 **The Value of Emancipatory Nursing Praxis and Caring Science in an Era of Legislative Censorship**. 269

14 **Reimagining Leadership: A Legacy Perspective** 287

15 **Reflective Practice, Unitary Caring Science, and Wisdom: The Heart of the Capacity to Grow** 303

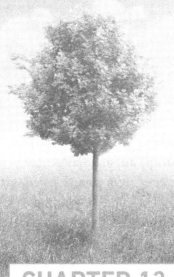

CHAPTER 13

THE VALUE OF EMANCIPATORY NURSING PRAXIS AND CARING SCIENCE IN AN ERA OF LEGISLATIVE CENSORSHIP

–Robin R. Walter, PhD, RN, CNE

LEARNING OBJECTIVES/SUBJECTIVES

- Analyze the implications of the current sociopolitical climate towards social justice, diversity, equity, and inclusion in higher education in general and nursing education specifically.

- Describe the learning process nurses experience in becoming social justice allies and equity advocates.

- Explain how a relational emancipatory pedagogy, grounded in Caring Science, can be used to educate nurses as social justice allies and equity advocates.

- Reflect on how social identity impacts nurse engagement with clients, coworkers, and peers.

OVERVIEW

This chapter opens with the current sociopolitical climate that seeks to suppress all forms of social justice teaching in public-funded K-12 schools, colleges, and universities across the United States. Against this backdrop, nursing has renewed its commitment to social justice, diversity, equity, and inclusiveness. On June 11, 2022, the American Nurses Association (ANA) unanimously adopted and released the *ANA Racial Reckoning Statement,* acknowledging the organization's past actions that "negatively impacted nurses of color and perpetuated systemic racism" (p. 1). This was a pivotal moment that heralded an overdue journey of healing since the structural, individual, and ideological racism that exists in nursing is rarely called out, and this silence has entrenched the idea of whiteness as the norm within nursing while marginalizing and silencing other groups and their perspectives (Burnett et al., 2020; Iheduru-Anderson, 2020). The American Association of Colleges of Nursing (AACN, 2021) released *The Essentials: Core Competencies for Professional Nursing Education,* which now defines social justice, diversity, equity, and inclusion as "competencies…[to be] fully represented and deeply integrated…in learning experiences across the curricula" (p. 5). Finally, the National League for Nursing (2019) calls on nurse educators to "assist students to reframe their understanding of the social determinants of health, recognizing that bias and stigmatization contribute to health disparities and that health issues…are not a choice, but rather the direct result of exposure to disparate financial, social, and environmental conditions" (p. 5). The question becomes, "How do nurse educators develop curricula and engage in learning experiences supporting these ideals at a time when the concepts and theories grounding them are, in effect, being censored across the nation?" This chapter answers that question with a nursing education curriculum grounded in Caring Science, scaffolded by relational emancipatory pedagogy, and implemented using emancipatory nursing praxis as a transformational learning theory. In this way, students and graduates of nursing programs will be positioned to actualize an inclusive, relational, and emancipatory approach to nursing and live the profession's commitment to equity and social justice.

THE PRECARIOUS STATE OF SOCIAL JUSTICE IN HIGHER EDUCATION

A primary assumption in a democracy is that we can have confidence in the people, so suppressing specific types of knowledge should not be forbidden unless there is a vital and compelling reason to withhold it (Porter, 2019). At the time of this writing (spring 2023), 33 states have introduced 670 bills, resolutions, executive orders, and other measures to censor the teaching of "divisive" theories and concepts, such as critical race theory, social justice, structural racism, and systemic disadvantages and inequities experienced by groups based on ethnicity, color, sexual preference, gender, citizenship, religion, etc. (UCLA School of Law Critical Race Studies Program, 2023). Additionally, 34 bills in 19 states would prohibit colleges from having diversity, equity, and inclusion offices or staff; ban mandatory diversity training; prohibit institutions from using diversity statements in hiring or promotion; or prohibit colleges from using race, sex, color, ethnicity, or national origin in admissions or employment (Lu et al., 2023). For example, Iowa now prohibits educators from teaching any topics that "assign fault, blame, or bias to a race or sex, or to members of a race or sex because of their race or sex, or claiming that, consciously or unconsciously, and by virtue of a person's race or sex, members of any race are inherently racist or are inherently inclined to oppress others, or that members of a sex are inherently sexist or inclined to oppress others," and "ascribing character traits, values, moral and ethical codes, privileges, status, or beliefs about a race or sex or to an individual because of the individual's race or sex" (Iowa House File 802, 2021, p. 3). Florida more explicitly banned collegiate discussion of anything that might make white students feel "discomfort" around the role racism has played in shaping American society. The Stop Wrongs to Our Kids and Employees (WOKE) Act, signed into Florida law in 2022, prohibits instruction on race relations or diversity that implies a person's status as either privileged or oppressed is necessarily determined by their race, color, national origin, or sex (Florida HB 7, 2022).

Engaging in social justice and equity advocacy, however, is a professional expectation of nurses nationally and globally, as described in the educational mandates of the AACN (2021), professional codes of the ANA (2010a, 2010b, 2010c), and the International Council of Nurses (2012). Buettner-Schmidt and Lobo (2011) defined the concept of social justice for nursing as the "full participation in society and balancing benefits and burdens by all citizens, resulting in a just ordering of society" (p. 948). Social justice is primarily concerned with identifying and redressing systems of oppression. These systems operate on individual, organizational, and societal levels to subjugate certain individuals or groups and privilege others based solely on actual or perceived membership in various social groups (e.g., race, sexual orientation, religion, class, socioeconomic status, gender, and physical ability). Consequently, some group members (e.g., white, heterosexual, upper-class, male) socially benefit from unearned privilege.

These privileges are referred to as "unearned" because they are not socially bestowed due to hard work, talent, virtue, or accomplishment. Instead, they result from inequitable social systems that confer dominance to some groups and subordination to all others.

Nurse engagement in social justice requires expanding the professional nursing role to include the role of equity advocates and social justice allies. As social justice allies, nurses function as members of a privileged, dominant social group working *with* those from an oppressed group to remedy the systemic denial of privilege and power based solely on social group membership. Functioning as an ally requires an ongoing commitment to listening to—and learning from—oppressed groups. The oppressed group members will ultimately decide who does (and does not) constitute an effective ally.

Emancipatory nursing praxis (ENP) offers nurses a substantive theoretical framework for developing the role of social justice ally across all areas of nursing education and practice. The alignment of a congruent science of nursing and pedagogy is key to actualizing this learning process across the nursing curriculum. What follows is an overview of ENP, and then a discussion of how Caring Science and relational emancipatory pedagogy offer a congruent conceptual guide for nurse educators seeking to develop future nurses as social justice allies and equity advocates.

EMANCIPATORY NURSING PRAXIS: OVERVIEW OF THE THEORY

Walter's (2017) ENP is a middle-range theory that explains transformational learning in becoming social justice allies. ENP identifies four stages of learning (becoming, awakening, engaging, and transforming) that are facilitated by two conditional contexts (reflexivity and relational). Taken together, the learning stages and contexts facilitate the acquisition of social justice competencies and role development as an ally. ENP details a reflective practice that supports and grounds nurses with the sense of self needed to enact real and meaningful contributions toward realizing a sustainable world (Rosa & Horton-Deutsch, 2017). A brief overview of these processes is helpful, as they can be used to guide nurse educators in the development of learning activities that meet students where they are in the process and move them toward actualizing their ability to transform structural inequities and unjust social relations (Coretta et al., 2021; Nye & Dillard-Wright, 2023).

BECOMING

Becoming is a process that reflects an individual's earliest memories and perceptions of social injustice or inequitable social situations; an initial exploration of perceptions and ways of being in the world (Walter, 2017). Intrapersonal characteristics and socio-environmental factors work in concert to provide a basic awareness that "something is not right" or "something needs to be done." The most frequent interpersonal characteristics identified in the *Becoming* stage of learning are recognizing unfairness, feeling a moral obligation to those less fortunate, wanting to make a difference, and wanting to be understood. Socio-environmental factors influencing this learning phase include parental and familial role modeling, faith-based experiences, direct or indirect experiences of marginalization or exclusion, and sensitizing social experiences.

AWAKENING

Awakening is the ENP learning process through which nurses come to identify or recognize their role or place in the larger societal-structural forces that impact the health and well-being of others (Walter, 2017). This learning phase demonstrates a change in how nurses see themselves in relation to others. This new awareness happens along several dimensions. One dimension is when formerly held beliefs, attitudes, and assumptions are compared to alternative beliefs, attitudes, and assumptions regarding the same situation. This comparison can help nurses position themselves contextually within larger social systems and identify intersecting sources of privilege and oppression in their own lives.

Another key dimension of *Awakening* involves dismantling and ultimately discarding culturally conditioned attitudes, perceptions, and assumptions that limit one's ability to live authentically. Budding nurse allies dismantled their socially conditioned understanding of gender, race/ethnicity, sexuality, and cultural competence. Reflection that is self-aware is marked by heightened intrapersonal awareness of feelings, emotions, and biases. Self-awareness, however, often stops short of contextualizing these perceptions within the larger context of how they have been culturally socialized and may leave developing nurse allies feeling overwhelmed. Critical, reflective dialogue with others mediates these disempowering attitudes and facilitates the initial process of deconstructing (dismantling) socially conditioned beliefs that perpetuate systems of oppression. Through dialogue, nurses can process experiences that confirm or challenge their new worldview and learn how to handle pressure from others to return to their former beliefs and behaviors.

ENGAGING

Engaging comprises the actions and interactions involved in doing social justice work as allies (Walter, 2017). It is a dynamic, evolving learning process in which nurses actively explore and cultivate the role of ally with the expressed intent of advancing transformative societal goals. A fundamental process of engaging in social justice is the identification and analysis of sources and balances of power. Social justice allies must identify the stakeholders in a given inequitable situation—those who benefit from the status quo and those who do not.

Identifying sources of power (and power imbalance) facilitates the ally's ability to engage in collective strategizing. This is also a critical, dialogic process of assessing, coalescing support, and planning the actions/interactions that will be required to move toward one or more social justice goals. Social justice engagement is collaborative-action driven, largely by members from the oppressed or marginalized groups with whom the nurse allies are affiliated. The role of the ally is to leverage their position of social advantage in ways that are not only beneficial to the oppressed group, but also seek to dismantle the system of oppression that created the inequity in the first place.

PRAXIS

Praxis was described by Paulo Freire as simultaneous "reflection and action upon the world in order to transform it" (1970, p. 33). In ENP, praxis involves paying attention to the ways in which our beliefs, assumptions, and behaviors foster or inhibit the ability to work with an individual or group in an emancipatory way. Stated another way, praxis fully integrates reflection with specific courses of action; the "praxis" in ENP is fundamentally relational.

TRANSFORMING

Transforming is experienced as an expansion of consciousness that fundamentally reconditions the nurse's thoughts, feelings, and actions (Walter, 2017). Three goal-directed processes include human flourishing, achieving equity, and transforming social relationships. Human flourishing is a condition of wellness and quality of life that everyone deserves. Achieving equity encompasses more than access to healthcare. It extends to all basic human necessities (education, housing, food security, employment, transportation) and full connectedness, belonging, and participation in society. Nurses learning to become allies see these conditions as foundational to human flourishing and which should be met before conception/birth. No individual should have to fight for equity once in the world but should be conceived and born into it. Finally, transforming social relationships encompasses more than simply adopting a new belief or a different way of thinking about and relating to others. *Transforming social relationships* constitutes the unfolding reality of learning how to engage authentically, in critical reflective dialogue, for the purpose of dismantling systems of oppression.

THE IMPORTANCE OF REFLEXIVITY

Nurses learning to become social justice allies move dynamically through the process of ENP via four dimensions of reflection: descriptive, self-aware, critical, and emancipatory.

- Descriptive reflection—first seen in *Becoming*—is a straightforward, retrospective accounting of events wherein emotive reactions are objectively reported, if at all.

- Reflection that is self-aware emerges in *Awakening* as a heightened awareness of personal feelings, emotions, and biases, but stops short of contextualizing these attitudes within the larger social context.

- Critical and emancipatory reflection characterizes the processes of *Engaging* and *Transforming*. This level of reflection-in-action promotes *praxis*, the ability to envision and take action toward possibilities of individual and collective self-determination.

The reflexivity that occurs as part of this dialogical process initially allows nurses to identify and deconstruct the personal beliefs, assumptions, and behaviors that inhibit their ability to work with an individual or group in an emancipatory way. This gives way to a collaborative reconstruction of attitudes and beliefs that generate new meaning-in-action (praxis). In this way, reflexive dialogue becomes more than a communication tool for change; it is "the very medium within which change occurs" (Ford & Ford, 1995, p. 542). ENP facilitates social change through a recursive process of social construction in which new realities are created, modified, and sustained via collaborative, relational processes.

USING RELATIONAL EMANCIPATORY PEDAGOGY TO DEVELOP EMANCIPATORY NURSING PRAXIS

ENP offers an explanation for how nurses learn to integrate social justice into their professional practice as allies. This type of learning is best facilitated by a pedagogical framework that is liberating, emancipating, and empowering. It requires restructuring educator and student roles to deeply relational ones, where knowledge is co-constructed rather than passed down. At all levels of nursing education, there is a need "to create and tolerate ambiguity, to challenge taken-for-granted assumptions, and to create an environment in which learners feel free to wrestle with ideas, challenge [educators] and other learners, share half-baked ideas, and engage in critical dialogue about the issues at hand" (Hills et al. 2021, p. 155). A relational emancipatory pedagogy addresses this need.

Relational emancipatory pedagogy was developed to support curriculum development in nursing grounded in Caring Science:

> A Caring Science curriculum seeks to create authentic, egalitarian, human-to-human relationships. This assumption is based on the notion that there is reciprocity between power, knowledge, and control and that, in order for there to be more equitable relationships, those with power need to give up and share control so that others may benefit and share their knowledge, thus their power. Authentic power is shared power; it is power with, not power over…It also means standing in one's own power, one's own truth and integrity, and authenticity without succumbing to another's…authoritarian control. (Hills et al., 2021, p. 44)

Foundational to relational emancipatory pedagogy is the belief that transformational learning occurs because of authentic caring relationships between educators and students. Four elements must be present for learning to occur: creating a culture of caring, creating collaborative caring relationships, engaging in critical dialogue, and reflection-in-action. The underlying processes for each of these elements support the learning processes in ENP.

CREATING A CULTURE OF CARING

Becoming a social justice ally is at once a deeply personal and profoundly relational process that begins with the uncomfortable but necessary reckoning of positionality in society. Understanding that our ideas, views, and opinions are not simply individual, but the product of internalized social and cultural messages taught from birth is essential to this process. We develop ideas about ourselves and others in terms of their race, class, gender, sexuality, ethnicity, religion, ability, and citizenship from the culture that surrounds us, and many of these ideas operate on an unconscious level (DiAngelo, 2017). Nursing culture is embedded within the dominant culture. Who we are and how we care are based on how we have been socialized into the dominant and nursing cultures. However, the values and expectations of the dominant culture may be at odds with the culture of nursing navigated by educators, students, and practitioners.

Current nursing culture in the United States and many other Western countries focus on "biomedical/technocure/behaviorist" priorities, where patients are seen as problems to be corrected rather than mysteries to behold and attend to (Hills et al., 2021, p. 169). Most service delivery models for acute and chronic care direct the focus of nursing care to managing treatments and adhering to schedules rather than developing a relational bond with clients that would create the space needed to express and explore feelings, experiences, and ways of dealing with their illness or trauma.

The risk here is the potential to objectify and dehumanize those with whom we are in caring-healing relationships as nurses. Objectification may impede nurses' progression in integrating social justice into their professional practice by stalling them in the *Becoming* phase. They are aware that something is wrong or unfair, but an awareness of the problem's root (social) cause and one's place (positionality) in that process is unclear (Walter, 2017). Creating a culture of caring in nursing academia is key to helping students transition from the *Becoming* to the *Awakening* phase of learning in ENP. For example, we as educators recognize the incongruence between the nursing culture taught in academia and experienced in clinical settings. A culture of caring can ground our efforts in helping students recognize the constrictive, oppressive institutional structures that make the clinical setting a challenging place to provide holistic, client-centered care. It also emboldens us to work with our students—at all levels of nursing education—to question practice that is not grounded in an empowering, emancipatory, and relational-humanistic framework. It is within the larger context of creating a caring culture that the three other elements of relational emancipatory pedagogy guide curriculum development.

CREATING COLLABORATIVE CARING RELATIONSHIPS

Creating caring relationships in the academy means "fostering egalitarian teaching/learning relationships based on trust, integrity, authenticity, caring, mutual respect, and shared power" (Hills et al., 2021, p. 167). Relationships are central to each aspect of developing and acting as an ally. Moving through the learning phases of *Awakening* to *Engaging* and into *Transforming* demonstrates how building authentic relationships across differences is itself an action that resists the systemic oppression that inherently divides people to maintain power for some and not others (Suyemoto et al., 2021; Walter, 2017).

Collaborative caring relationships have the same goal, but require different things from educators and students. It is the educator's responsibility to create the space for these relationships to develop, and it is the student's responsibility to decide how to respond (Hills et al., 2021, pp. 176, 178). Educators need to consider factors that may make students reticent to engage with new information about how they benefit from social inequities related to the intersection of race, gender, able-bodiedness, ethnicity, sexual orientation, religion, and socioeconomic class in their lives. DiAngelo (2017) identified these barriers as the need to avoid being judged; feeling complicit in the suffering of others; the fear of losing one's privileged status; and feeling powerless to change the status quo.

Educators may observe students engaging in defensive behaviors, such as focusing on personal experiences of marginalization or oppression, rather than exploring the unearned benefits of their privileged social identities. Students may also fail to acknowledge interpretations of course materials from alternate perspectives, or they may engage in avoidant or disruptive behaviors when certain topics are covered (e.g., class absences, unexpected changes in the level of in-class participation, texting during class, or engaging in side conversations during class; Bishop, 2015). Students may be in denial that any form of oppression exists, or if they do acknowledge some aspects, they "tend to think it can be dealt with quickly and easily by education and good intentions, and . . . certainly do not see themselves as perpetrators" (Bishop, 2015, p. 88). Students may also cite exceptions to the rules to discredit the role of privilege in maintaining oppression. For example, students may cite accomplished Black individuals (e.g., President Obama, Oprah Winfrey, Condoleezza Rice) to dismiss the advantages accorded to whites relative to people of color. This calls for a deeper exploration of how the very nature of an exception may, instead, function to prove the rule.

More often, however, educators' attempts to discuss equity, diversity, and inclusion may be met with silence. Although there may be several reasons students choose not to participate in class discussions, there is evidence that apprehension about discussing sensitive issues plays a significant role. Students have expressed concern about being criticized by peers, with those from non-dominant groups feeling particularly at risk (Kolowich, 2018; Walls & Hall, 2018). This dynamic is inconsistent with a collaborative caring relationship largely due to power dynamics operating in the classroom. Hills et al. (2021) argue that power relations in the classroom can be discussed and negotiated. In the scenarios discussed in this section, negotiating ground rules with students before entering into discussions about sensitive topics would be consistent with creating a space where everyone is meaningfully engaged. The guidelines typically address matters of open-mindedness; tolerance of inadvertent offense (assuming good intentions); active listening; using respectful language; avoiding personal attacks; allowing people to make mistakes; being aware of nonverbal, dismissive cues; and not asking anyone to serve as a spokesperson for their ethnicity or group (Kite et al., 2021).

ENGAGING IN CRITICAL DIALOGUE

Critical dialogue is often the most difficult aspect of teaching equity advocacy and social justice in nursing because "it requires that we challenge our own and others' assumptions, engage in healthy debate and dialogue, and be caring and respectful of each other, all at the same time" (Hills et al., 2021, p. 168). In the *Awakening* phase, participants described engaging in critical dialogue on three levels: positionality, dialogue, and dismantling (Walter, 2017). *Positionality* involves comparing currently held beliefs, attitudes, and assumptions with alternative ones. In exploring these differences with others, participants were able to position themselves within larger societal hegemonic systems and began identifying sources of privilege, dominance, and oppression in their own lives. Budding nurse allies sought out those with a different lived experience than themselves and began a relational-dialogical process of self- and peer-teaching and learning to understand a different reality. This led participants to begin *dismantling* —identifying, breaking down, and ultimately discarding culturally conditioned assumptions that were seen as limiting the ability to live authentically in relationships with others with different life experiences.

Walker and Wellington (2022) posit that there are three tenets for successfully engaging in critical dialogue: acknowledging vulnerabilities, mutual trust, and radical openness. In practice, acknowledging vulnerabilities starts with educators recognizing and claiming their own vulnerabilities. Teaching about social justice, structural racism, diversity, and inequity is not for the faint of heart. As educators, we need to engage in not only the same self-reflection we require of students but also in our intellectual and emotional competencies to teach this content. Effective critical dialogue is built on mutual trust between educator-student and student-student dyads. Trust is not static in academic settings; it must be continuously built upon by ongoing actions that reinforce and recommit to it. Once this trust is established, participants are more likely to exhibit *radical openness:* the ability to expose their limitations and collaborate in challenging and strategizing ways to redress acts of social exclusion and injustice. Implementing these tenets of critical dialogue empowers those in collaborative caring relationships to stretch beyond the mere convergence of beliefs and ideas into a space of intentional, emancipatory actions.

REFLECTION-IN-ACTION

Reflection-in-action "attends to the development of mindfulness, of catching oneself *in the moment* in learning, processing, and critiquing oneself" (Hills et al., 2021, p. 611). As nurses navigate through the learning phases of *Engaging* and *Transforming,* the type of reflection they use changes from internal, quiet introspection to action-oriented, social, and political (Walter, 2017). Praxis embodies this type of reflection and was described by Friere (1970,

p. 51) as "reflection and action upon the world in order to transform it." Nurses begin to pay attention to the ways in which their beliefs, assumptions, and behaviors foster or inhibit their ability to collaborate with an individual or group in an emancipatory way. Stated another way, praxis fully integrated their critical reflections with specific actions toward transformative, emancipatory social goals. Reflection-in-action is a relational, experiential way of being in the world.

Kolb (1984) defines *experiential learning* as knowledge that is generated from reflection on personal experiences. Privilege-focused learning activities such as readings, formal written assignments, projects, service learning, and in-class activities allow students to think critically about the relationship between privilege and oppression. Williams and Melchiori (2013) found that when experiential learning is combined with structured reflection, students are more effective in identifying and challenging socially conferred privilege. What is interesting about their teaching methods is that many of these seemingly passive, receptive learning activities are not stand-alone. They are always performed in concert with face-to-face feedback and collaborative student reflection with faculty.

Their approach to service learning as a strategy for examining social class privilege is particularly resonant with ENP's focus on the deconstructive and reconstructive aspects of critical, reflective dialogue. First, they identify a common student assumption that service learning is a type of charity endeavor: "Students may think they are serving people who are unable to help themselves" (Williams & Melchiori, 2013, p. 176).

Viewing service learning as this type of helping activity diminishes the reciprocal power that can be possible between the students and community members (Wise & Case, 2013). Once this assumption is laid bare, faculty are able to help students deconstruct their service learning experiences and question the privileged discourses that reinforce oppression based on social class. Community partners and their constituents are positioned as co-educators and equal stakeholders in the students' service-learning experience. They are involved in "creating the service-learning assignments . . . and provide input on the students' final grades" (Williams & Melchiori, 2013, p. 176). They devote multiple class sessions to reflective dialogue with students during the service-learning experience. These ongoing, collaborative, dialogic reflections help students to reconstruct their experiences by acknowledging their social class privilege and consciously deciding to use it to ameliorate disadvantage rather than maintain oppressive structures and social interactions.

NURSES AS SOCIAL JUSTICE ALLIES: LIVING THE CARING SOCIAL MANDATE

Jean Watson, after acknowledging a deeply embedded yet subjugated social justice model of caring in nursing, once asked, "At a time when there are those of us who are longing to respond, can we find hope from within our midst?" (Watson, 2008, p. 59). ENP offers evidence that social justice engagement continues to emerge and evolve as a profoundly caring and transformational force within the profession of nursing. It is a process that can be integrated into the nursing curriculum through a relational emancipatory pedagogy grounded in Caring Science. Actions taken from an allied position are inherently relational, as educators and students collaborate to support, amplify, and advance others experiencing marginalization and foster understanding or awareness in people with privilege.

Nurses around the globe are reclaiming the profession's sacred social mission as they commit to the emancipatory practices defining their roles as social justice allies. They ascribe to a long-held "paradigm that recognizes societal factors as primary pathogenic forces in . . . major health problems" (Flaskerund & Nyamathi, 2002, p. 139). They courageously examine and dismantle their witting and unwitting roles in perpetuating systems of oppression that lead to social inequity and health disparities. They *stand-with,* rather than *stand-in* for the marginalized, stigmatized, and vulnerable who are often oppressively blamed for their own circumstances.

This recommitment to our social mandate is happening at a time in history when health disparities, inequities, and atrocities against human rights and the environment continue despite international mandates seeking to redress them. The lack of uniform progress in achieving the United Nations' (UN) 2001–2005 Millennium Development Goals (MDG) has been met with a renewed call to action in the 2015–2030 Sustainable Development Goals (SDG). The 17 SDGs and 169 benchmark targets build on the MDGs and seek to complete what was not achieved: environmental sustainability; food and water security; gender equality; the empowerment of women, girls, and vulnerable/marginalized populations worldwide; and a "resolve to free the human race from the tyranny of poverty" (UN, 2015, p. 1; UN, 2016). These are social, economic, and environmental expectations for all countries, not just resource-poor, developing nations. As nurses, we are called professionally and ethically to identify and redress social injustice locally and globally. We must expand our professional role as advocates to include the role of social justice ally:

> We are running out of time. Each new generation of nursing students we produce as novice nurses entering the health care arena without an analysis of power and structure . . . and the intersection of gender, class, and sexuality (among other domains of life) with health, perpetuates the strength of

ineffective systems and structures of healthcare delivery . . . and leads to increased constraints on individual agency and (global) sustainability. (Kagan, 2014, p. 323)

REFLECTIVE SUMMARY

This chapter highlighted the renewed imperative to educate nurses as equity advocates and social justice allies. It also showed the way forward, despite current political and legislative censorship of teaching this content. The key is to firmly ground our social justice, diversity, equity, and inclusion teachings within nursing science, nursing pedagogy, and nursing learning processes. Caring Science, relational emancipatory pedagogy, and ENP provide nursing education with a way forward at a time when the values we hold sacred in our profession are being censored. Allies engage in social justice from positions of privilege, and as we have discussed, privilege intersects with oppression to create complex social identities for each of us. It is fitting to close this chapter with a quote and an invitation to reflect on your social identity and the myriad ways it may prepare you to become an ally. The quote is by Adrienne Rich (1986, p. 199):

> When those who have the power to name and to socially construct reality choose not to see you or hear you, whether you are dark-skinned, old, disabled, female, or speak with a different accent or dialect than theirs, when someone with the authority of a teacher, say, describes the world and you are not in it, there is a moment of psychic disequilibrium, as if you looked into a mirror and saw nothing.

In closing, realize that educating nurses to become social justice allies will raise many more questions than it will answer. Integrating social justice into professional nursing practice requires concerted effort, ongoing reflection, and mindfulness of how privilege impacts your thoughts, beliefs, actions, and interactions that—knowingly and unknowingly—perpetuate the oppression of others. Becoming a social justice ally is a lifelong process of authentic collaboration of the "privileged" with the "other," toward the ultimate goal of emancipation for both.

LEARNING NARRATIVE

The primary goal of this chapter was to demonstrate the science, pedagogy, and learning processes educators could use in teaching nurses to become social justice allies. Raising awareness and deepening students' consciousness of social justice, diversity, and equity will inevitably engage ideas and experiences new to many students that may be difficult to understand. There will be rebuttals and objections to some of these ideas by educators and students alike. Many of these objections, however, are predictable. This learning activity asks you to critically, reflectively, and collaboratively wrestle with possible answers to the following rebuttals commonly offered by individuals who are in the early stages of learning about social justice (adapted from DiAngelo, 2017):

Citing exceptions to the rule

- "Barack Obama was elected President, so racism has ended in the US."

- "I have a friend who is Latina, and she is the CEO of the company."

- "My professor is openly gay, and he still got tenure."

Appealing to a universalized humanity

- "Why can't we all just be humans?"

- "We all bleed red."

- "It's focusing on our differences that divides us."

Insisting on immunity from cultural socialization

- "I was taught to see everybody the same."

- "My parents raised me to be colorblind."

- "My parents told me that it didn't matter that I was a girl. I could be anything I wanted."

- "That's not my experience."

Ignoring intersectionality

- "I'm oppressed as a lesbian, so I might be white, but I have no privilege."

- "I think the true oppression is poverty. If we address that, then the other oppressions will disappear."

Refusing to recognize structural and institutional power

- "Women are just as sexist as men."

- "People of color are racist too."

REFLECTIVE QUESTIONS

1. What are my individual and social group identities and how does that affect my current life experiences?

2. What are my own personal biases about others and how can I be prepared to monitor, address, and/or manage these biases? How can I make the unconscious things I have been socialized to believe more conscious so that I can wrestle with them?

3. How can I understand that being more aware of what I have been socialized to believe, no matter how embarrassing and shameful those beliefs are, is liberating for the oppressed and the privileged?

4. What does it mean to be a social justice ally? How can I work systemically to foster more justice and equity? How can I advocate for social justice, identifying ways to create change and promote social justice in our communities and the greater society?

5. How do systems of oppression function in society, and how is that system maintained and perpetuated? How does this play out on individual, institutional, and societal levels? How does this play out consciously/intentionally and unconsciously/unintentionally?

6. Reflect on your practice setting. Who is not being heard or represented? How does your reflection on your own privilege and oppression inform a new way of seeing this situation?

REFERENCES

American Association of Colleges of Nursing. (2021). *The essentials: Core competencies for professional nursing education.* https://www.aacnnursing.org/Portals/42/AcademicNursing/pdf/Essentials-2021.pdf

American Nurses Association. (2010a). *Code of ethics for nurses.* American Nurses Publishing.

American Nurses Association. (2010b). *Nursing: Scope and standards of practice.* American Nurses Publishing.

American Nurses Association. (2010c). *Nursing's social policy statement.* American Nurses Publishing.

American Nurses Association. (2022). *Journey of racial reconciliation: Our racial reckoning statement.* https://www.nursingworld.org/~4a00a2/globalassets/practiceandpolicy/workforce/racial-reckoning-statement.pdf

Bishop, A. (2015). *Becoming an ally: Breaking the cycle of oppression* (3rd ed.). Fernwood Publishing.

Buettner-Schmidt, K., & Lobo, M. L. (2011). Social justice: A concept analysis. *Journal of Advanced Nursing, 68*(4), 948–958. https://doi.org/10.1111/j.1365-2648.2011.05856.x

Burnett, A., Moorley, C., Grant, J., Kahin, M., Sagoo, R., Rivers, E., Deravin, L., & Darbyshire, P. (2020). Dismantling racism in education: In 2020, the year of the nurse & midwife, "it's time." *Nurse Education Today, 93,* 104532. https://doi.org/10.1016/j.nedt.2020.104532

Coretta, J., Murillo, C. L., Chew, A. Y., & Barksdale, D. J. (2021). Simulation in PhD programs to prepare nurse scientists as social justice advocates. *Nursing Education Perspectives, 42*(6), E60–E62. https://doi.org/10.1097/01.NEP.0000000000000835

DiAngelo, R. (2017). *Is everyone really equal? An introduction to key concepts in social justice education* (2nd ed.). Teachers College Press.

DiAngelo, R. (2018). *White fragility: Why it's so hard for white people to talk about racism.* Beacon Press.

Flaskerund, J. H., & Nyamathi, A. M. (2002). New paradigm for health disparities needed. *Nursing Research, 51*(3), 139–140. https://doi.org/10.1097/00006199-200205000-00001

Florida HB 7. (2022). *Individual freedom.* https://www.flsenate.gov/Session/Bill/2022/7

Ford, J. D., & Ford, L. W. (1995). The role of conversations is producing intentional change in organizations. *The Academy of Management Review, 20*(3), 541–570. https://doi.org/10.2307/258787

Freire, P. (1970). *Pedagogy of the oppressed.* Continuum International Publishing Group.

Hills, M., Watson, J., & Chantal, C. (2021). *Creating a caring science curriculum* (2nd ed.). Springer Publishing Company, LLC.

Iheduru-Anderson, K. C. (2020). The White/Black hierarchy institutionalizes White supremacy in nursing and nursing leadership in the United States. *Journal of Professional Nursing.* Advance online publication. https://doi.org/10.1016/j.profnurs.2020.05.005

International Council of Nurses. (2012). *The ICN code of ethics for nurses.* Author.

Iowa House File 802. (2021). *An Act providing for requirements related to racism or sexism trainings at, and diversity and inclusion efforts by, governmental agencies and entities, school districts, and public, postsecondary educational institutions.* Governor Approval Letter, June 8, 2021. https://www.legis.iowa.gov/legislation/BillBook?ba=HF%20802&ga=89

Kagan, P. (2014). Afterword. In P. Kagan, M. Smith, & P. Chinn (Eds.), *Philosophies and practices of emancipatory nursing: Social justice as praxis* (pp. 323–326). Routledge.

Kite, M. E., Case, K. A., & Williams, W. R. (2021). *Navigating difficult moments in teaching diversity and social justice.* American Psychological Association.

Kolb, D. A. (1984). *Experiential learning: Experience as the source of learning and development.* Prentice Hall.

Kolowich, S. (2018, Sept. 13). U. of Nebraska wondered whether conservative students were being silenced. Here's what it found out. *The Chronicle of Higher Education, 64*(5). https://www.chronicle.com/article/U-of-Nebraska-Wondered/244517

Lu, A., Elias, J., June, A. W., Charles, J. B., Marijolovic, K., Roberts-Grmela, J., & Surovell, E. (2023, May 15). DEI legislation tracker. *The Chronicle of Higher Education.* https://www.chronicle.com/article/here-are-the-states-where-lawmakers-are-seeking-to-ban-colleges-dei-efforts

National League for Nursing. (2019, April). *A vision for integration of the social determinants of health into nursing education curricula.* https://www.nln.org/docs/default-source/uploadedfiles/default-document-library/social-determinants-of-health.pdf?sfvrsn=aa66a50d_0

Nye, C. M., & Dillard-Wright, J. (2023). Queering the classroom: Teaching nurses against oppression. *Journal of Nursing Education, 62*(4), 193–198. https://doi.org/10.3928/01484834-20230208-02

Porter, B. (2019). *Forbidden knowledge: Things we should not know.* Academica Press.

Rich, A. (1986). Invisibility in academe. In A. Rich (Ed.), *Blood, bread, and poetry: Selected prose 1979–1985* (pp. 198–201). W. W. Norton & Company.

Rosa, W., & Horton-Deutsch, S. (2017). The importance of reflective practice in creating the world that we want. In W. Rosa (Ed.), *Global nursing global health: Our contributions to sustainable development*. Springer.

Suyemoto, K. L., Hochman, A. L., Donovan, R. A., & Roemer, L. (2021). Becoming and fostering allies and accomplices through authentic relationships: Choosing justice over comfort. *Research in Human Development, 18(1-2)*, 1–28. https://doi.org/10.1080/15427609.2020.1825905

UCLA School of Law Critical Race Studies Program. (2023). *CRT Forward*. https://crtforward.law.ucla.edu/

United Nations. (2015). *The Millennium Development Goals report 2015*. http://www.un.org/millenniumgoals/reports.shtml

United Nations. (2016). *Sustainable Development Goals: 17 goals to transform our world*. http://www.un.org/sustainabledevelopment/sustainable-development-goals

Walker, A., & Wellington, D. E. (2022). Using critical dialogue to drive feedback, reflection, and anti-racist action in education. *Voices from the Middle, 29*(4), 31–36.

Walls, J .K., & Hall, S. S. (2018). A focus group study of African American students' experiences with classroom discussions about race at a predominantly White university. *Teaching in Higher Education, 23*(1), 47–62. https://doi.org/10.1080/13562517.2017.1359158

Walter, R. R. (2017). Emancipatory nursing praxis: A theory of social justice in nursing. *Advances in Nursing Science, 40*(3), 225–243. https://doi.org.10.1097/ANS.0000000000000157

Watson, J. (2008). Social justice and human caring: A model of caring science as a hopeful paradigm for moral justice for humanity. *Creative Nursing, 24*(1), 1–8. https://doi.org/10.1891/1078-4535.14.2.54

Williams, W. R., & Melchiori, K. J. (2013). Class action: Using experiential learning to raise awareness of social class privilege. In K. A. Case (Ed.), *Deconstructing privilege: Teaching and learning as allies in the classroom* (pp. 169–187). Routledge.

Wise, T., & Case, K. A. (2013). Pedagogy for the privileged: Addressing inequality and injustice without shame or blame. In K. A. Case (Ed.), *Deconstructing privilege: Teaching and learning as allies in the classroom* (pp. 17–33). Routledge.

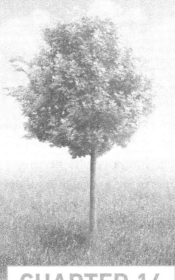

CHAPTER 14

REIMAGINING LEADERSHIP: A LEGACY PERSPECTIVE

–Daniel J. Pesut, PhD, RN, FAAN

LEARNING OBJECTIVES/SUBJECTIVES

- Define the concept of legacy leadership to inform personal and professional reflection about career contributions to nursing education, practice, research, and policy.

- Describe five practices of legacy leadership to gain insight into ways of leading, being, and doing to activate a legacy leadership plan.

- Appreciate the role of personal strengths, values, and contribution appraisals to gain insights about one's vision, mission, and legacy.

- Determine a legacy through reflection-in and -on legacy leadership principles and practices.

- Reimagine one's professional nursing journey to enact legacy leadership principles and practices.

OVERVIEW: A PERSONAL REFLECTION

The purpose of this chapter is to describe and discuss principles and practices of legacy leadership and to invite personal and professional reflection on one's legacy contributions to nursing education, practice, research, and policy. Reflecting on one's purpose, values, and contributions to the profession supports intentions and guides action into the future. Here, the principles of legacy leadership in the context of reflective practice and Caritas processes, values, best practices associated with legacy leadership, and strategies for reimagining leadership with legacy perspective in mind are described. This chapter also covers the importance of self-knowledge in regard to one's personal strengths, values, and contributions related to legacy as well as exercises and learning activities to discern personal strengths, values, and contributions.

Throughout my professional nursing career, I have been committed to advancing the profession of nursing through creativity, innovation, and the development of knowledge, skills, and abilities related to self-regulation, creative thinking, clinical reasoning, leadership development, and futures thinking (Pesut, 2016a, 2016b, 2019a, 2019b). Most of my career was devoted to teaching and leadership development in nursing (Allison-Napolitano & Pesut, 2015). To be honest, while engaged in the practice of nursing I did not consciously think about legacy mapping or intentionally set out to create a legacy. Now, after 48 years in nursing, I am retired and have had the opportunity to reflect on my career and realize the impact and influence I had through time. Such reflection has contributed to my personal and professional wisdom. I also have come to appreciate the value of my own and others' sense-making regarding a leadership legacy perspective (Linderman, 2021; Linderman et al., 2015; Pesut, 2001, 2014, 2016b, 2019b, 2022; Pesut & Thompson, 2018). Such sense-making and knowledge transfer are worthwhile, and I hope that the thoughts and ideas presented here will positively influence the reader's ability to reimagine leadership with a legacy perspective. Perhaps if I had written a Sage Letter (FutureMe, n.d.) to my younger self my leadership insights and learnings would have been more intentional.

THEORETICAL FRAMEWORKS TO SUPPORT LEGACY LEADERSHIP REFLECTION

These three leadership theories and caring practices we discuss in the following section help reimagine leadership with a legacy perspective.

CASTLE PRINCIPLES

Leadership expert Lance Secretan (2010), author of the book *The Spark, the Flame, and the Torch,* suggests the essence of leadership is mastery, chemistry, and delivery. *Mastery* involves learning what one must do well to accomplish objectives. *Chemistry* involves empathy to build relationships and inspire others to achieve goals. *Delivery* consists of deep listening and service in meeting people's needs.

Secretan also conceived the CASTLE principles (2010):

- Courage: Reaching beyond the boundaries of our existing limitations, fears, and beliefs.

- Authenticity: Being genuine, transparent, and aligned with our inner voice in all aspects of life.

- Service: Willing, and actively supporting, the good of the other.

- Truthfulness: Being honest and transparent in all thoughts, words, and actions.

- Love: Relating to others by touching their hearts in ways that add to who we both are as people.

- Effectiveness: Achieving desired outcomes successfully.

Secretan also challenges people to develop a Why-Be-Do statement. He prompts people to become clear about their destiny and clarify what is important to them (their Why), who they will Be, and what they will Do in terms of their destiny, calling, and legacy.

REFLECTIVE LEADER ATTRIBUTES

Reflective practice scholar Christopher Johns defines leadership as mindful, insightful caring, ever vigilant of its authenticity in being of service to others within a community of practice that lifts everyone to higher levels of morality and growth, focused towards achieving shared goals and personal aspiration (Johns, 2016). John's definition of leadership calls attention to the importance of attributes that contribute to developing as a powerful reflective leader.

According to Johns (2000), the powerful, reflective self is born as one develops these attributes:

- **Embrace commitment:** A belief in oneself and in the value of practice. Requires openness, curiosity, and a willingness to challenge norms and the status quo.

- **Acknowledge contradiction:** Requires negotiation of the tensions that exist between the ideals and the realities of practice.

- **Manage conflict:** Manages tensions that exist between competing commitments and uses that tension and energy to create new options.

- **Accept challenge and support:** Conflict can be helpful if challenges are linked with support. Acknowledging challenges and negotiating support are key leadership skills.

- **Engage in catharsis:** Works through negative feelings.

- **Nurture creativity:** Holds the tension of contradictions and opposites long enough for something new to emerge from the tension.

- **Foster connection:** Links new insights with past learning, brings past learning to new situations, and connects the dots associated with pattern recognition and intuition.

- **Practice caring:** The energy that fuels desirable practice as an everyday reality.

- **Strive for congruence:** The alignment of thoughts, feelings, and actions is facilitated through reflective practice.

- **Construct personal knowing:** Spin and weave the threads of personal knowledge and experience with theory to construct knowledge that builds nursing intelligence, scholarship, and a caring consciousness.

MCDOWELL-WILLIAMS CARING LEADERSHIP MODEL

Williams and colleagues (2011) developed a model of leadership integrating Watson's (2008) caring theory and Kouzes and Posner's (2007) leadership theory by integrating the five practices of exemplary leadership (model the way, inspire a shared vision, challenge the process, enable others to act, and encourage the heart) with Watson's 10 Caritas Processes (see Chapter 1). These theories complement each other and provide an effective basis for shared governance in both academic and clinical facilities, and support the use of reflective practice as an essential element of leadership as a caring process.

The McDowell-Williams Caring Leadership Model (Williams et al., 2011) advises leaders to adopt the following core values:

- Lead with kindness

- Lead with compassion

- Lead with equality

- Generate hope
- Generate faith
- Co-create
- Actively innovate
- Share insights
- Be reflective
- Appreciate the value of wisdom
- Create a protected space
- Practice mutual respect
- Create caring environments
- Offer help and trust
- Attend to issues of self-care

PRINCIPLES AND PRACTICES OF LEGACY LEADERSHIP

Leadership scholars James Kouzes and Barry Posner note, "…legacies are not the result of wishful thinking. They are the results of determined doing. The legacy you leave is the life you lead. We live our lives daily. We leave our legacy daily. The people you see, the decisions you make, and the actions you take—they are what tell your story" (Kouzes & Posner, 2006, p. 180). Dr. Pamela Hinds and colleagues (2015) have proposed legacy mapping to plan for and document meaningful work in nursing. Legacy mapping begins with two questions:

- What do you want to improve in nursing through your efforts?
- What would you like to be best known for?

Hinds and her colleagues have developed a systematic way to create a career legacy map with intention and purpose. *Legacy planning* is an interactive process that integrates aspects of career goal planning, attends to issues of meaning and purpose in terms of self and others, and is a shared experience between mentors and mentees as well as between leaders and followers. Legacies can be planned and made explicit with a legacy map. O'Connor (2019) has developed a career legacy toolkit to help advanced practice nurses understand the context, components, and elements of a career trajectory. Brooks and colleagues (2004) as well as Shane Yount (2007) provide strategies and questions to support reflection about creating and maintaining a leadership legacy.

As executive coaches, Dr. Jeannine Sandstrom and Dr. Lee Smith (2017b) note, "Legacy in leadership is not about leaving something behind. It is about influencing others enough to cause change, a shift from unconsciously doing leadership to consciously being a leader and leaving your legacy now" (Sandstrom & Smith, 2017b, p. 21). Legacy leadership is a philosophy, a model, and a proven process for bringing out individual best, developing other leaders in an organization, establishing organizational leadership culture, and positively impacting the bottom line.

Sandstrom and Smith (2001, 2008) articulate the definitions, values, and best practices and principles that incorporate and accomplish the rewards of legacy leadership. Legacy is created by leaders who aspire to:

- Develop people with maximization of people's leadership talents, abilities, and characteristics in mind.

- Serve others first, then themselves.

- Hold vision and values.

- Create trust, innovation, and creativity.

- Influence inspiration.

- Champion differences and build community.

- Calibrate organizational dynamics with responsibility and accountability in mind.

These practices require core competencies and specific ways of being (be-attitudes) that result in simple, sophisticated, elegant, and successful approaches to leadership. The philosophy and model are derived from concepts, principles, and practices of transformational and servant leadership, leader-member exchange theory, path-goal theory, and systems theory (Sandstrom & Smith, 2008). One can easily see the legacy leadership model resonates and reflects Caritas Processes and is built on foundations of reflective practice and attention to personal work related to clarification of one's strengths, values, and contributions to a greater good.

THE BE-ATTITUDES OF LEGACY LEADERSHIP

Every legacy practice involves a set of core competencies, best practices, and specific ways of being and doing. Legacy leadership requires living today with the behaviors, competencies, and attitudes of a great leader who will be remembered tomorrow. In addition to these principles, Sandstrom and Smith (2001) outline what they call the *be-attitudes* of legacy leadership. Check out the essential concepts in the Legacy Leadership Framework at the Coachworks website (https://coachworks.com/legacyleadership/pdfs/LL_At-A-Glance_0508.pdf). Table 14.1 outlines several of the conditions and success factors that support legacy leadership.

TABLE 14.1 CONDITIONS AND SUCCESS FACTORS OF LEGACY LEADERSHIP

LEADERSHIP TRAIT	POSITIVE TRAITS TO SUPPORT SUCCESS	NEGATIVE ATTRIBUTES THAT PREVENT SUCCESS
Vision and Values	• Clear compelling vision • Values statement • Business objectives • Strategic design • Road map and milestones • Communication throughout the company • Ways to measure all	• Lack of commitment and modeling of values • Missing communication • Lack of measurements • Focus on short-term activity vs. long-term commitment
Collaboration and Innovation	• Creative environment • Commitment to innovation • Processes for collaboration • High levels of trust • Process for capturing outcome	• Mindset for change avoidance • Lack of trust • Lack of inspiration by leader • Lack of methods for discovery • Fear of creative tension
Influence and Inspiration	• Positively inspired leaders • Abilities and processes to engage others from strengths • Personal connections • Stories that inspire	• Focus on numbers not people • Not knowing what influences • Fear or mistrust • Previous negative history with the influencer
Difference and Community	• Processes for identifying strengths and styles • Comfort with differing perspectives • Practice inclusion versus exclusion	• Belief systems and biases • Stereotyping • Rubber stamp mentality • Avoidance of vulnerability • "Us against them" thinking

continues

TABLE 14.1 CONDITIONS AND SUCCESS FACTORS OF LEGACY LEADERSHIP (CONT.)		
LEADERSHIP TRAIT	POSITIVE TRAITS TO SUPPORT SUCCESS	NEGATIVE ATTRIBUTES THAT PREVENT SUCCESS
Responsibility and Accountability	• Calibration processes versus discipline • Measurements and rewards • Measurements against road maps and milestones	• Leader not holding self or others accountable • "Either/or" thinking • Qualifiers that diminish • Exclusion of customer in the measurement mix

Adapted from Sandstrom & Smith, 2017b

The following sections will help you take a moment to reflect on these five be-attitudes of legacy leadership.

HOLDS VISION AND VALUES

The first be-attitude of legacy leadership is that a legacy leader is a holder of vision and values. This involves direction and commitment. This means the leader is a values-driven, whole systems thinker who is other-oriented and a guardian. The leader effectively communicates and sustains processes to achieve the vision and upholds the values throughout the enterprise area of responsibility. The leader believes in the value of developing others. Such a leader has a well-defined vision and goals and a set of guiding principles to elicit a reputation for excellence and pride.

CREATES COLLABORATION AND INNOVATION

The second be-attitude of legacy leadership is about creating collaboration and innovation. This supports a positive environment of working relationships. A legacy leader is a trust builder, an intuitive listener, possibility minded, change-neutral, and mentally agile. They are aware of when change needs to occur and when it does not. They are masterful at facilitating creative and innovative thinking, conversation, and dialogue. This be-attitude requires shifts from judgment to curiosity, from suspicion to trust, from ordinary to extraordinary, from a focus on the past to a focus on the future, and from fear of change to embracing the new.

INSPIRES AND INFLUENCES

The third be-attitude of legacy leadership is about inspiration and influence. This requires connecting with individuals and attention to relationships, and a conscious understanding of one's impact and influence. Attention to mentoring and inspiring self and others is vital to this be-attitude. The essence of this practice is a focus on humility and a focus on people and positive intentions to build the success of the organization with the greater good in mind.

ADVOCATES DIFFERENCES AND COMMUNITY

The fourth be-attitude requires one to be an advocator of differences and community. This involves distinction and inclusion, being community-minded, and being a champion who can unite and include people while discerning and appreciating the issues at hand, ever mindful of the importance of dialogue and the spirit of the community aspirations toward a greater good.

CALIBRATES RESPONSIBILITIES AND ACCOUNTABILITY

The fifth be-attitude of a legacy leader is a calibrator of responsibility and accountability. This relates to execution and performance. Legacy leaders are results-oriented, vigilant, and committed to achieving organizational goals and outcomes. They are attuned to an organization's external and internal environments, constantly scanning trends and recalibrating action considering ongoing developments. They constantly focus on what is working and not working and strive to improve people, processes, and outcomes in service of goal achievement. These be-attitudes presuppose that one is clear about one's strengths, values, and contributions.

CREATING LEGACY INSIGHTS THROUGH STRENGTHS, VALUES, AND CONTRIBUTIONS APPRAISALS

Leadership experts Robert and Shawn Quinn (2015) believe "lift" is one of leaders' fundamental contributions to organizations. Lift is accomplished based on the following reflective questions:

- What results do I want to create?

- What would my story be if I were living the values I expect of others?

- How do others feel about this situation?

- What are three strategies I could use to accomplish my purpose?

The key to success in answering these questions is knowing your strengths, values, and contributions. Legacy insights are gained with attention to personal and professional appraisals that help identify and strategically make use of your strengths, values, and contributions in creating a leadership legacy.

As a coach and educator, I encourage people to learn about and know their top five signature strengths. Rath and Conchie (2008) have fine-tuned a strengths assessment that helps people discern their strengths and relate the strengths they possess to the needs followers have; namely, trust, compassion, hope, and stability. Knowing your strengths helps to clarify your personal vision and mission. Such knowledge is also useful in terms of understanding how to best work with people to build trust, compassion, stability, and hope. In addition to strengths, another important source of information that helps clarify your gifts is a values inventory.

The Values in Action (VIA) Survey from the VIA Institute on character assesses 24 character strengths that provide insight and guidance to individuals interested in knowing more about themselves and what they value (https://www.viacharacter.org/survey/account/Register). The strengths are grouped by the virtue categories of wisdom, courage, humility, justice, temperance, and transcendence. Knowledge of character strengths stimulates legacy leadership insight. Taking strengths, values and character assessments helps one clarify talents, gifts, and contributions they can make in the world. As one comes to appreciate the nuances of strengths and character, one can be clearer about the values, beliefs, talents, skills, and contributions they bring to an organization or project. Tom Rath (2020) has developed an assessment that identifies ones' contributions (https://contribify.com/about), which he believes are the answer to life's greatest question: What is my purpose? He outlines three domains of contribution: create, relate, and operate. Contributions related to initiating, challenging, teaching, and visioning are within the creative domain. The related domain includes contributions of connecting, energizing, perceiving, and influencing. Within the operating domain, the contributions and talents of organizing, achieving, adapting, and scaling are major.

Reflection to understand your contributions, values, and strengths helps you activate legacy principles and practices and enact legacy leadership with the realization that legacy leadership is not about leaving something behind; it is about influencing others enough to cause change, a shift from unconsciously doing leadership to consciously being a leader and living a legacy in the now (Sandstrom & Smith, 2017b). Taking the time to write yourself a Sage Letter (FutureMe, n.d.) may prompt you to reimagine leadership with a legacy perspective in mind.

APPLICATION FOR PERSONAL AND PROFESSIONAL PRACTICE

Determine your strengths, values, and contributions:

- Complete the strengths finders survey (Rath & Conchie, 2008): https://store.gallup.com/p/en-us/10369/strengths-based-leadership

- Complete the VIA's Character Strengths Survey: https://www.viacharacter.org/survey/account/Register. See how your top values dovetail and support your leadership strengths. (VIA Institute on Character, n.d.)

- Complete the contribify profile (Rath, 2020): https://contribify.com/book/lifes-great-question

- Invest in and study the legacy leadership application workbook authored by Sandstrom, J., & Smith, L. (2017a).

- Write yourself a Sage Letter. Imagine that you are 70 years old looking back on your career. Write a letter to your younger self and explain the lessons you learned, the reputation you developed and the legacy that you created during your working years. Or consider writing a letter to the future self you aspire to become. Explore this resource: http://www.futureme.org.

REFLECTIVE SUMMARY

The purpose of this chapter was to describe and discuss principles and practices of legacy leadership and to invite personal and professional reflection on one's legacy influence in nursing education, practice, research, and policy. Principles of legacy leadership in the context of reflective practice and Caritas processes were described and discussed. The importance of self-knowledge about one's personal strengths, values, and contributions related to legacy were highlighted. Exercises, tools, and assessment activities to discern personal strengths, values, and contributions were shared. Questions to prompt reflection about one's leadership legacy were presented. The author shared a personal learning narrative and resources that summarize his reflections about his leadership legacy in nursing.

LEARNING NARRATIVE

I had the opportunity to contribute a chapter to a book edited by Dr. Billy Rosa (2016), *Nurses as Leaders: Evolutionary Visions of Nursing Leadership.* The book is an excellent resource full of inspiration and stories of many nursing leaders and their contributions through time. Each chapter is a learning narrative. The title of my chapter was "Transformed and In Service: Creating the Future Through Renewal." In this chapter, I share my professional journey and path to becoming a nurse. I also share some legacy contributions related to my time as President of the Honor Society of Nursing, Sigma Theta Tau International (2003–2005). My presidential call to action was "Create the Future Through Renewal" (Pesut, 2004). I challenged Sigma members to consider the most meaningful activities that support personal and professional renewal. One of several outcomes I identified for the 2003–2005 biennium was the creation of a resource paper on reflective practice in nursing (Freshwater et al., 2005). The foreword I wrote to that report details my logic about the importance of reflective practice and personal and professional renewal. I also believe it crystalizes my leadership legacy intentions both at the time, and today. I wrote:

> Personally, and professionally, I believe reflection is a means of renewal. My logic goes something like this: As self is renewed, commitments to service come forward more easily. Renewed commitments to service require attention to mindfulness and reflective practice. Mindful reflective practice begets questions that support inquiry. Such inquiry guides knowledge work and evidence-based care giving. Caregiving supports society as knowledge, values, and service intersect. Knowledgeable people and especially knowledgeable nurses provide care that society needs. Creating a caring society is the spirit work of nursing. Creating a caring society starts with nurses caring for themselves and becoming, through reflection, more conscious and intentional in their being, thinking, feeling, doing, and acting. Reflection is a form of "inner work" that results in the energy for engaging in "outer service." Reflection in-and-on action supports meaning-making and purpose management in one's professional life. The nursing scholars who have participated in the development of this resource paper are to be commended. They have devoted many long hours to the creation of this document. They have role modeled for all of us the creation and development of a learning community dedicated to enhancing knowledge, learning, and service. They created a global transcendent team and have demonstrated the value and benefits of global cooperation around a very important professional developmental concept and practice for nurses. I admire and appreciate the

work and effort this team has put forth and am pleased to introduce their work to the members of the honor society and nurses throughout the world. There are many stimulating and provocative ideas in this resource paper. If reflective practice is new to you, I hope that the ideas and resources you discover will stimulate your curiosity and enable you to see your work in nursing through new ways. If reflective practice is already familiar to you, I hope that you support and encourage others to experiment with the notions, information, and resources gathered in this paper. As we collectively reflect on the professional purpose of nursing, I am certain the spirit of nursing will be renewed. As members of the Honor Society of Nursing, Sigma Theta Tau International, each of us has a responsibility to enact the virtues of love, honor, and courage that are part of our heritage. As we develop our capacity and commitment for reflection, we will affirm that spirit of nursing and make nursing-care differences in the lives of people for whom we care.

I invite readers to access the report (freely available in the Sigma Repository at https://www.sigmarepository.org/) and appreciate the legacy leadership it represents 18 years later. In fact, the people who worked on that task force have created a program of scholarship and their own legacies related to reflective practice in the nursing profession (Freshwater et al., 2009; Horton-Deutsch & Sherwood, 2017; Sherwood & Horton-Deutsch, 2015; Wei & Horton-Deutsch, 2022). The knowledge work and programs of scholarship about reflective practice initiated in 2005 continue today and are an example of leadership reimagined with a legacy perspective in mind.

REFLECTIVE QUESTIONS

1. How do I enact the legacy leadership principles and practices in my work?

2. How do my strengths, values, and contributions influence my thinking about legacy leadership?

3. What lessons am I teaching in each interaction I have?

4. What stories will people share about me in the future?

5. What will others learn from those stories?

6. What is more important to me, the results I achieve or how I achieve them?

7. Have I made the impact I want in my work?

8. What will colleagues remember about me as someone who made a difference in their lives?

9. How have I put a system in place that enables people to feel connected and a sense of belonging, commitment, and dedication to their work accordingly?

REFERENCES

Allison-Napolitano, E., & Pesut, D. J. (2015). *Bounce forward: The extraordinary resilience of nurse leadership.* American Nurses Association.

Brooks, M., Stark, J., & Caverhill, S. (2004). *Your leadership legacy: The difference you make in people's lives.* Berrett-Koehler.

Freshwater, D., Horton-Deutsch, S., Sherwood, G. D., & Taylor, B. J. (2005). *The scholarship of reflective practice.* https://sigma.nursingrepository.org/handle/10755/621207

Freshwater, D., Taylor, B., & Sherwood, G. (2009). International textbook of reflective practice in nursing. *Neonatal Network, 28*(3), 31–32.

FutureMe. (n.d.). *Write a letter to your future self.* https://www.futureme.org/

Hinds, P. S., Britton, D. R., Coleman, L., Engh, E., Humbel, T. K., Keller, S., Kelly, K. P., Menard, J., Lee, M. A., Roberts-Turner, R., & Walczak, D. (2015). Creating a career legacy map to help assure meaningful work in nursing. *Nursing Outlook, 63*(2), 211–218. https://doi.org/10.1016/j.outlook.2014.08.002

Horton-Deutsch, S., & Sherwood, G. D. (2017). *Reflective practice: Transforming education and improving outcomes* (2nd ed.). Sigma Theta Tau International.

Johns, C. (2000). *Becoming a reflective practitioner.* Blackwell Science.

Johns, C. (2016). *Mindful leadership: A guide for the health care professions.* Palgrave Macmillan.

Kouzes, J., & Posner, B. (2006). *A leader's legacy.* Jossey-Bass. https://www.legacyleadership.com/model.html

Kouzes, J. M., & Posner, B. Z. (2007). *The leadership challenge* (4th ed.). Jossey Bass.

Linderman, A. (2021). *The Katharine J. Densford International Center for Nursing Leadership: A tribute to the three directors.* University of Minnesota School of Nursing. University of Minnesota Digital Conservancy. https://hdl.handle.net/11299/226602

Linderman, A., Pesut, D., & Disch, J. (2015). Sense making and knowledge transfer: Capturing the knowledge and wisdom of nursing leaders. *Journal of Professional Nursing, 31*(4), 290–297. https://doi.org/10.1016/j.profnurs.2015.02.004

O'Connor, L. (2019). Career legacy cartography portfolio for advanced practice nursing. In L. O' Connor (Ed.), *The nature of scholarship, a career legacy map and advanced practice* (pp. 93–138). Springer. https://doi.org/10.1007/978-3-319-91695-8_6

Pesut, D. J. (2001). Healing into the future: Recreating the profession of nursing through inner work. In N. Chaska (Ed.), *The nursing profession: Tomorrow and beyond* (pp. 853–865). Sage Publications, Inc.

Pesut, D. J. (2004). Create the future through renewal. *Reflections on Nursing Leadership, 30*(1), 24–25, 56.

Pesut, D. J. (2014). Avoiding derailment: Leadership strategies for identity, reputation, and legacy management. In J. Daly, S. Speedy, & D. Jackson (Eds.), *Leadership & nursing contemporary perspectives* (2nd ed., pp. 251–261). Elsevier.

Pesut, D. J. (2016a). Innovation leadership. In S. Ketefian (Ed.), *Shaping nursing science and improving health, the Michigan legacy* (pp. 245–250). University of Michigan Press. http://dx.doi.org/10.3998/mpub.9497632

Pesut, D. J. (2016b). Transformed and in service: Creating the future through renewal. In W. Rosa (Ed.), *Nurses as leaders: Evolutionary visions of leadership* (pp. 165–178). Springer.

Pesut, D. J. (2019a). Anticipating disruptive innovations with foresight leadership. *Nursing Administration Quarterly, 43*(3), 196–204. https://doi.org/10.1097/NAQ.0000000000000349

Pesut, D. J. (2019b). *Nursing foresight leadership.* University of Minnesota School of Nursing Katharine J Densford International Center for Nursing Leadership. University of Minnesota Digital Conservancy. https://hdl.handle.net/11299/201644

Pesut, D. J. (2022). Wisdom leadership: A developmental journey. In H. Wei & S. Horton-Deutsch, *Visionary leadership in healthcare* (pp. 443–461). Sigma Theta Tau International.

Pesut, D., & Thompson, S. A. (2018). Nursing leadership in academic nursing: The wisdom of development and the development of wisdom. *Journal of Professional Nursing, 34*(2), 122–127.

Quinn, R. W., & Quinn, R. S. (2015). *Lift: the fundamental state of leadership.* Berrett-Koehler Publishers.

Rath, T. (2020). *Life's great question: Discover how you contribute to the world.* Tom Rath.

Rath, T., & Conchie, B. (2008). *Strengths based leadership.* Gallup Press.

Rosa, W. (Ed.). (2016). *Nurses as leaders: Evolutionary visions of leadership.* Springer Publishing Company.

Sandstrom, J., & Smith, L. (2001). *Legacy leadership at a glance.* https://coachworks.com/legacyleadership/pdfs/LL_At-A-Glance_0508.pdf

Sandstrom, J., & Smith, L. (2008). *Legacy leadership.* Coachworks Press.

Sandstrom, J., & Smith, L. (2017a). *Legacy leadership: The application workbook.* Coachworks Press.

Sandstrom, J., & Smith, L. (2017b). *Legacy leadership: The leaders guide to lasting greatness* (2nd ed.). Coachworks Press.

Secretan, L. (2010). *The spark, the flame, and the torch.* The Secretan Center, Inc.

Sherwood, G., & Horton-Deutsch, S. (2015). *Reflective organizations: On the front lines of QSEN & reflective practice implementation.* Sigma Theta Tau International.

VIA Institute on Character. (n.d.). *About the VIA Institute on Character.* https://www.viacharacter.org/about

Watson, J. (n.d.). *10 Caritas Processes.* Watson Caring Science Institute. https://www.watsoncaringscience.org/jean-bio/caring-science-theory/10-caritas-processes/

Watson, J. (2008). *Philosophy and science of caring* (Revised new ed.). University of Colorado Press.

Wei, H., & Horton-Deutsch, S. (2022). *Visionary leadership in healthcare.* Sigma Theta Tau International.

Williams, R. L., McDowell, J. B., & Kautz, D. D. (2011). A caring leadership model for nursing's future. *International Journal for Human Caring, 15*(1), 31–35. https://doi.org/10.20467/1091-5710.15.1.31

Yount, S. (2007). *Leaving your leadership legacy: Creating a timeless and enduring culture of clarity, connectivity, and consistency.* OakleePress.

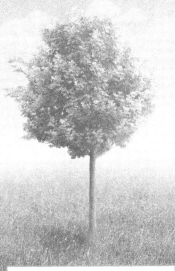

CHAPTER 15

REFLECTIVE PRACTICE, UNITARY CARING SCIENCE, AND WISDOM: THE HEART OF THE CAPACITY TO GROW

–*Sara Horton-Deutsch, PhD, RN, FAAN, ANEF, SGAHN*
Gisela van Rensburg, DLitt et Phil, RN, RM, RPN, RCN, RNE, RNA, ROrthN, FANSA

LEARNING OBJECTIVES/SUBJECTIVES

- Describe reflective practice and Caring Science's underlying ethical, moral, and philosophical worldviews.

- Appreciate the essential nature of reflection for personal and professional growth.

- Value individual and relational practices in reflection.

- Explore ways to connect more deeply and wisely with others.

- Unite personal, relational (professional), and organizational ways of understanding our way of being, doing, and becoming in the world.

"You have to act as if it were possible to transform the world radically. However, you must do it all the time."

–Angela Y. Davis

OVERVIEW

This final chapter intends to open a heart space for learners to meet their unique gifts, talents, and wisdom. It will not provide answers but practices, resources, and notes on life to inspire an inner wisdom journey that radiates into relations with others and throughout organizations. Grounded in Unitary Caring Science, it invites learners to tap into the most profound and wisest part of themselves.

SUPPORTING THEORETICAL FRAMEWORKS AND EVIDENCE

Like other chapters, Unitary Caring Science forms the foundation for this narrative. A theory that invites and encourages a deeply introspective human experience, an opportunity to wonder, to open to a spiritual phenomenon that sages worldwide have spoken to for thousands of years. Grounded in a philosophical-ethical, epistemological-methodological context for praxis and healthcare policy, Unitary Caring Science offers a worldview rooted in caring/love (Caritas) and values (Veritas; Watson, 2018, 2021).

Through this lens, the discipline of nursing holds its unique, timeless values, heritage, traditions, and knowledge development and translation toward sustaining health and humanity. The discipline informs and matures professional nursing practice; however, when the profession loses sight of its disciplinary context, it risks losing its identity and way amid external forces such as institutional demands. According to Watson (2018), the discipline of nursing holds the following:

- An ontology of the whole person, mind-body-spirit

- A philosophical orientation toward an ethical covenant with humanity to sustain caring, healing, and health for all

- The orientation to knowledge development, including theories and what counts as knowledge beyond conventional medical epistemologies

- Nursing's research traditions, diverse and evolving approaches to knowledge development

- Expanded, creative, and innovative methodologies and methods consistent with human illness experiences and caring-healing health

- Grand, middle-range, and situation-specific theories to provide an inclusive evolved worldview. Through this lens, social-moral justice, whole person/system processes and outcomes, human caring, and ecological caring are one. Vitally, this reflects a distinctive disciplinary position.

So, in the simplest of terms, what does this mean?

- As nurses, we see and care for the whole person. We recognize that we are all connected, and when something happens to one of us, there is a rippling effect affecting all.

- Nurses have an ethical pledge and commitment to care for all human beings despite race, ethnicity, gender identity, religious preference, or socio-economic status.

- We embrace an expanded worldview of what counts as knowledge, comprising *empirics* (the science of nursing) and *esthetics* (the art of nursing); personal knowledge in nursing; ethics-moral knowledge in nursing (Carper, 1978); and the more recently added *emancipatory knowing* (Chinn & Kramer, 2018), where we critically examine social, political, and institutional structures to uncover injustices and inequities and ask critical questions to address them.

- We remain open to innovative and evolving ideas to improve health, wholeness, and humanity.

- By holding this expansive worldview, the discipline of nursing continues to develop theories and knowledge that contribute distinctively to human and planetary health and well-being.

Notably, the Unitary Caring Science worldview connects the theorist to the practitioner, where knowledge supports practical in-practice solution-seeking and growth. Throughout this text, numerous approaches to reflection have been introduced where nurses generate new knowledge based on their experiences in practice following various reflective practice frameworks and models from Dewey (1938) to Schön (2016). These models provide a framework for the nurse to bridge the education-to-practice gap, where nurses modify and generate new knowledge based on their experiences in practice.

Reflective practice, viewed through the perspective of Unitary Caring Science, extends these approaches, inviting the development and refinement of an intuitive, less structured system built on the cultivation of values, consciousness, and informed moral knowledge and skills to engage in doing and being as a nurse that services humankind. To enter practice through this theoretical lens requires a reflective stance, engaging in ever-evolving consciousness of what it means to be a nurse, developed through the creative use of Caring Science micropractices that are informed by the 10 Caritas Processes.

Practice furthermore requires a professional orientation that follows its professional norms (rules of behavior) and values (desired behavior) within an ethical-legal framework. This orientation refers to the professional identity consisting of certain attributes, which include a caring approach, the art and intuition that nurses should possess. Historically, altruism, as the moral foundation of care, was the primary characteristic of the nursing philosophy, while human dignity was a core nursing value (Fagermoen, 1997; Nahra, 2020). The profession gradually evolved into a self-sacrificing, devotional, and altruistic profession.

Recently, the image of nursing has become more complex with more pressure from patients, the profession itself, and the public. The Unitary Caring Science worldview, through its notion that knowledge supports practical in-practice solution-seeking and growth, places more emphasis on intuition, cultivation of values, consciousness, and informed moral knowledge and skills. Therefore, a sound professional nursing identity that aligns with its norms and values within an ethical-legal and clinical framework is essential. Such an identity that is characterized by a "set of attributes, beliefs, values, motives, morals, ideals and experiences by which nurses define themselves in their professional lives" (Moola, 2017, p. 1), forms their social identity, sense of belonging, and own self-conception (Browne et al., 2018; Tsakissiris, 2015). Professional identity is the nurse's concept of nursing and functioning as a nurse (Goodolf & Godfrey, 2020). Ontologically, the fundamental nature of the nursing identity manifests in practice.

Over the past 35 years, nursing education has increased its emphasis on knowledge, skills, and technological competencies at the expense of ontological competencies and caring literacy skills grounded and rooted within the discipline and profession. Without this foundation, nurses often become dispirited and worn down from caring for others at the expense of themselves. In addition, nurses' professional identity is closely interwoven with discipline skills, and knowledge and becomes the moral compass, reflecting an image of ethical behavior guiding quality care. Reflective practice and Unitary Caring Science necessitate nurses to slow down and attend to self-caring and practices that guide their evolution and consciousness for their lives and work in the world (Watson, 2018).

REFLECTIVE PRACTICE AND UNITARY CARING SCIENCE

Reflection has been explored since ancient times by Western and Eastern philosophers like Buddha, Plato, and Lao-Tzu. These perspectives all have in common the willingness to learn more about one's fundamental nature, essence, and purpose. As a practice, self-reflection invites inquiry into the human condition and the philosophical consideration of awareness, consciousness, and intellectual growth.

Vitally, Unitary Caring Science's values and principles are rejuvenated through an ongoing relationship with reflection and reflective practice. In turn, reflecting through the lens of Unitary Caring Science brings one into communion with the heart and the daily practices of living and caring. In this light, reflection is viewed as a mode of caring and connecting with the flow of intention. The commitment of practitioners who reflect through this lens supports a society furthered by the emergence of consciousness, embodied by ethical gravity that grounds the human spirit in awareness of being and becoming. Reflective practice is the art of being with another, listening, noticing, assimilating, and integrating that which serves and letting go of that which does not. As a dynamic process of mental-emotional-spiritual growth, it provides the space and profoundly knows the impediments that prevent self and systems from reaching a desired state of balance. As reflecting through the lens of Unitary Caring Science expands, it simultaneously expands the opportunity for wisdom (Horton-Deutsch & Rosa, 2019).

REFLECTIVE PRACTICE, CARING SCIENCE, AND WISDOM

How do we go about encouraging the heart to grow? How do we embody wisdom? In essence, reflective practice and Unitary Caring Science provide a path through nurturing new ways of being/doing/becoming. As an exemplar, the 10 Caritas Processes serve as a guide for reflecting on being/doing/becoming, leading to ever-evolving caring literacy. Caring literacy is about deepening our ways of attending to and cultivating how to *Be* deeply human/humane and how to *Be-caring* (Watson, 2017), to be fully present, engaged, and attentive to another. Similarly, Mark Nepo (2020) calls us to face our experiences directly, and Parker Palmer (1993) calls us to be committed to the best potential of the human spirit by staying faithful to what is possible. So at a time when so many external forces keep us on the surface, how can we enter our becoming today? Engaging in reflective practices through the lens of Unitary Caring Science draws us below the surface. To remain awake, to attend to our becoming, we can ask ourselves: *What works for me, in which circumstances, in what respects, and how?*

The following sections provide exemplars of individual, relational, and group/organizational reflective practices that draw us below the surface. They invite us to remain awake, to attend to our way of being/doing/becoming. These practices invite us to engage in reflection through the lens of Unitary Caring Science to discover our embodied wisdom and expand our capacity to grow. They move the theory to a living tradition and form the foundation for a different way of being in the world, one that models and holds a vision for work that needs to be done for humanity and the planet.

INDIVIDUAL PRACTICES

Earlier chapters, particularly Chapters 2, 4, and 6, introduced ways in which to reflect using the 10 Caritas Processes and before, during, and after Caring Moments. Three additional practices that dive deeper below the surface of our being include a courageous caring moment, Jean Watson's Seven Sacred Sutras, and noble truths.

COURAGEOUS, CARING MOMENT

What is a courageous, caring moment? Nepo (2020) says courage is to focus on the heart of what matters in each moment, and Watson defines the caring moment as the essence of nursing, as a transpersonal experience that encompasses nursing's art form (2018). Thus, it takes courage to care in each moment; mainly when it is hard. Nischwitz (2022) invites us to consider whether courage is the outcome of caring enough.

Watson shares how we courageously care in each moment: "We do this through heart-centered consciousness, integrating head, heart, and soul, into our very presence; we radiate our Love into the infinity of the universe, affecting the whole: the collective continuing soul consciousness beyond physical death from this world. So, one person's healing, one person's caring is contributing to the caring and healing of the world" (Watson, 2021, p. 244). So how do we remember to bring our heart-centered consciousness into each interaction with others? To do this we must remember to:

- Pause and slow down

- Let time unfold (which tests our courage)

- Stand by our core values

- Unlock our fears

- Let the story we are in continue

- Live close to the moment that is forming everything
- When it is time, speak our truth from the heart

COURAGEOUS CARING MOMENT

Think of a time when you experienced a courageous caring moment, a time you were able to rise above the hurt, disappointment, conflict, and uncertainty.

Questions for Reflection

- *Where did your courage come from?*
- *What core value(s) was present?*
- *Now think about the story/situation...*
  - *What did you feel?*
  - *What did you see?*
  - *What did you do?*
  - *What did you say?*
  - *How did you love?*

Questions for Deeper Reflection

- *Why do you think this moment continues to stand out to you now?*
- *What difference did this make then?*
- *What difference has it made through time for you, your organization, family, community, and the world?*

SEVEN SACRED SUTRAS

In ancient Hindu teaching, a *sutra* is an aphorism, an observation of general truth, or a concise statement of scientific principle. It is frequently a word or brief string of words of utmost brevity that can be committed to memory (Britannica, n.d.). Watson (2021, p. 4) defines *sutras* as "energetically laden words or phrases that point to spiritual truths...beyond the simple aphorisms themselves." She offers Seven Sacred Sutras to access the sacred, to practice facing oneself, to stop the mind, and to open the self to unknowns and mystery.

They are offered as contemplative meditation, to face oneself and enter a sacred spiritual space. Contemplating each one in silence for just a moment is an opportunity to connect to source, soul, and sacred.

Contemplate your sutras. What words guide you to your truth? How might the practice of your sutras help you to be more present, develop insight and wisdom, and find peace and contentment?

JEAN WATSON'S SEVEN SACRED SUTRAS

Stillness

Silence

Solitude

Spirit

Simplicity

Service

Surrender

NOBLE TRUTHS

Using a lens of Unitary Caring Science and applying one's wisdom requires virtues such as those sutras. *Virtues* are qualitative characteristics with meritocratic dignity ennobled based on one's achievements. They include honor, knowledge, protecting, flourishing, change, fairness, conflict, balance, courage, discipline, fidelity, hospitality, industriousness, perseverance, self-reliance, truth, and control.

Reflective practices, based on virtuous moral qualities, lay a foundation for being/doing/becoming that leads to an ever-evolving caring literacy. Caring literacy is about developing our ways of nurturing how to *Be* deeply human/humane and how to *Be* caring. Possessing noble virtues as part of caring literacy means one admires and respects oneself and others in an unselfish and morally good way, based on high moral principles, thus enhancing a sense of belonging.

Being courageously caring is to set aside fears, allow ourselves to be vulnerable, and explore ways to stand up for ourselves and others, or important causes. Reflecting on acts of courage must embrace the self, not only our patients. It includes kindness, accountability, uniqueness (with pride), commitment, forgiveness, authenticity, and attentiveness. Acknowledge and embrace caring moments. Understand how to be in the moment. It is an action of choice. Make a conscious effort to preserve human caring. Caring endorses our professional identity.

Noble virtues, originally introduced in Chapter 2, are sets of moral and situational guidelines within which one functions. Various models exist with different virtues and they are related to the Eightfold path of Buddhism (Solomon & Higgins, 1997). Caring for the self and others, guided by the eight ancient principles outlined in the sidebar, can steer us when reflecting on our positions as nurses and change agents.

NOBLE VIRTUES

1. *Right view:* This refers to the respect that we show our patients, the community, and our colleagues. When assessing a patient, it should be done objectively and without any prejudice.

2. *Right thought:* Ensure all information, actions, or incidents are reported diligently and correctly. Do a comprehensive assessment and do not rush. Respect the human dignity of all your patients, their loved ones, and your colleagues.

3. *Right speech:* Always act professionally and as a role model when addressing patients, community members, or colleagues. Choose your words carefully and make sure the person understands you. It often is not what you say but how you say it.

4. *Right action:* Ensure that your conduct is always professional. This requires competent nurses who are committed to continuous professional development. The fact that you have completed your course does not mean that you are going to stop improving your competence or learning new skills.

5. *Right living:* This refers to one's actions, thoughts, and speech. Engage in actions that do not cause any harm, physically or psychologically; always be honest (e.g., when reporting on the condition of a patient). Ensure that all actions are meaningful.

6. *Right effort:* Our professional conduct must be of such a nature that we are seen as leaders in the professional community. We must ask ourselves how much effort we are putting into what we are doing and how we are doing it. The right effort will require deliberate self-development.

7. *Right mindfulness:* In realizing this we should be mindful of what we are thinking, saying, and doing. Have a positive attitude and treat everyone with respect.

8. *Right concentration:* The last element refers to the cognitive processes. Through reflection-on-action and reflection-in-action, the right knowledge will be developed.

RELATIONAL PRACTICES

This book explores ways to reflect together including reflective listening, dialogues, and incorporating liberating structure activities. Healing and wisdom circles extend these practices by bringing a group of individuals together to support each other in personal growth, healing, and self-discovery. The purpose of these circles is to create a safe space where individuals can share their experiences, feelings, and insights without judgment.

Healing circles are a traditional form of healing that have been used by various cultures throughout history. The practice of gathering in a circle to address physical, emotional, and spiritual needs has been around for centuries. The history of healing circles is rooted in the idea that physical, emotional, and spiritual healing can be achieved through community support and intentional practices that promote wellness and balance (Baldwin & Linnea, 2010; Macy, 2007). Applying the principles and practices of Unitary Caring Science to the healing circle, Griffin and colleagues (2021) created Caritas circles where caregivers come together to learn about Caring Science and share the emotional side of being a healthcare professional.

As originally explored in Chapter 4, both healing and Caritas circles are spaces that allow reflection on one's surroundings and experiences. They provide a safe and accepting environment in which one explores their healing while opening one's heart to others, leading to intra and interpersonal growth. As a circle, we work together to discover the best ways to address or remove hindrances and burdens and promote emotional, mental, and physical well-being. Participants can share their struggles, traumas, and challenges with others who can offer support, empathy, and guidance. Healing/Caritas circles can be particularly helpful for those who have experienced significant emotional or physical trauma, as the group setting can provide a sense of safety and community that can aid in the recovery process.

Healing/Caritas circles take place in welcoming and conducive environments that create a warm atmosphere within which all can open their hearts, *Be* deeply human/humane, and *Be* caring. Different activities and ways of engagement that can enhance our way of being/ doing/becoming are applied. Activities include guided visualization, music, reading, guided meditation, the use of silence, and poetry.

When we are on our own, we can also hold a circle (Circle of One) for the different voices from within. We can be a team on our own, embracing the different roles or dimensions of our being. This is the time we look inside (emic perspective) and listen carefully to what is most important to us at that moment, following our intuition. Communication is a silent circle that is about communication with body, mind, and spirit and may come as sensations, visualizations, imagery, or voices. The voices may come as conflicts in terms of the different roles we play in life, the range of emotions we experience, or physical conflicts within the body.

The planning, introduction, intentions, check-in, and check-out processes are planned processes. The focus is on everyone in the room having a voice. Underlying intentions are that everyone is comfortable, the space is sacred, there are common bonds between members, there is intention, and members are "present." Each circle has a host and a guardian. The host protects the "center" of the circle by opening and closing the circle. The guardian protects the energy of the group and the group dynamic. All participants share responsibility for holding the circle and for their healing. A tangible action is used to initiate a pause or closing (i.e., ringing a bell or blowing out a candle).

The core of a healing circle is heart-sharing. Heart-sharing may include symbolic actions by holding an object, touching the chest as a symbol of touching the heart, or silence. This sacred time involves vulnerability, authenticity, and self-discovery. This is where one moves towards one's healing and wholeness.

Healing/Caritas circles are powerful social support engagements, emotional support activities, learning opportunities, network-building engagements, and healing sessions. The magic lies in the whole-heartedness of the group. Learning takes place through a variety of interactions:

- Asking deeply relevant and authentic questions that matter in one's own life

- Asking open and honest questions to each other that matters to others

- Answering honestly and from one's own experience

- Reflecting deeply to ensure one understands the self and others

Healing circles are about inner wisdom as well as finding collective and universal wisdom. Moving from a healing circle to a wisdom circle is moving from intentional self-care, presence, integrated mindfulness, heart-sharing, and deep reflection to co-creating shared visions, values, and beliefs and embracing caring moments. To move to a wisdom circle there must be intentional care, authenticity, clarity, and self-leadership.

WISDOM CIRCLES

Wisdom circles are safe, respectful engagements where learning takes place through wise interactions. Transformative relationships are created. Wisdom circles provide a framework and intentions to create such spaces. Wisdom circles facilitate groups of people into the spirit of choice-creation to face and solve complex issues together. Through such circles, the transformative relationships nurture transformative processes that are used to allow for critical reflection and building resilience creatively and collaboratively. Choice-creation sparks into existence a new entity of "we the people" and a capability of ultimate responsibility for the health and well-being of ourselves and our colleagues. It allows for networking by building communities of practice. Through wisdom circles, we can address a complex issue, advocate for our choices and processes of healing, speak with feeling, experience breakthroughs at different times and in different ways, and create choices rather than make decisions as leaders alone.

Wisdom circles offer spaces that are safe from judgment (we need not agree or disagree), freeing participants to speak from their vision, values, and beliefs rather than as representatives or from a particular role. Wisdom circles follow energy generated by the members. It is not a problem- or solution-finding engagement. Diversity is seen as an asset, rather than simply ascertaining different views.

Reflection within a wisdom circle, using the lens of Unitary Caring Science, allows the discovery of embodied wisdom and allows our capacity to grow. Critical reflection forms the core of a wisdom circle and leads to group conclusions in the form of "co-census" rather than consensus. Choices are made rather than decisions. The spirit of "we" through a process of enhanced individuality allows people to become more knowledgeable, capable, and unique. Through this living tradition, the foundation for a different way of being in the world evolves and contributes to the process of healing and building resilience (Van Rensburg et al., 2022).

Overall, the practice of engaging in healing and wisdom circles is to create a space where individuals can feel supported, heard, and validated in their experiences, and to foster personal growth and healing through shared knowledge and wisdom.

ORGANIZATIONAL PRACTICES

In organizations, reflective practice can be used to improve individual and organizational performance by creating spaces for individuals to regularly reflect on their and the organization's work, identify areas for improvement, and develop strategies for addressing these areas. Reflective organizational practices promote continuous learning and development among employees. By encouraging individuals to regularly reflect on their experiences, organizations can help members gain a deeper understanding of their work and identify areas for growth. This can lead to increased innovation, improved decision-making, and better outcomes for the organization.

Reflective practice is also important for promoting individual and organizational resilience. By reflecting on challenging experiences, employees can develop a greater sense of self-awareness and learn strategies for responding to difficult situations. This can help individuals and organizations to better navigate change, uncertainty, and adversity.

Reflective practice can also promote a culture of learning and development within organizations. By encouraging individuals to share their reflections and insights with others, organizations can create a collaborative environment where knowledge and experience are valued and shared.

APPRECIATIVE INQUIRY

Appreciative inquiry is a positive approach to organizational development that focuses on identifying and building upon an organization's strengths and successes rather than focusing solely on its weaknesses and challenges. This approach encourages individuals and organizations to identify what is already working well and to build upon those strengths to create positive change and growth (Hammond, 2013). Appreciative inquiry is in alignment with the premises and practices of Unitary Caring Science, where the focus is on caring literacy and solutions rather than what is broken. For example, a health system practiced through the lens of Unitary Caring Science focuses on the creation of healthy and healing work environments over nursing staff retention.

Appreciative inquiry typically involves a 5-D cycle: define, discover, dream, design, and deliver or destiny.

- **Define** what to inquire about or choose a topic. This initial step is the opportunity to choose to live and lead through the lens of Unitary Caring Science to be guided by the 10 Caritas Processes (which are outlined in Chapter 1).

- **Discovery** allows individuals and organizations to reflect on their successes and strengths and identify what is currently working well. Discovery integrates Caritas Process 1 (sustaining humanistic-altruistic values of loving-kindness, compassion, and equanimity for self and other) and Caritas Process 6 (creative problem-solving/solution-seeking via the use of all ways of knowing).

- **Dream** gives individuals and organizations an opportunity to envision a future state that builds upon those strengths and successes. This phase applies Caritas Process 3 (being sensitive to self and others by cultivating spiritual practices beyond ego to transpersonal presence), Caritas Process 6 (creative problem-solving/solution-seeking), and Caritas Process 10 (opening to spiritual, mystery, unknowns).

- **Design** is when individuals and organizations create a plan for achieving that future state. Caritas Process 6 (creative problem/solving-solution-seeking), Caritas Process 7 (engaging in transpersonal teaching and learning within the context of a caring relationship, staying within another's frame of reference—shifting toward coaching model for expanded health/wellness), and Carita Process 10 (opening to spiritual, mystery, unknowns) speak to this phase.

- **Deliver/destiny** allows individuals and organizations to implement the plan and monitor progress, and using the Caritas Process 10, remain open to mystery and the unknowns.

Appreciative inquiry and the 10 Caritas Processes can be used to address a wide range of organizational challenges, including team building, leadership development, quality improvement projects, strategic or future planning, and other change management activities. One of the central benefits is that together they serve to create a positive, relational, optimistic mindset among individuals and organizations. By focusing on strengths, successes, and creative solutions, individuals within organizations are more likely to feel valued, motivated, and energized, and to approach challenges with a sense of hope, possibility, and opportunity.

EMERGENT STRATEGIES

Emergent strategies arise through a process of learning and adaptation in response to changes in the environment. They are not predetermined or planned, but instead emerge as the organization learns more about its environment and adapts its approach accordingly (Brown, 2017). Some common characteristics of emergent strategies include:

- **Flexibility and adaptability:** Emergent strategies are flexible and adaptable because they are based on ongoing feedback and learning from the environment. They allow organizations to respond quickly to changing conditions and adjust their course of action as needed.

- **Bottom-up approach:** Emergent strategies often emerge from the bottom-up, rather than being imposed from the top down. They are the result of decentralized decision-making and the collective intelligence of the organization's members.

- **Incrementalism:** Emergent strategies are often developed incrementally, through a series of small adjustments and adaptations over time. This allows organizations to experiment with different approaches and gradually build momentum toward a larger goal.

- **Emergence from complex systems:** Emergent strategies are often the result of complex systems, where the behavior of the system is greater than the sum of its parts. This can result in surprising and unpredictable outcomes, which can be both a challenge and an opportunity.

- **Continuous learning:** Emergent strategies require continuous learning and experimentation, as organizations must constantly monitor their environment and adapt their approach accordingly. This means that emergent strategies are never truly complete or final but are always evolving based on new information and feedback.

Emergent strategies and Unitary Caring Science share some alignment, particularly in their emphasis on adaptability, continuous learning, and holistic approaches. Unitary Caring Science emphasizes the interconnectedness of all beings and the environment, recognizing that health and healing are dynamic processes that involve the whole person and their environment. Similarly, emergent strategies are flexible and adaptable, allowing organizations to respond quickly to changes in their environment, and to continuously learn and adapt their approach.

Both emergent strategies and Unitary Caring Science recognize the importance of holistic approaches that consider the whole person, their environment, and their unique experiences and needs. Emergent strategies are developed over time, through a series of small steps and experiments, rather than as a single grand plan. Similarly, Unitary Caring Science encourages nurses and healthcare professionals to approach care holistically, considering the physical, emotional, and spiritual needs of the patient.

Finally, both emergent strategies and Unitary Caring Science emphasize the importance of continuous learning and growth. Emergent strategies are based on a process of continuous learning and adaptation, rather than a fixed plan or set of assumptions. Similarly, Unitary Caring Science encourages nurses and healthcare professionals to continuously learn and grow, and to cultivate practices that promote mindfulness, compassion, and wisdom.

APPLICATION FOR PERSONAL AND PROFESSIONAL PRACTICE

Embracing personal, relational, and organizational ways of expanding our being, doing, and becoming in the world through the lens of Unitary Caring Science and wisdom practices serves as a guide for personal and professional growth. By recognizing and embracing the interconnectedness of all beings, and by cultivating practices that promote mindfulness, compassion, and wisdom, we develop a deeper understanding of ourselves, our relationships, and our place in the world. This understanding helps us to make more informed decisions, build trusting-caring relationships, and work towards a common purpose in our personal and professional lives.

Personal understanding of our way of being, doing, and becoming in the world informs how we approach our personal and professional lives. This understanding includes our values, beliefs, goals, and aspirations. By reflecting on our understanding, we can align our actions with our core values and make choices that are consistent with our aspirations and goals.

Relational ways of expanding our being, doing, and becoming occur through attending to how we relate to others, including meeting them where they are, allowing for the expression of positive and negative feelings, and understanding the social and cultural context. By recognizing and appreciating the diversity of experiences and perspectives among our colleagues, patients, their families, and other stakeholders, we develop more trusting-caring relationships, foster inclusivity and diversity, and collaborate more effectively. A relational understanding also helps us to understand how our actions and decisions influence others, and how we can collectively work to create a healing environment.

An organizational understanding involves how we understand the mission, vision, and values of the organizations we work with, as well as their culture, structure, and processes. This understanding helps us to align our personal and professional goals with those of the organization and to work towards a common purpose. It also allows us to more readily recognize when values and goals are not in alignment. By understanding the organizational context, we have the opportunity for innovation and improvement, work collaboratively with others to implement change, or make our own change to discover a better fit.

REFLECTIVE SUMMARY

Reflective practice and Unitary Caring Science share underlying ethical, moral, and philosophical worldviews that value the interconnectedness of all beings and recognize the importance of a holistic approach to care. Reflection is essential for personal and professional growth, as it allows us to examine our experiences, values, and beliefs, and to align our actions with our aspirations and goals. Reflective practitioners value both individual and relational practices, as our relationships with others are an integral part of our personal and professional lives. By exploring ways to connect more deeply and wisely with others, we can build more trusting-caring relationships and collaborate more effectively. Finally, applying personal, relational, and organizational ways of expanding our way of being, doing, and becoming in the world aligns with the values and principles of Unitary Caring Science, emphasizing a moral and philosophical foundation for care, continuous learning, and a holistic approach that considers the whole person and their environment.

LEARNING NARRATIVE

Using the 5-D cycle of appreciative inquiry, the 10 Caritas Processes, and emergent strategies as a guide, plan to deliver a healing or wisdom circle. Some individual and group reflection questions to get started are in this learning narrative.

Individual reflection:

- Why are you calling a circle?
- Where does hosting this circle fit into your life?
- How does it serve your soul/your own wholeness?
- Whom would you enjoy co-hosting the circle with?

Group reflection:

- Share your ideas of what makes an effectively functioning relationship between co-hosts.
- How can you support each other?
- What is the intention of the circle?
- Whom would you like to welcome into the circle and how will you invite and reach out to them (if known/if unknown)?
- Where will you host the circle?
- How would you like to prepare the physical space to ensure circle members will feel welcome and safe?

REFLECTIVE QUESTIONS

1. How does my understanding and appreciation for the value of experiential knowledge expand in an environment that promotes reflective practices?

2. In what ways do I already practice reflectively? How can I deepen practice through the lens of Unitary Caring Science?

3. How do reflective practice and Unitary Caring Science guide me to embodied wisdom?

4. What are the needs of educational and practice settings to promote reflection and Unitary Caring Science in teaching, learning, and service?

5. How am I continually nurturing and cultivating my ways of being and becoming more human? How congruent are my practices with the principles of Unitary Caring Science?

6. How can I use individual, relational, and group/organizational reflective practices to expand caring consciousness and embodied wisdom?

REFERENCES

Baldwin, C., & Linnea, A. (2010). *The circle way: A leader in every chair.* Berrett-Koehler.

Britannica. (n.d.). Sutra. In *Britannica online dictionary.* https://www.britannica.com/topic/sutra

Brown, A. M. (2017). *Emergent strategies: Shaping change, changing worlds.* A.K. Press.

Browne, C., Wall, P., Batt, S., & Bennet, R. (2018). Understanding perceptions of nursing professional identity in students entering an Australian undergraduate nursing degree. *Nurse Education in Practice, 32,* 90–96. https://doi.org/10.1016/j.nepr.2018.07.006

Carper, B. (1978). Fundamental patterns of knowing in nursing. *Advanced Nursing Science, 1*(1), 13–23. https://doi.org/10.1097/00012272-197810000-00004

Chinn, P., & Kramer, M. (2018). *Knowledge development in nursing* (10th ed.). Mosby.

Dewey, J. (1938). *Logic: The theory of inquiry.* Henry Holt and Company.

Fagermoen, M. S. (1997). Professional identity: Values embedded in meaningful nursing practice. *Journal of Advanced Nursing, 25*(3), 434–441. https://doi.org/10.1046/j.1365-2648.1997.1997025434.x

Goodolf, D. M., & Godfrey, N. (2020). A think tank in action: Building new knowledge about professional identity in nursing. *Journal of Professional Nursing, 37*(2), 493–499. https://doi.org/10.1016/j.profnurs.2020.10.007

Griffin, C., Oman, K. S., Ziniel, S. I., Kight, S., Jacobs-Lowry, S., & Givens, P. (2021). Increasing the capacity to provide compassionate care by expanding knowledge of caring science practices at a pediatric hospital. *Archives of Psychiatric Nursing, 35*(1), 34–41. https://doi.org/10.1016/j.apnu.2020.10.019

Hammond, S. (2013). *The thin book of appreciative inquiry* (3rd ed.). Thin Book Publishing Co.

Horton-Deutsch, S., & Rosa, W. (2019). Reflective practice and Caring Science. In W. Rosa, S. Horton-Deutsch, & J. Watson (Eds.), *The handbook for Caring Science.* Springer.

Macy, J. (2007). *Widening circles.* New Catalyst Books.

Moola, S. (2017). The evolution of a professional identity as perceived by Saudi student nurses. *Global Journal of Health Science, 10*(2), 1–10.

Nahra, C. (2020). Altruism and moral enhancement. *Kriterion, 61*(147), 633–648. https://doi.org/10.1590/0100-512X2020n14704cn

Nepo, M. (2020). *Finding inner courage.* Red Wheel.

Nischwitz, J. (2022). *Jeff Nischwitz.* http://www.nischwitzgroup.com/

Palmer, P. (1993). *To know as we are known: Education as a spiritual journey.* Harper.

Schön, D. (2016). *The reflective practitioner: How professionals think in action.* Routledge.

Solomon, R. C., & Higgins, K. M. (1997). *A passion for wisdom: A brief history of philosophy.* Oxford University.

Tsakissiris, J. (2015). *The role of professional identity and self-interest in career choices in the emerging ICT workforce.* Queensland University of Technology. https://eprints.qut.edu.au/91646/1/Jane_Tsakissiris_Thesis.pdf

Van Rensburg, G., Horton-Deutsch, S., Monroe, C., & Borges, W. (2022). *From healing circle to wisdom circle: A process of moving from insiders to outsiders to insiders.* Presented at the Sigma Research Congress, Edinburgh, Scotland.

Watson, J. (2017). Global advances in human caring literacy. In S. Lee, P. Palmieri, & J. Watson (Eds.), *Global advances in human caring literacy* (pp. 3–11). Springer.

Watson, J. (2018). *Unitary caring science: The philosophy and praxis of nursing.* University of Colorado Press.

Watson, J. (2021). *Caring science as sacred science* (Rev. ed). Lotus Library.

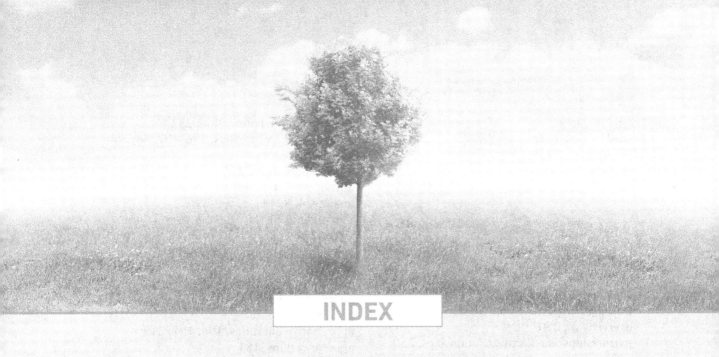

INDEX

NOTE: Pages marked with an *f* are figures; pages marked with an *t* are tables

1-2-4-All, 219
6-word stories, 157*f*
55-word stories, 158*f*

A

AACN Essentials, 68, 69, 116, 189, 227, 228, 241, 243, 261
academic education, 249, 250
    evidence, 255–259
    learning perspectives on, 250–255
    overview of, 250
    partnerships as reflective relationships, 259–260
    personal experience, 260–261
    professional experience, 260–261
    social justice in higher education, 270–272
    theoretical frameworks, 255–259
accountability, 295
acting, 90
actions, 25, 166
    reflection-beyond-action, 173
    reflection-for-action, 260
    reflection-in-action, 31, 173, 216–220, 279–280
    reflection-on-action, 31, 173, 187, 216–220
    wise, 220–222
adaptability, 316
Advancing Healthcare Transformation: A New Era for Academic Nursing (2016), 251
advocacy
    differences and community, 295
    strategies, 169
agency, importance of, 12
ambitions, 15
American Association of Colleges of Nursing (AACN), 20, 163, 183, 251, 270. *See also* AACN Essentials
American Nurses Association (ANA), 68, 70, 270
American Nurses Association Racial Reckoning Statement, 132
American Nurses Credentialing Center Magnet Recognition Program, 258
American Psychiatric Nurses Association, 219
ANA Racial Reckoning Statement (2022), 270

Annie E. Casey Foundation, 232
annual nurse evaluations, 196–197. *See also* evaluation
antigay prejudices, 236
anti-oppression, 240
anxiety, 4, 8, 44
    avoiding, 11
    death, 8
    performance, 121
application for development, 36–37
appraisals, 295–297
appreciative inquiry (AI), 100, 119, 186–187, 315–326
appreciative questions, 196, 197, 219
apprenticeships, 184
art, 35
artificial intelligence (AI), 4, 10
assessment
    feedback, 193–195
    redesigning, 193–195
    self-assessments, 197–198
assignment of rubrics, 194
attributes of leadership, 289–290
authenticity, 7, 11, 79, 289
    communications, 13
    connections, 28–30
    listening, 48
    presence, 49–52
authentic presence (Caritas Process #2), 68–69, 79
authoritarian behaviors, 231
autoethnographic data, 48
awakening, 273, 275

B

Bartels, Jonathan, 154
base interventions, 94
be-attitudes of leadership, 292–295
Be-caring, 307
becoming, 7, 272–273, 275
behaviors
    authoritarian, 231
    caring, 237–238

nursing, 73
   shifting, 216*f*
being, authenticity of, 7
beliefs, 33
belonging, 45
Belonging-Being-Becoming, 45
biases
   cognitive bias simulation training, 171–172
   recognition of, 231
Blake, William, 46
bottom-up approach, 316
brave learning places, 131–132
bravery, encouraging, 131
breadcrumbing, 237
Buddhism, 310
building trusting caring relationships (Caritas
   Process #4), 69

C

care
   development of, 121–127
   end-of-life care, 168
   healthcare delivery of, 252
   person-centered, 238
careers, risks, 8
caring, 46, 90
   behaviors, 237–238
   building trusting caring relationships (Caritas
      Process #4), 69
   compassionate care, 117
   consciousness of, 56
   courageous caring moments, 308–309
   cultures of, 276–277
   developing caring practices, 91
   development, 30–32
   intentions, 54*t*
   limitations of, 76
   listening as form of, 153–154
   literacy, 70, 81, 310
   McDowell-Williams Caring Leadership Model,
      290–291
   reflective practice, 48–58
   relationships, 57, 277–278
   role of reflection, 115 (*see also* reflection)

social mandates, 281–282
   theories, 92
Caritas Council, 81
Caritas literacy, 3, 4–5, 6, 7, 50, 230
   10 Caritas Processes, 9–10
   consciousness, 7
Carnegie Foundation, 184
case studies, 33, 181
CASTLE principles, 289
censorship, 269
   overview of, 270
   social justice in higher education, 270–272
centering, 75
change agents, educators as, 34–36
Charon, Rita, 150
check-in, 82
check-out, 83
chronic disease care, 253
Circle of One, 312
circles
   healing, 313
   wisdom, 313–314
clearness committees, 220–222
climate change, 23
clinical environments, listening in, 78–81
clinical experiences, 252
clinical instructor training, 167
clinical judgment, 27
Clinical Judgment Model, 26*f*
clinical learning, collaboration in, 184–187
coaches, 37
cognitive bias simulation training, 171–172
cognitive disablement, 237
collaboration, 131, 170, 179, 196, 294
   AACN Essentials, 227
   caring relationships, 277–278
   in clinical learning, 184–187
   developing relationships, 191–194
   overview of, 180–181
collaborative learning, 255
committees, clearness, 220–222
common humanity, 118
communications, 170, 312
   authenticity, 13
   journaling, 147–148
   listening, 147 (*see also* listening)

communities, 249
  academic education, 249, 250 (*see also* academic education)
  building, 58, 314
  definition of, 257
  Quaker, 220
  reflective academic-practice learning, 260
  reflective learning, 57–58, 259, 261
  stories and, 146 (*see also* stories)
  thinking and being, 256
compassion, 46, 51, 90
  authentic presence and, 50
  development of, 121–127
  role of reflection, 115 (*see also* reflection)
  self-compassion, 117
compassionate care, 117
competence, 28
competencies
  mastering, 253
  quality, 179, 183–184 (*see also* quality)
  Quality and Safety Education for Nurses (QSEN), 167
  safety, 183–184 (*see also* safety)
complexities of diversity of thought, 231–237
complexity, definition of, 10
complexity science, 209, 210–211
complex systems, emergence from, 316
components of nursing practice, 116–117
connections, 47
  authenticity, 28–30
  communities, 258 (*see also* communities)
  purpose, 75
  Unitary Caring Science, 305
consciousness, 54t
  10 Caritas Processes, 72
  of caring, 56
  of self, 98f
consensus, 214
constant reflection, 34
content, reflective practice, 37
context, 99, 164–165
continuous learning, 316
contradictions, 25, 182–183
contributions, 295–297
Conversation Café website, 217
conversations, restarting, 217–218
Core Competencies for Interprofessional Collaborative Practice report (2016), 170

courage, 289
courageous caring moments, 308–309
COVID-19, 4, 5, 23, 59, 145
  death anxiety, 8
  disruptions, 10
  education and, 253
  resilience, 9
  self-care, 197
  stress, 95
creative spaces, 43
  10 Caritas Processes, 47–48 (*see also* 10 Caritas Processes)
  for caring reflection, 52–55
  creating safe places, 50
  overview of, 44–45
  personal practice, 58–59
  professional practice, 58–59
  reflective learning communities, 57–58
  for reflective practice, 48–58
  support of framework and evidence, 45–46
creative tension, 32, 182
critical Caritas consciousness, 3, 4–5, 231
critical dialogues, 279
critical reasoning, 21, 27
critical reflection model, 25, 34, 182
critical theory, 6, 13
critical thinking, 38, 131, 149, 231
cultures
  of caring, 276–277
  contemporary workplace, 232
  definition of, 208
  promoting, 133
  shifting, 216f

D

death, anxiety, 8
decision-making, 185, 221
deep learning, 38
deeply listening, 78. *See also* listening
Describe, Examine, and Articulate Learning (DEAL) model, 119–120
descriptive practice model, 182
descriptive reflection, 25
design thinking, 256

development
  application for, 36–37
  of awareness of empathy, 242
  of care, 121–127
  of caring, 30–32
  of caring practices, 91
  of caring reflective practitioners, 30–32
  of collaborative relationships, 191–194
  of communities (*see* communities)
  of compassion, 121–127
  of educators, 35
  of emancipatory nursing praxis (ENP), 275–282
  of habits, 148
  of knowledge (*see* knowledge development)
  of leadership, 169
  of mindfulness, 95–98
  of practice, 32–33, 92–93, 189–190
  of professional identity, 92–93, 124, 182
  of relationships, 117
  of self-awareness, 95–98
  of stories, 50
  of trust, 71
dialogic reflection model, 25, 182
dialogues, 13, 279, 311. *See also* communications
discernment, 220–222
discipline
  of nursing, 304 (*see also* nursing)
  practice-based, 92
discomfort, 131
disease prevention, 252
disillusionment, 183
dissatisfaction, 93
diversity
  definition of, 233
  justice, equity, diversity, and inclusion (JEDI), 240
diversity, equity, and inclusion (DEI), 232, 233, 234, 239–240
diversity of thought, 227
  caring behaviors, 237–238
  complexities of, 231–237
  education, 234–235
  empathy, 233–234
  labels, 235–237
documentation, 73
dominance, 154

E

Educating Nurses (2010), 20, 184
education
  10 Caritas Processes, 36
  AACN Essentials, 227
  academic (*see* academic education)
  appreciative inquiry (AI), 100, 119, 186–187
  authentic connections, 28–30
  caring reflective practitioners, 30–32
  clinical instructor training, 167
  cognitive bias simulation training, 171–172
  COVID-19 and, 253
  discipline of, 306
  diversity, 234–235
  emancipatory, 22, 23
  frameworks, 21–30
  graduate nursing education, 168–170
  interprofessional education (IPE), 170–171
  learning and teaching (Caritas Process #7), 69
  learning experiences, 11
  learning to listen, 71–78
  liberatory, 230
  models of reflective practice, 23–26
  narratives, 151
  nursing, 254*f*
  online, 10
  pluralistic possibility model, 238–239
  practice-based discipline, 92
  practice development, 32–33
  prelicensure nursing education, 167–168
  program overview, 116
  recreating nursing, 148–149
  redesigning, 26–27
  self-directed learning, 37
  simulation-based learning, 162–163, 166–172 (*see also* simulation-based learning)
  telehealth, 172
  transformation, 20, 28
  transformative learning theory, 21–23
  Unitary Caring Science, 30
educators, 37
  as change agents, 34–36
  development, 35
  diversity, equity, and inclusion (DEI), 239
  evaluation, 196–197

pedagogies, 144
restrictions on subjects to teach, 271 (*see also* censorship)
effectiveness, 289
Eightfold path (Buddhism), 310
elements of Ignatian Pedagogy, 165*f*
emancipatory education, 22, 23
emancipatory knowing, 305
emancipatory nursing praxis (ENP), 269
awakening, 273, 275
becoming, 27, 272–273
caring relationships, 277–278
caring social mandates, 281–282
critical dialogues, 279
cultures of caring, 276–277
development, 275–282
engaging, 273–274, 275
importance of reflexivity, 275
overview of, 272–275
reflection-in-action, 279–280
transforming, 274–275
emergent strategies for shaping futures, 211–214, 316–317
emotional intelligence, 97, 98*f*, 186
emotional labor, 8
emotions, 35, 153
expressing feelings (Caritas Process #5), 69
hiding from, 49
risks, 94
empathy, 233–234
development of awareness of, 242
pluralistic possibility model, 241–243
empirics, 305
end-of-life care, 168
engaging, 273–274, 275
equanimity, 76
equity, 232, 240
The Essentials: Core Competencies for Professional Nursing Education (AACN, 2021), 252, 270
The Essentials of Nursing Practice (AACN, 2021), 238
esthetics, 305
Ethic of Face (Watson), 46
Ethic of Hand (Watson), 46
ethics, 4, 9
Watson's Unitary Caring Science, 46–47

evaluation, 166, 179
educators, 196–197
responses to reflection papers, 192–193
evidence
academic education, 255–259
leadership, 288–291
listening, 68–70
pluralistic possibility model, 229–231
role of reflection, 117–121
simulation-based learning, 163–166
stories, 143–148
support for, 5–7, 45–46
transformative learning theory, 181–184
Unitary Caring Science, 304–306
well-being, 91–93
working together, 208–209
experiences, 165
experiential learning, 163–164, 181, 184, 194
Experiential Learning Theory, 28, 38, 208–209
expressing feelings (Caritas Process #5), 69

F

family narratives, 151–153
fear, 4
feedback, 153, 196
assessments, 193–195
feminism, 51
fifty-five word stories, 158*f*
flexibility, 316
foresight, 250–255, 251*f*
formats, stories, 155. *See also* stories
frameworks, 188
AACN Essentials, 227 (*see also* AACN Essentials)
education, 21–30
Experiential Learning Theory, 38, 208–209
Heart of Caring, 119
liberatory education, 231
phases of, 24–25
and reflective practice, 33–36
support for theoretical, 5–7, 45–46
theoretical (*see* theoretical frameworks)
Unitary Caring Science, 9, 11, 12 (*see also* Unitary Caring Science)

Freire, Paulo, 6, 230, 239, 274
Fricker, Miranda, 237
The Future of Nursing 2020–2030 report, 234, 257
Future of Nursing report (2021), 162
futures, shaping, 211–214

G

Gadamer, Hans-Georg, 12
gaslighting, 237
ghosting, 237
Gibran, Kahlil, 56
go-go-go mentality, 129
Google Scholar, 257
G.R.A.C.E, 52, 53
Grace and Grit (Wilber), 47
grading systems, 194
graduate nursing education, 168–170
grief, 44
growth, 13, 97*f*
    promoting, 117
    support, 55
    Unitary Caring Science, 303 (*see also* Unitary Caring Science)
guided reflection, 145*f*
    for learning from stories, 156*t*
Guiding Principles for Academic-Practice Partnerships (2012), 259

H

habit development, 148
handoff tools, 71
healing, 46, 312
    circles, 313
    intentions, 54*t*
    narratives, 143
    support, 55
Healing Circles, 81, 82*f*, 312–313
healing environments (Caritas Process #8), 69, 72
healthcare, 252. *See also* care; caring
    delivery of, 258
    education and, 254*f*

Heart of Caring framework, 119
heart-sharing, 313
heterosexism, 236
higher education, 270–272. *See also* academic education; education
Hinds, Pamela, 291
hindsight, 250–255, 251*f*
Hinduism, 309–310
history of phobias, 236, 237
holding space, 53, 77. *See also* creative spaces
homophobia, 236
hooks, bell, 118, 230
hospice care, 253
Housen, Abigail, 102
human rights, 22

I

identity, 89
    developing professional, 92–93, 124, 182
    overview of, 90
    well-being, 90 (*see also* well-being)
Ignatian Pedagogy, 164–166
    elements of, 165*f*
improving practice, 150–156
    organizational cultures, 208
    organizational relationships, 210–211
inclusion, 232, 234
    justice, equity, diversity, and inclusion (JEDI), 240
incrementation, 316
individual practices, 308–311
inequality, 234
influence, 295
infodemic, 4
innovation, 294
inquiry strategies, 169
insight, 250–255, 251*f*
insights, leadership, 295–297
in-situ simulations, 171
inspiration, 295
Institute for Healthcare Improvement Quadruple Aim, 116
integrity, 221
intentions, 74
    caring, 54*t*

healing, 54*t*
listening, 55–57, 68 (*see also* listening)
setting, 78
interactions
    courageous caring moments, 308–309
    recreating, 214–216
interactive pedagogies, 22
International Council of Nurses, 116
Interprofessional Collaborative Practice
    Competencies, 170
interprofessional education (IPE), 170–171
interruptions, 154
interventions, 25, 94
isolation, 237

J

job risks, 8
Johns, Christopher, 181–183, 289
journaling, 147
justice, equity, diversity, and inclusion (JEDI),
    240

K

kindness, 58
knowledge development, 3, 4–5, 81
    limitations of, 48
    in nursing, 305
    practical knowledge, 92
    relational learning and, 14–15
    tacit knowledge, 24, 32, 92
Knowles' Adult Learning Theory, 163–164
Kouzes, James, 291

L

labels
    diversity of thought, 235–237
    pluralistic possibility model, 235–237

languages. *See also* Caritas literacy
    of medicine, 50
    pluralistic possibility model, 235–237
Lao Tzu, 57
leadership, 98*f*, 287. *See also* management
    attributes, 289–290
    be-attitudes of, 292–295
    CASTLE principles, 289
    creating insights, 295–297
    development, 169
    evidence, 288–291
    McDowell-Williams Caring Leadership Model,
        290–291
    overview of, 288
    personal experience, 297
    principles and practices of, 291–292
    professional experience, 297
    theoretical frameworks, 288–291
    traits, 293*t*–294*t*
learners
    narrative pedagogies and, 144
    practice development, 32–33, 189–190
learning. *See also* education
    co-creating, 141 (*see also* stories)
    co-creating safe learning spaces, 146–148
    collaboration in clinical, 184–187
    collaborative, 255
    communities (*see* communities)
    continuous, 316
    from experiences, 163–164, 181
    experiential, 184, 194
    Experiential Learning Theory, 38, 208–209
    guided reflection, 145*f*
    how students want to learn, 240
    how to ask questions, 197
    to listen, 71–78
    from mistakes, 181
    narratives, 151
    from narratives, 99–101
    perspectives on academic education, 250–255
    reflective (*see* reflective learning)
    simulation-based, 161 (*see also* simulation-
        based learning)
    situated, 166
    stories (*see* stories)
    transformative learning theory, 181–184, 209
    writing to learn, 101

learning and teaching (Caritas Process #7), 69
learning environments, listening in, 81–83
learning experiences, 11, 67. *See also* education; listening
learning narratives, 38–39
legacy leadership. *See* leadership
legacy planning, 291
legislative censorship, 269. *See also* censorship
liberating structures, 214–220
    menus, 215*f*
liberatory education, 230, 231
limitations of caring, 76
listening, 67, 90, 257, 311
    authenticity, 48
    check-in, 82
    check-out, 83
    clearness committees, 221
    in clinical environments, 78–81
    co-creating learning, 141 (*see also* stories)
    deeply listening, 78
    doing to being, 78
    evidence, 68–70
    as form of caring, 153–154
    heart-sharing, 82–83
    holding space, 77
    intentions, 55–57
    in learning environments, 81–83
    learning to, 71–78
    to other, 76–77
    overcoming frenzy, 73
    reflecting deeply, 83
    right relation with self, 74–76
    to self, 74
    support, 68
    theoretical frameworks, 68–70
    ways of, 71–72
love, 47, 90, 289
loving-kindness, 51

meaning, quest to find, 44
medicine
    language of, 50
    narratives, 150–156
meditation, 133, 309–310
menus, liberating structures, 215*f*
metacognition, 231
Mezirow, Jack, 6
micropractices, 78
    co-creating safe learning spaces, 146–148
    critical thinking, 149
    multiple perspectives, 149
    quality, 187–188
    safety, 187–188
Millennium Development Goals (MDGs), 281
mindfulness, 57, 118
    development of, 95–98
mirroring, 98
mistakes, learning from, 181
models
    Clinical Judgment Model, 26*f*
    critical reflection, 25, 34, 182
    Describe, Examine, and Articulate Learning (DEAL), 119–121
    descriptive practice, 182
    dialogic reflection, 25, 182
    McDowell-Williams Caring Leadership Model, 290–291
    pluralistic possibility (*see* pluralistic possibility model)
    of reflective practice, 23–26
    self-care plans, 122–123
    Tanner's Model of Clinical Judgment, 164
models of reflective practice, 23–26
morality, 4
morals
    courage, 4, 8–10
    knowledge, 306
multiple perspectives, 149

M

management, responding to, 98. *See also* leadership
McDowell-Williams Caring Leadership Model, 290–291

N

narratives
    co-creating learning, 141
    families, 151–153

guided reflection, 145*f*
improving practice, 150–156
learning from, 99–101
medicine, 150–156
patients, 151–153
reasoning, 100
recreating nursing education, 148–149
reimagining self, 99–103
resources, 152*t*–153*t*
storytelling, 119
National Academies of Sciences, Engineering, and Medicine (NASEM), 162, 234, 254, 255
National Advisory Council on Nurse Education and Practice, 232
National Institutes of Health (NIH), 232
National League for Nursing, 270
navigating work environments, 93–95
Neff, Kristen, 118
negative emotions, 153. *See also* emotions
Nightingale, Florence, 237
noble truths, 310–311
Noddings, Nel, 118
noticing, 24
nursing
    art of, 70
    attending to self, 95–99
    behaviors, 73
    components of practice, 116–117
    definition of, 68, 70
    developing caring practices, 91
    discipline of, 304
    education, 254*f*
    educator evaluation, 196–197
    knowledge development in, 305
    languages, 50
    pausing before entering, 79
    practice development, 189–190
    recreating nursing education, 148–149
    reimagining self, 99–103
    retirement, 162
    shortages, 251
    student wellness courses, 125*t*–127*t*, 128*t*–129*t*
    sustaining professionalism, 183
    well-being, 90 (*see also* well-being)
Nursing: Philosophy and Science of Caring (Watson), 35

O

1-2-4-All, 219
online education, 10
ontological competencies, 7
organizational cultures, 208
organizational practices, 314
organizational relationships, 210–211
others, 99
    listening to, 76–77
    relating to, 98–99

P

pain, 44
palliative care, 253
pandemics, 4, 168. *See also* COVID-19
partnerships, 249
    academic-practice, 250–255
    definition of, 257
    as reflective relationships, 259–260
patients
    encounters, 79*f*
    narratives, 151–153
pausing, 154. *See also* listening
    before entering, 79
    micropractices, 80
peace, micropractices, 80
pedagogies
    development of care/compassion, 121–127
    educators, 144
    guided reflection, 145*f*
    Ignatian Pedagogy, 164–166
    improving practice, 150–156
    interactive, 22
    narratives, 143–148 (*see also* narratives)
    reflexive pedagogy, 131
    relational emancipatory pedagogy, 275–282
    stories, 142–143 (*see also* stories)
Pedagogy of the Oppressed (Freire), 6
peers, 37
performance anxiety, 121
personal practice, 81
    academic education, 260–261
    application for development, 36–37

authentic connections, 28–30
creative spaces, 58–59
frameworks, 21–30
leadership, 297
models of reflective practice, 23–26
overview of, 20–21
pluralistic possibility model, 238–243
redesigning education, 26–27
role of reflection, 132–134
self-assessments, 197–198
simulation-based learning, 172–173
stories, 155–156
Unitary Caring Science, 30, 317–318
value of, 118–121
well-being, 109
working together, 222–223
personal transformation, 12
person-centered care, 238
perspectives, recognizing, 37
phases of frameworks, 24–25
planning, legacy, 291
plans, self-care, 122–123
pluralistic possibility model, 227
    caring behaviors, 237–238
    complexities of diversity of thought, 231–237
    diversity, equity, and inclusion (DEI), 239–240
    education, 234–235, 238–239
    empathy, 233–234, 241–243
    evidence, 229–231
    labels, 235–237
    languages, 235–237
    overview of, 227
    personal experience, 238–243
    professional experience, 238–243
    self-awareness, 241–243
    self-awareness through STEAM, 244
    theoretical frameworks, 229–231
politics, 270. *See also* censorship
positive emotions, 153. *See also* emotions
Posner, Barry, 291
power
    of silence, 154–155
    of stories, 150–151
practical knowledge, 92
practice
    across state lines, 168
    communities (*see* communities)

components of nursing, 116–117
context of, 93–95
development, 189–190
improving, 150–156
interprofessional education (IPE), 170–171
of leadership, 291–292
making sense of, 109*t*
organizational practices, 314
overview of, 180–181
simulation-based learning, 161 (*see also* simulation-based learning)
practice-based discipline, 92. *See also* academic education
practice development, 32–33, 92–93
praxis, 12
    emancipatory nursing praxis (ENP), 269 (*see also* emancipatory nursing praxis [ENP])
    Freire, Paulo, 274
prejudices, 236. *See also* biases; diversity of thought
prelicensure nursing education, 167–168
premise reflection, 34
presence
    authenticity, 49–52
    micropractices, 80
Princeton University Trustee Report (2013), 233
principles, 213
    of leadership, 291–292
problem-solving, 259
processes
    10 Caritas Processes, 9–10, 36, 45, 307
    design thinking, 256
    reflection, 31, 34
    transformation of education, 28
    transformative learning theory, 21–23
    TRIZ process, 219–220
professional identity, developing, 92–93, 124, 182
professional practice, 81
    academic education, 260–261
    application for development, 36–37
    authentic connections, 28–30
    creative spaces, 58–59
    frameworks, 21–30
    leadership, 297
    models of reflective practice, 23–26
    overview of, 20–21

pluralistic possibility model, 238–243
redesigning education, 26–27
role of reflection, 132–134
self-assessments, 197–198
simulation-based learning, 172–173
stories, 155–156
sustaining professionalism, 183
Unitary Caring Science, 30, 317–318
well-being, 109
working together, 222–223
prompts, 188, 188*t*
The Prophet (Gibran), 56
protocols, 213–214
psychological hardiness, 8
PubMed, 257
purpose
connections, 75
quest to find, 44

Q

Quadruple Aim, 132
Quaker communities, 220
quality, 179
competencies, 183–184
micropractices, 187–188
overview of, 180–181
praxis and reflection, 182
tools for improving, 117
Quality and Safety Education for Nurses (QSEN),
167, 183, 238, 258
questions
appreciative, 196, 197, 219
learning how to ask, 197
Quinn, Robert, 295
Quinn, Shawn, 295

R

racism, 23, 234, 236
Rath, Tom, 296
rational thinking, 93
reasoning, narratives, 100

redesigning
assessment, 193–195
education, 26–27
reflection, 24, 99, 165
as an asset, 96
collaboration in clinical learning, 184–187
constant, 34
creative spaces for caring, 52–55
critical, 25
as critical thinking, 38
cultural contexts, 13
descriptive, 25
dialogic, 25
growth, 97*f*
guided, 145*f*
for learning from stories, 156*t*
mirroring, 98
processes, 31, 34
purpose of, 33
recreating, 214–216
and relationships, 10–12
role of, 115 (*see also* role of reflection)
simulation-based learning, 161 (*see also*
simulation-based learning)
social contexts, 13
summary of, 13–14
through stories, 142 (*see also* stories)
time and space to reflect, 185
well-being and, 109
reflection-before-action, 31
reflection-beyond-action, 173
reflection-for-action, 260
reflection-in-action, 31, 173, 216–220, 279–280
reflection-on-action, 31, 173, 187, 216–220
reflection papers, responding to, 192–193
reflective academic-practice learning
communities, 260
reflective inquiry, 27
reflective learning communities, 57–58, 259, 261
reflective mindful practices, 98. *See also*
mindfulness
reflective models, 31*t*
reflective practice, 30–32
content, 37
contradictions and, 182–183
creative spaces for, 48–58
frameworks and, 33–36

individual practices, 308–311
informing narrative pedagogies, 145
overview of, 180–181
strategies, 187
summaries, 38
Unitary Caring Science and, 305, 307–311 (*see also* Unitary Caring Science)
wisdom, 307–308
reflective practice models, 23–26
reflective relationships, partnerships as, 259–260
reflective work, reviewing, 195–196
reflexive pedagogy, 131
regenerative care, 253
reimagining self, 99–103
relating to others, 98–99
relational emancipatory pedagogy, 275–282
caring relationships, 277–278
caring social mandates, 281–282
critical dialogues, 279
cultures of caring, 276–277
reflection-in-action, 279–280
relational learning, 12, 13
knowledge development and, 14–15
relational practices, 311–317
relationships
building trusting caring relationships (Caritas Process #4), 69
caring, 57, 277–278
developing collaborative, 191–194
development, 117
flow, 53
organizational, 210–211
partnerships as reflective, 259–260
reflection and, 10–12
repatterning support, 55
resilience, 9, 197
resources, narratives, 152t–153t
responding, 90
management, 98
to reflection papers, 192–193
responsibilities, 295
restarting conversations, 217–218
restorative care, 253
retirement from nursing, 162
reviewing reflective work, 195–196
right action, 9. *See also* ethics
right relation with self, 74–76, 77

Rilke, Rainer Maria, 56
risks
emotions, 94
jobs, 8
Rogers, Martha, 57
role of reflection, 115
component of nursing practice, 116–117
development of care/compassion, 121–127
evidence, 117–121
overview of, 116
personal practice, 132–134
professional practice, 132–134
self-care plans, 122–123
social change, 131–132
student wellness courses, 125t–127t, 128t–129t
theoretical frameworks, 117–121
value of personal experiences/stories, 118–121
rubrics, 194

S

safe places, 50, 51. *See also* creative spaces
co-creating safe learning spaces, 146–148
social change, 131–132
time and space to reflect, 185
wisdom circles, 313–314
safety, 179
competencies, 183–184
micropractices, 187–188
overview of, 180–181
praxis and reflection, 182
Sandstrom, Jeannine, 292
SBAR (situation, background, assessment, and recommendation), 155
scaffolding, 101
The Scholarship of Reflective Practice, 37, 100
science, 35, 185
complexity science, 209
organizational relationships, 210–211
Secretan, Lance, 289
self, 99
attending to, 95–99
listening to, 74
reimagining, 99–103
right relation with, 74–76, 77

self-assessments, 197–198
    personal experience, 197–198
    professional experience, 197–198
self-awareness, 12, 95–98, 186, 231
    pluralistic possibility model, 241–243
    through STEAM, 244
self-care, 133
    building practices, 81
    COVID-19, 197
    plans, 122–123
    promoting, 117
    student wellness courses, 125t–127t,
        128t–129t
    well-being and, 103–108
self-compassion, 117
self-directed learning, 37
self-knowledge, 155
self-management, 186
self-reflection, 67
    learning to listen, 71–78
    listening in clinical environments, 78–81
    overview of, 68
self-talk, 121
sensations, thoughts, emotions, actions,
    mentalizing (STEAM), 244
service, 289
Seven Sacred Sutras, 309–310
shaping futures, 211–214
sharing stories, 141. *See also* communities; stories
shortages, nursing, 251
silence
    co-creating learning, 141 (*see also* stories)
    power of, 154–155
simulation-based learning, 161
    clinical instructor training, 167
    cognitive bias simulation training, 171–172
    education, 166–172
    evidence, 163–166
    graduate nursing education, 168–170
    Ignatian Pedagogy, 164–166
    in-situ simulations, 171
    interprofessional education (IPE), 170–171
    Knowles' Adult Learning Theory, 163–164
    overview of, 162–163
    personal experience, 172–173
    prelicensure nursing education, 167–168
    professional experience, 172–173

Tanner's Model of Clinical Judgment, 164
    telehealth, 172
    theoretical frameworks, 163–166
situated cognition theory, 166
situated learning, 166
six-word stories, 157f
skill development, 7
Smith, Lee, 292–294
social change, role of reflection, 115, 131–132.
    See also reflection
social justice, 22
    in higher education, 270–272
    Watson, Jean, 281
social mandates, caring, 281–282
spiritual knowing, 96
stand-in, 281
stand-with, 281
Stop Wrongs to Our Kids and Employees
    (WOKE) Act (2022), 271
stories, 99–101. *See also* narratives
    development of, 50
    evidence, 143–148
    fifty-five word, 158f
    guided reflection for learning from, 156t
    improving practice, 150–156
    overview of, 142–143
    personal experience, 155–156
    power of, 150–151
    professional experience, 155–156
    recreating nursing education, 148–149
    sharing, 141
    six-word, 157f
    theoretical frameworks, 143–148
    value of, 118–121
    writing, 147
storytelling, 119, 150–151
strategies
    advocacy, 169
    emergent strategies for shaping futures, 316–
        317
    inquiry, 169
    listening, 155 (*see also* listening)
    reflective practice, 187
    shaping futures, 211–214
    visual-thinking, 101–103
stress, 4, 8, 94, 95
students, wellness courses, 125t–127t, 128t–129t

support
    of framework and evidence, 45–46
    listening, 68
supportive care, 253
surrender, 47
sustainability, 15
Sustainable Development Goals (SDGs), 281
sustaining professionalism, 183

T

tacit knowledge, 24, 32, 92
Tanner's Model of Clinical Judgment, 164
teaching, learning and (Caritas Process #7), 69
teamwork, 170, 208. *See also* working together
10 Caritas Processes, 9–10, 36, 45, 47–48
    authentic presence (#2), 68–69, 79
    building trusting caring relationships (#4), 69
    consciousness, 72
    expressing feelings (#5), 69
    healing environments (#8), 69, 72
    learning and teaching (#7), 69
    ways of listening, 72
technology-enhanced learning (TEL), 14
telehealth, 172
Te Tiriti o Waitangi principles, 14
theoretical frameworks
    academic education, 255–259
    leadership, 288–291
    listening, 68–70
    pluralistic possibility model, 229–231
    role of reflection, 117–121
    simulation-based learning, 163–166
    stories, 143–148
    support for, 5–7
    transformative learning theory, 181–184
    Unitary Caring Science, 304–306
    well-being, 91–93
    working together, 208–209
theoretical framing, 217
theories
    caring, 92
    critical theory, 6
    Experiential Learning Theory, 38, 208–209
    Knowles' Adult Learning Theory, 163–164

situated cognition theory, 166
    Theory of Human Caring, 44
    transformative learning theory, 6, 21–23,
        181–184, 209
Theory of Human Caring, 44
time and space to reflect, 185
Tolle, Eckhart, 73
tools
    handoff, 71
    simulation-based learning, 163
    stories (*see* stories)
touchstones, 78, 79
training
    clinical instructor, 167
    cognitive bias simulation, 171–172
traits of leadership, 293t–294t
transformation, 13
    education, 20, 28
    support, 55
transformative learning theory, 6, 13, 21–23, 209
    evidence, 181–184
    and reflective practice, 33–36
    theoretical frameworks, 181–184
transforming, 274–275
transpersonal care, 72, 73
TRIZ process, 219–220
trust, 213
    building trusting caring relationships (Caritas
        Process #4), 69
    cultures of, 131
    development of, 71
    eroding, 154
truthfulness, 289

U

uncertainty, 10
understanding ourselves, 12
Unitary Caring Science, 9, 11, 12, 13, 30, 44, 45,
        229, 303
    appreciative inquiry (AI), 315–326
    censorship, 269 (*see also* censorship)
    centering, 75
    connections, 305
    developing caring practices, 91

emergent strategies for shaping futures, 316–317

evidence, 304–306

holding space, 77

individual practices, 308–311

organizational practices, 314

personal experience, 317–318

professional experience, 317–318

and reflective practice, 33–36

reflective practice and, 307–311

relational practices, 311–317

self-reflection, 67 (*see also* self-reflection)

theoretical frameworks, 304–306

ways of listening, 72

well-being, 90

wisdom and, 307–308

University of Auckland, 14

University of Pennsylvania School of Nursing, 256

V

values, 33, 294

of personal experience, 118–121

of stories, 118–121

Watson's Unitary Caring Science, 46–47

Values in Action (VIA) Survey, 296

Veterans Affairs Nursing Academic Partnership, 259

videos, YouTube, 129

virtual simulation, 167. *see also* simulation-based learning

virtues, 310–311

vision, 294

visual literacy, 101

visual-thinking strategies, 101–103

Vygotsky, Lev, 101

W–X

Waipapa ki Uta: The Landing Place, 15

Watson, Jean, 46, 49, 304

authentic presence, 49

building practices, 78

on compassion, 71

on equanimity, 76

healing environments, 72

on human dignity, 55

Seven Sacred Sutras, 309–310

social justice and, 281

Watson's Unitary Caring Science, 44, 45. *See also* Unitary Caring Science

communities, 57–58

ethics, 46–47

reflective practice, 48–58

support of framework and evidence, 45–46

values, 46–47

WCSI Caritas Coach Education Program (CCEP), 52, 57

well-being, 90, 252

attending to self, 95–99

evidence, 91–93

navigating work environments, 93–95

personal practice, 109

professional practice, 109

reimagining self, 99–103

relating to others, 98–99

self-care and, 103–108

theoretical frameworks, 91–93

WikiEducator, 131

wisdom

circles, 313–314

reflective practice, 307–308

Unitary Caring Science, 303 (*see also* Unitary Caring Science)

wise actions, 220–222

wishful thinking, 291

work environments, 232

clearness committees, 220–222

navigating, 93–95

working together, 207. *See also* collaboration; relationships

evidence, 208–209

liberating structures, 214–220
organizational relationships, 210–211
overview of, 208
personal experience, 222–223
professional experience, 222–223
shaping futures, 211–214
theoretical frameworks, 208–209
writing
    journaling, 147–148
    to learn, 101
    prompts, 188*t*
    stories, 147–148

Y–Z

Yenawine, Phillip, 102
Yount, Shane, 292
YouTube, 129

Zimmer, Ben, 236